Praise for
Miranda Esmonde-White and Essentrics

"I've been doing Essentrics two to three times a week for the past twenty years to date. As an athlete, I used it to aid in recovery and to add speed and balance to my game. . . . It allowed me to train harder and perform better."

—Jonathon Power, World Squash Champion

"Miranda combined scientific principles with intuition in creating Essentrics, a workout that rebalances the full musculoskeletal system using flexibility training to increase strength. Essentrics complements any fitness routine and offers huge potential for health promotion and disease prevention."

—Emilia Zarco, chair of the Department of Health and Sport Sciences at Adelphi University

"I've been doing Essentrics for more than ten years. As a former dancer, I fell in love with the technique and how it made my body feel. Over the years I've grown to appreciate what the technique does to calm my entire nervous system. Every morning on set I do a fifteen-to-forty-five-minute Essentrics warm-up in my trailer. It helps me tune into my body, align my posture, and tap into a mindful state."

—Sarah Gadon, actor, *Alias Grace* and *True Detective*

THE
MIRACLE *of*
FLEXIBILITY

A HEAD-TO-TOE PROGRAM TO INCREASE STRENGTH, IMPROVE MOBILITY, AND BECOME PAIN FREE

MIRANDA ESMONDE-WHITE

SIMON ELEMENT

New York   London   Toronto   Sydney   New Delhi

SIMON
ELEMENT

An Imprint of Simon & Schuster, Inc.
1230 Avenue of the Americas
New York, NY 10020

First Simon Element hardcover edition March 2023

SIMON ELEMENT is a trademark of Simon & Schuster, Inc.

For information about special discounts for bulk purchases, please contact Simon & Schuster Special Sales at 1-866-506-1949 or business@simonandschuster.com.

The Simon & Schuster Speakers Bureau can bring authors to your live event. For more information or to book an event, contact the Simon & Schuster Speakers Bureau at 1-866-248-3049 or visit our website at www.simonspeakers.com.

Photography by Natasha Launi & Alexandre Paskanoi
Illustrations by Amy Wetzler

Manufactured in China

3   5   7   9   10   8   6   4   2

Library of Congress Cataloging-in-Publication Data has been applied for.

ISBN 978-1-6680-0016-8
ISBN 978-1-6680-0017-5 (ebook)

I dedicate this book to the creator, with gratitude
and awe for giving us the miracle of the human body.

CONTENTS

INTRODUCTION: WHAT IS ESSENTRICS?   xi

SECTION I

1: THE BALANCED BODY   3

2: REDEFINING STRETCHING   9

3: THE MUSCULOSKELETAL TRIFECTA   15

4: THE POOR POSTURE EPIDEMIC   21
    Anatomy and Posture   24
    Basic Spine Movements   35
    Techniques for Good Posture   37

SECTION II

5: NEUROMUSCULAR TECHNIQUES   41

6: GETTING STARTED   45
    Equipment   45
    Correct/Incorrect Positions   48

7: THE WARM-UP   57
    Warm-Up   58
    The Essentrics Warm-Up Routine   69

8: THE ESSENTRICS SEQUENCES   77
    Category 1: Forward Flexion   78
    Category 2: Diagonal Rotation   88
    Category 3: Side to Side   102
    Category 4: Upper-Body Extension   112
    Category 5: Full-Body Figure Eights   117

Category 6: Pliés   121
Category 7: Hands, Arms, and
    Shoulders   129
Category 8: Legs and Hips   136
Category 9: Feet, Ankles, and Calves   144
Category 10: Chair/Barre Stretching   150
Category 11: Floor Strengthening   163
Category 12: Floor Stretching   173

9: ESSENTRICS ROUTINES FOR
EVERY DAY   185
    Morning Routine   186
    Evening Routine   189
    Travel Days   192
    Walking the Dog   195
    Stress Relief   198
    Relaxation   201
    Increase Your Energy   204
    Stimulate Your Brain   208
    Routine for Kids   212

10: ESSENTRICS ROUTINES FOR
TARGETED TRAINING   217
    Beginner Flexibility   217
        Floor   217
        Chair   221
    Advanced Flexibility   224
    Cooldown or Recovery   227
    Upper-Body Toning   230
    Lower-Body Toning   233
    Explosive Power   237
    Routine for Speed   241

Agility   244

Balance   248

Jumping Higher   252

Spine Mobility   255

11: ESSENTRICS ROUTINES FOR SPORTS   259

American Football   259

Ballet and Gymnastics   262

Baseball   266

Basketball   269

Cycling   273

Dance   277

Diving   281

Figure Skating   285

Golf   288

Hiking   291

Hockey   294

Horseback Riding   298

Martial Arts   302

Racket Sports (Tennis, Squash, Badminton,
    Racquetball, Pickleball)   305

Rowing, Kayaking, Canoeing   309

Running   313

Skiing   316

Snowboarding   319

Soccer   323

Surfing   326

Swimming   330

Volleyball   334

Yoga and Pilates   337

12: ESSENTRICS ROUTINES FOR THE WORKPLACE   341

On Your Feet All Day   341

At a Desk All Day   344

Manual Labor/Construction/
    Landscaping   347

Flight Attendants   350

Housekeeping   354

Hairdressing   358

13: ESSENTRICS ROUTINES FOR CHRONIC PAIN   363

Back Pain   363

Knee Pain   367

Foot and Calf Pain (Plantar Fasciitis
    and Achilles Tendonitis)   370

Hip Pain   374

Shoulder Pain   378

Fibromyalgia and IBS   381

Neck Pain   385

Finger, Wrist, and Elbow Pain   388

14: ESSENTRICS ROUTINE FOR BETTER POSTURE   391

Posture Routine   392

AFTERWORD   429

MEET THE MODELS   431

ACKNOWLEDGMENTS AND THANKS   435

NOTES   439

INDEX   443

THE
MIRACLE *of*
FLEXIBILITY

INTRODUCTION
What Is Essentrics?

If you're reading this book, you're probably someone who loves to move, like me—and who wants to keep moving for life.

Or you're someone who wishes you were moving more, who feels that the hours you spend immobilized over your phone or your laptop are harming your health, but who hasn't yet found a complete, full-body workout that you can fit into your day that leaves you feeling energized and pain-free.

I'm about to tell you about a stretching and fitness revolution that will keep you moving, energized, and pain-free for life. It began with a simple insight: many exercise programs, including the ones I used to teach at my own studio, actually leave you with less mobility and restricted joints, which lead to premature aging and injury. Throwing out the idea of "no pain, no gain," I spent years studying how we're actually designed to move and creating a full-body program that stretches and strengthens all the muscles in a balanced way, enhances the range of motion of every joint, and unglues stuck connective tissue. The result is Essentrics, a groundbreaking practice of gentle movement, respecting the muscle chains and joint mobility of the body, that scientists from Harvard, Adelphi, and McGill Universities have validated as a way to keep us strong, flexible, and fit for life, as well as providing immense benefits for brain and digestive health.

From my own experience I know high-impact activities like running, team sports, and tennis are fun, social, take us out into the fresh air, and exercise our bodies. As exhilarating as these activities are, they're also hard on us. Work, too, whether we're sitting at a desk or constantly on our feet, creates wear and tear on our joints and muscles. We need to protect our bodies from permanent damage so we can live fulfilling, pain-free lives at any age.

We tend to reward men or women who display the strength and ability to keep going despite pain. Athletes, professional and amateur, push through pain and injury to finish marathons or triathlons, or to participate in sports like football, where the concussion and prescription drug use statistics are infamous.[1] We've seen talented athletes sidelined by severe pain and injuries and high-intensity training participants who have suffered muscle damage so severe that the proteins and electrolytes released into their bloodstream as a result put them into kidney failure.[2] But we don't seem to learn the lesson that this kind of exercise prematurely ages the body; we just keep pushing ourselves to the breaking point. I danced with the National Ballet of Canada and know from personal experience that professional dancers ignore extreme pain and injuries up to the point at which their bodies can go no further.

Most fitness programs are designed to push young bodies to the limit; they are not designed to keep people injury- or pain-free. Quite the contrary: Pain is the gold standard for judging whether a workout is relevant. Over the years I've seen many people drop gym memberships because their bodies can't handle the stress and pain. I've seen people stop exercising altogether because of injuries that led to chronic pain and surgeries. Unfortunately, many people equate exercising to pain and a sense of personal failure, and they don't want to try again.

With Essentrics, I've discovered a way to be fit without ending up in pain. Suffering from chronic pain and healing slowly are not inevitable, even as we live well into our eighties and even nineties and beyond; we want those years to be as much fun and full of activity as the first part of our lives. But if we're in pain when we're young, it's unlikely that we'll be pain-free as we age. I'm here to show you how you can and should be pain-free and fully active for all the years of your life.

Injuries are another thing that age us. The human body is designed to last well into our nineties without overuse injuries or joint damage. Some fitness experts say the body gets stronger when it heals after injury. My long experience and the thousands of people I've worked with have shown me that this is not true: Injuries that occur in childhood and young adulthood often haunt people's bodies throughout their entire lives. Injuries from repetitive strains or acute trauma often lead to increased risk of recurrent injuries or chronic pain if the source of the trauma is continuously reproduced.[3]

This is the problem: Life, many workout regimens, and many sports involve repetitive, high-impact movements that unbalance the 206 bones, 650 muscles, 360 joints, and connective tissue (fascia) of the human body. When you unbalance the body, you will injure it.[4]

In 2010 I was presenting a flexibility workshop at canfitpro, a major fitness convention in Toronto, Canada. I asked the two hundred participating coaches and fitness instructors to raise their hands if they were in pain. Ninety-six percent of the hands went up. If that many instructors were in pain, think of how their clients felt! Unfortunately, to this day in the fitness industry, some level of pain and injury are considered normal, acceptable, and even celebrated as evidence that you've worked hard. The pain, you're often told, is *good pain, strengthening pain.* For the record, there is no such thing as good pain. Pain is a neurological message telling us that something is wrong. Despite what some experts say, pushing through pain will not ultimately make you stronger. Yes, for a time, your muscles will get stronger—until they start to break down.

Muscles make up one-third of the musculoskeletal system, which comprises three interdependent yet independent systems: the muscular system, the skeletal system, and connective tissue. Ignore one of these systems at your peril; this is when injury and pain occur. But when you work these systems as a trinity, pain and injury are rare. When your primary focus is strengthening muscles, you often stress the connective tissue that supports and protects those muscles, causing conditions like tendonitis and inflamed ligaments.[5] This is why the repetitive actions found in many workouts systematically destroy the cartilage, a connective tissue, in the joints.[6] Many people believe that much of the pain and immobility we endure are natural results of growing older, but there's nothing natural about them. They're actually the consequences of unbalancing our bodies.[7]

In the 1990s, many of the students at my fitness center who were turning forty began to complain to me that the high-impact aerobics routines we taught at the time were causing them injuries and pain. They asked me to create a workout that didn't hurt, *but they still wanted results*. They wanted the good posture, elongated look, and stamina of a ballet dancer. As a former dancer, I thought I knew how to create both strength and length in muscles, but that assumption soon proved wrong, and I found myself doing an abrupt turn away from dance and fitness into the world of neurology, biology, science, and anatomy.

The program I created—now called Essentrics—was based on the ways our bodies are actually designed to move, which involves having full range of motion in all 360 joints, equal strength in all 650 muscles, and well-hydrated, malleable connective tissue. The best part of my discovery was that this objective could be achieved by doing a daily twenty- to thirty-minute workout that used gentle, active movements to stretch and strengthen the whole body, including joints, ligaments, and fascia. This discovery was so contrary to everything I had previously learned that it took me years of receiving testimonials from students and clients (tens of thousands of them by now) and the results of scientific studies to believe that the benefits of Essentrics were real.[8]

I studied anatomy, neurology, and physiology to reinforce my intuitive understanding of how the various parts of our body interact with one another. I looked at how the body was created to move and quickly realized that so many of our habits, workouts, types of physical labor, and sports distort our musculoskeletal system, and that this was the problem. We often do exactly the opposite of what the body needs to be physically fit.

When I began teaching classes based on these principles, my own horrendous chronic back pain disappeared. A recent X-ray showed that, at seventy-two, my lower spine had definite signs of arthritis, but I still have no pain—the reward for practicing what I preach for the past twenty-five years.

WHAT IS ESSENTRICS?

Essentrics is an injury-free, pain-free, age-supporting way to exercise. *It's exercise in a healing mode.*

Time and again, I've witnessed the way the human body performs as a self-healing machine. With the correct method of exercising, it can self-repair.

Each workout (ranging from twenty to sixty minutes) is designed to engage all 650 muscles and 360 joints in the human body, with an emphasis on stretching and moving the full-body fascia. To achieve this, we use gentle, rotational, massage-like movements that slowly return every joint to its original full natural range of motion. Unlike many other programs, Essentrics' primary goal is to stretch *all* the muscles equally, so there are no tight muscles to tug on other muscles, creating imbalances and injury.

It's extremely important to *never* use external weights while doing Essentrics. You can strengthen yourself and stay fit simply by lifting the bones and muscles of your own body. Range-of-motion sequences in the Essentrics program use the principle of eccentric training, which is *lengthening while strengthening.* The joints of the human body are not designed to handle excessive weight and can be overstretched and damaged if you add external weights to Essentrics movements.

These sequences and workouts meet the demands of a wide spectrum of users, from people who are already in shape to people who are completely out of shape, from athletes to people of all ages who just want to be able to bend enough to slip on their shoes and remain independent.

Essentrics works by rebalancing the muscles to enhance functional mobility. I know this not only because it has transformed my own body but also from the thousands of testimonials I mentioned. Essentrics increases strength and flexibility without injury or pain using, among other techniques, eccentric training, which lengthens *and* strengthens. In addition to rebalancing every muscle and joint in the body, Essentrics improves posture by placing a special focus on the alignment and placement of the body. It can slow or even reverse symptoms of biological aging,[9] from relieving arthritis and a multitude of aches and chronic pains to boosting energy. Clients in their twenties and thirties who work out the Essentrics way talk about how much better they feel in their bodies and how much more fun they have participating in their favorite sports. People in their sixties, seventies, and eighties report that they feel decades younger.[10] Just twenty minutes of Essentrics every day can give you a strong, vibrant body free of pain and injury.

You may find it hard to believe that fitness can be easy and much less time-consuming than most fitness experts recommend. I had trouble believing that also. But it's true: with Essentrics, your body can be both pain-free and powerful.

I

CHAPTER 1
The Balanced Body

It's our birthright to live in a pain-free, fully mobile body, and to have effortless flow in every movement we make. We're born with incredible potential for healing and regeneration.[1] We function most efficiently when all the many parts of our bodies are in balance.[2] Whether our body has been damaged through diet, disease, a sedentary lifestyle, or excessive training, we can reverse much of the harm and trigger the healing process simply by rebalancing the musculoskeletal system.

We are all born with a natural range of joint motion, but we lose that range of motion as we remold our muscles and fascia every day through how we choose to move or not to move. Muscles can become imbalanced and stiff from sports or other activities, or from a life of sitting at a desk, on a couch, or in a car. As we get older, the choices we make can suddenly catch up to us. Activities that used to be effortless suddenly become difficult. We feel stiff and tight and notice that we don't move as easily as we used to, we can't play sports the way we did when we were younger, running has become painful, or that basic daily chores are challenging and exhausting. Even for people in their forties, getting up off the floor can become a major task, along with putting on pants and socks, pulling on sweaters, and tying shoes. The good news is that none of these limitations are destined to happen, and most are reversible through the full-body rebalancing range of motion exercises I outline in this book.

Rebalancing the body requires the engagement of the full musculoskeletal system, which includes the muscles, the bones and joints, and the connective tissues (peri-fascia, fascia, tendons, ligaments, cartilage, and lymph). I call the three systems in balance a trifecta. To create that balance, we need to simultaneously strengthen and stretch all our muscles as we move through the range of motion of our 360 joints. This may sound like an impossible feat, but it's actually quite simple, as you'll see in the sequences in the exercise section.

Within the concept of a balanced body, muscles play an important role and should not be extremely weak or extremely strong. Muscles have the potential to be strengthened from 0 percent to 100 percent, with a zone of total weakness at the lowest end of the scale and one of maximum strength at the top. In between the two extremes is a middle zone hovering closer to the 50 percent mark that I call the Golden Medium, and yes, this is the range within which the body is at its healthiest. Below you'll find descriptions of the three zones, along with simple quizzes that will help you establish which zone you're in. Your goal is to try to stay as close to the Golden Medium as possible.

ZONE ONE

Weak from a Sedentary Lifestyle

Many people who sought out Essentrics were in Zone One, and quickly transformed their health and are now in the Golden Medium. Zone One includes people who live a sedentary lifestyle and rarely exercise. They use between 1 and 25 percent of their potential muscle strength, which means that their muscles are often too weak to support good posture. They have accelerated muscle and fascia atrophy—if you don't use it, you really do lose it. They have difficulty climbing or descending stairs, and/or getting on and off a toilet or chair. They often have poor circulation, heal slowly, and have low levels of energy. Their connective tissue sticks due to dehydration, which can lead to chronic joint inflammation, often requiring joint replacement. Ironically, a sedentary lifestyle causes

the identical shrinkage, imbalance, and damage to muscles, tendons, and ligaments that extreme exercise does. This group tends to age prematurely.

Do you feel stiff all over?
Yes ___ No ___

Do you have low-grade chronic pain in one or several joints (for example, hips, shoulders, knees, or ankles)?
Yes ___ No ___

Do you have trouble walking at least fifteen minutes every day?
Yes ___ No ___

Do you have trouble adhering to a regular exercise program?
Yes ___ No ___

Do you find excuses to not get off your chair?
Yes ___ No ___

Are you too tired to visit friends?
Yes ___ No ___

Do you have trouble getting on and off a chair rapidly and with ease?
Yes ___ No ___

Do you have trouble running up and down stairs?
Yes ___ No ___

Have you changed your wardrobe to clothes that are easier to put on and take off?

Yes ___ No ___

Do you huff and puff when you get off a chair or do basic chores like housework, gardening, or getting dressed?

Yes ___ No ___

Does it take you a long time to recover from illnesses, even a cold?

Yes ___ No ___

Does it take you a long time to heal from cuts, burns, and bruises?

Yes ___ No ___

Have you had or do you expect to have a joint replacement?

Yes ___ No ___

Have you had steroid shots to relieve pain?

Yes ___ No ___

Do you take pain medication on a regular basis?

Yes ___ No ___

Do you need regular massages to relieve your pain?

Yes ___ No ___

If you answered yes to most of these questions, you're in Zone One.

The Golden Medium

This is the zone that Essentrics is trying to achieve for your body. People in this zone have the full natural range of motion in all their joints. They've developed between 26 and 75 percent of their potential muscle strength. Those muscles are strong and flexible enough to handle any sporting activity they choose, as well as maintain good posture all day. People in this zone are generally healthy, heal rapidly, have good energy, rarely suffer from chronic pain, and live fully active lives. These people perform regular moderate exercise to maintain strong and mobile muscles, and rarely (though occasionally, for the fun of it) push their body to its extreme limits. These people look younger than their years and feel fit. They age slowly and remain active well into their senior years.

Do all your joints move through their designated ranges of motion?

Yes ___ No ___

Are you basically pain-free?

Yes ___ No ___

Do you have lots of energy throughout the day?

Yes ___ No ___

Do you have good posture?

Yes ___ No ___

Do you heal from cuts, bruises, and other minor injuries quickly?

Yes ___ No ___

If you answered yes to most of these questions, you're in Zone Two.

Have you had or do you expect to have a joint replacement?

Yes ___ No ___

Have you had steroid shots to relieve pain?

Yes ___ No ___

Do you take pain medication on a regular basis?

Yes ___ No ___

Do you need regular massages to relieve your pain?

Yes ___ No ___

If you answered no to these questions, you're still in Zone Two.

ZONE THREE

Extreme or High-Performance Living

I've trained thousands of people in this zone who had the best intentions of developing a healthy, fit body but got out of balance; Essentrics helped them achieve the Golden Medium. People in this zone regularly push themselves to their limits, driving their body through pain and damage, sometimes to the point of collapse from exhaustion or injury. Most people who participate in competitive sports or extreme physical activity—weight lifting, distance running, high-intensity training programs, professional sports, or dance training, for example—fall into this zone. These types of activities shorten muscle length and limit range of motion. Muscle imbalances can then distort alignment, stressing the joints, ligaments, and muscles to the point of chronic inflammation, chronic pain, permanent joint damage, and premature aging.

Do you train by pushing your muscles to their maximum more than four times a week?

Yes ___ No ___

Do you have chronic pain?

Yes ___ No ___

Do you have recurring injuries?

Yes ___ No ___

Are your muscles losing their flexibility?

Yes ___ No ___

Do you have limited range of motion in your spine? Shoulders? Hips? Knees?

Yes ___ No ___

Do you feel extremely stiff and in pain when you get out of bed?

Yes ___ No ___

Do you enjoy or feel proud of your pain?

Yes ___ No ___

Do you tell people that pain and injury don't stop you?

Yes ____ No ____

Do you suffer from chronic back pain?

Yes ____ No ____

Have you had steroid shots to relieve pain?

Yes ____ No ____

Have you had or do you expect to have a joint replacement?

Yes ____ No ____

Do you take pain medication on a regular basis?

Yes ____ No ____

Do you need regular massages to relieve your pain?

Yes ____ No ____

If you answered yes to most of these questions, you're in Zone Three. (Most athletes and people who regularly participate in physically strenuous activity are in Zone Three.)

In order to rebalance your body, you must change your focus from training individual muscles to improving the range of motion of each joint.[3] Every joint is attached to the body by many muscles. If one of those muscles is weak, stiff, or injured, it will affect the range of motion of the entire joint.

To simplify this concept, let's look at the hip joint. It's attached to and uses all these muscles and more: the gluteus group, hamstrings, quadriceps, psoas, piriformis, gracilis, and long adductors, and to the IT band. When people focus on strengthening their glutes, quads, and hamstrings, they can't be sure they've strengthened those muscles equally, for one, and they also ignore all the other muscles in the hip joint that are used to move their hips and legs. In time, the stronger muscles slowly overwhelm the weaker muscles, pulling the joint out of its socket. When this happens, the ligaments, which act as stabi-

lizers to keep the joint in place, become overstretched and weakened and can't do their job.

No matter your age, an unbalanced joint will be painful. When we flip our focus from strengthening individual muscles to improving the range of motion of the joints through multidirectional, whole-body movements, we're able to pull the joints back into alignment, and the pain disappears.[4] Depending on the degree of muscle-fascia imbalance, relief can occur immediately or over time. When we move the entire joint, the individual muscles are integrated as a system to support a continuous flow of movement. As the system works in synergy, the muscles of the joint are equally recruited to make the movement happen. This is why range-of-motion exercises are the safest, most efficient, and most painless way to strengthen your body.

Essentrics may give the illusion of being an easy workout, but people are always amazed at the strength they develop by doing it. It seems easy because all the muscles are doing the work. It's like having fifty people doing a job instead of ten: the job is finished more quickly, and no one is exhausted.

The bonuses to rebalancing your joints are amazing posture, massive energy, and a pain-free body.

CHAPTER 2

Redefining Stretching

What is stretching? Stretching is the action we take in order to decrease the feeling of stiffness and increase our flexibility. The feeling of stiffness is caused when muscles shorten around their attached joint, limiting the joint's ability to move easily or comfortably. The action of stretching the muscles pulls a tight joint apart with the objective of relieving the feeling of stiffness, tension, or pain. Unfortunately, in many cases the relief is temporary, which causes many people to lose faith in the potential of stretching.

We have viewed stretching through a very small lens, believing it can offer limited, short-term relief of stiffness and pain. Our new definition of stretching offers the potential to unleash explosive power and strength, reduce injuries, help slow the aging process, increase energy, and open the possibility of living in a pain-free body.

These objectives cannot be achieved by focusing on muscle flexibility alone. They can only be achieved when, in addition to muscles, we focus on full-body range of motion of the joints. This will automatically stretch, strengthen, and rebalance the body.

Some programs claim to be full-body workouts, but they aren't. Some claim to rebalance the body, but they don't. Many gyms are equipped with flexibility equipment. Unfortunately, no machine can calibrate an individual person's sensitivities enough to adjust to every client's level or potential flexibility. Traditional stretching, the kind we're taught to do before we begin to exercise, targets specific muscle groups, and recommends that a stretch be held for twenty to sixty seconds. Studies by the University of Australia, among others, support my experience that such traditional, static stretching yields few benefits and can even impair performance if done prior to exercising.[1]

There is significant evidence that holding a stretch for a minute or more temporarily decreases strength and speed for up to an hour, likely due to changes in the neuromuscular signaling from brain to muscle and loss of contractile ability.[2] Or simply because it unbalances a joint! The result is impaired performance. In a recent study conducted at the University of Nevada, Las Vegas, athletes generated less force from their leg muscles after static stretching than they did after not stretching at all. Other studies have found that static stretching decreases muscle strength by as much as 30 percent. "There is a neuromuscular inhibitory response to static stretching," says Malachy McHugh, the director of research at the Nicholas Institute of Sports Medicine and Athletic Trauma at Lenox Hill Hospital in New York City.[3] The straining muscle becomes less responsive and stays weakened for up to thirty minutes after stretching, which is not what an athlete needs before a rigorous training session.

Despite this, static stretching is the most common form of stretching used today. In fact, according to a 2016 study of 605 personal trainers in the US—virtually all of whom had certifications from the American College of Sports Medicine[4] or the National Strength and Conditioning Association—80 percent still prescribed traditional static stretching to their clients. It's discouraging to me that, despite decades of research showing its inefficacy, static stretching remains one of the prominent forms of flexibility training.

Yoga is a wonderful mind-body program that originated in India and that has been mislabeled as a flexibility program. Yoga was designed not to work through the full range of motion of all the joints but to help focus and calm the mind. To do so, it uses many static poses that practitioners are meant to hold. It can be painful to hold a pose for a long period of time, but after a while the body becomes numb and blocks out the pain. That's the point: to discipline the participant's mind to overcome the pain and discomfort caused by deliberately stressing joints when holding poses. Unfortunately, this also unbalances joints, which explains some of the most common injuries related to Westerners' yoga practice: carpal tunnel syndrome, back pain, and chronic shoulder pain. I know many

people who love yoga and find great benefit in regular practice; adding a program like Essentrics will make sure your muscles and joints stay in balance while maintaining full mobility.

Pilates, which many people also think of as a flexibility program, was created during World War I by Joseph Pilates as a rehabilitation program. Pilates was a true healer, and he created a powerful healing and strengthening technique that is still popular with professional ballet dancers, athletes, and physiotherapists. However, unlike Essentrics, it was not designed to be a full-body program. If you love Pilates, then to maintain the flexibility and mobility in your entire body and prevent injuries, an Essentrics workout is the ideal complement. Most of the Pilates classes offered today were not created by Joseph Pilates (who did not trademark his technique) but by hundreds of fitness instructors who are not obliged to follow his wise concepts. To get the best out of Pilates, people need to work with highly skilled therapists or trainers who safely supervise and guide them in the use of the equipment that Pilates designed. Common injuries from participating in Pilates workouts are shoulder, neck, and back pain. Adding Essentrics workouts to a Pilates regimen will help safeguard practitioners from such injuries, and, again, will balance the body.

Physiotherapy exercises are designed to target specific injuries and heal them; they are not suggested for use as a stand-alone workout. Under the guidance of a physiotherapist the injured area is targeted with rehabilitation exercises, but once the healing has occurred, it's time to return to a full-body program. I studied with a sports physiotherapist for several years, and I've incorporated many physiotherapy techniques into the Essentrics program.

It's very simple to judge whether a program is a full-body regimen: if it doesn't use the full range of motion of every joint, engage movement on every plane, twist and bend, reach to the ceiling and floor with both slow and rapid movements, and use fingers, toes, and every other joint, then it isn't full-body. So far, Essentrics is the only program that can make that claim, because I created it with that purpose in mind.

As I was developing Essentrics, I realized that the secret to flexibility (and a permanent increase in flexibility) is in rebalancing the joints. The flexibility in the dozens of muscles that are involved in the range of motion of any given joint will be automatically increased when the range of motion is improved. A healthy joint is one capable of moving effortlessly through its designated full range of motion. If a joint can rotate, bend, or swing effectively, then the muscles and fascia connected to that joint will be fully flexible, too, and there is no need to add individual muscle flexibility exercises. This is the trifecta in action: the muscles, connective tissue, and bones and joints working in harmony.

When joints cannot move through their designated range of motion, they need to be restored with range-of-motion exercises that automatically rebalance the muscles and connective tissue.[5] Muscle flexibility is the by-product of a healthy range of motion, not the other way around.

Flexibility and hyperextension (or hypermobility) are two unrelated issues. Hyperextension/hypermobility is most often a genetic connective tissue condition in which the person has varying degrees of hyperextended or hypermobile joints. In most cases, the hyperextension is not extreme enough to cause an imbalance in joint stability. In rare cases when it's extreme, a flexibility program is not advised.[6] I've almost never come across dangerous hyperextension, but when I do I recommend beginner ballet, because it's a slow and deliberate strengthening method.

We've been looking in the wrong place to relieve stiffness, which has less to do with individual muscles and everything to do with range of motion. When we feel stiff, it's most likely that the range of motion of a joint has been reduced because the muscles and connective tissue around the joint are shrinking, shortening, and atrophying, limiting their movement. By doing range-of-motion exercises, you can prevent the muscles of that joint from shrinking and atrophying, making the stiffness disappear. Any improvement in our range of motion makes everyday activities easier. The best part is that a positive chain reaction takes place: The more the joints are liberated, the more we'll use them, and the more we use them, the less likely they are to stiffen.

We also know from experience that people

The human body is complex and needs a complex workout to effectively keep it fully mobile. We need to move but we need to move wisely and deliberately. There are many transformative benefits of improving the range of motion of all your joints, from toes to shoulders. Some are:

- Getting rid of scar tissue
- Releasing contracted muscles frozen in spasm. A spasm usually involves the contraction of an overworked muscle to force us to stop overusing it. The surrounding muscles stiffen to "splint" and protect the overworked muscle. If you've ever experienced the leg cramps known as charley horses, you know how painful this can be!
- Relaxing muscles
- Improving posture
- Improving mobility. The more mobile we are, the more we can move and the stronger our muscles will become.
- Stimulating healing
- Improving energy
- Improving circulation

have trouble sticking with traditional stretching or flexibility programs. Most complain that they don't get satisfactory results, or that stretching takes too long and is boring. Human beings are driven by immediate gratification, and when they don't get it, they often simply quit. When it comes to many stretching programs, the instant gratification part is missing because most flexibility techniques focus on stretching specific tight muscles. But many scientific studies have shown that stretching one muscle at a time simply doesn't produce lasting benefits;[7] any muscle is only as flexible as the tightest muscle on its team. For example, it's impossible to permanently increase the flexibility of the hamstring by isolating it with traditional targeted stretching, because any tension or stiffness in the other muscles and fascia of the hip joint, such as the glutes or psoas muscles, will limit the hamstring's ability to maintain its flexibility. In order for the hamstring to maintain its flexibility, the entire chain of muscles related to the hamstring—the quadriceps, psoas, gluteus group, quadratus lumborum, and others—must be simultaneously stretched.

To redefine stretching, we must see the body as a whole and not as individual parts, and work to return all those parts to their natural range of motion simultaneously. Essentrics shows how easily and rapidly this can be accomplished. Not only are your muscles awakened and stimulated when you twist, turn, reach, and bend in an Essentrics workout but your brain, your emotions, and your imagination are also. The effort of focusing on doing what are referred to as "complex movements" (as opposed to the simple, repetitive movements involved in something like running or walking, which don't require conscious thought) gives you a holiday from everyday life issues. A break from stressful thoughts always puts you in a better mood, so by the end of a workout both your body and your mind feel happier. I've found that within days of starting Essentrics, most people begin looking forward to their sessions.

Another element in the quest for a more flexible and mobile body is exercising the connective tissue. With its slow pace, rotational movements, and focus on range of motion, Essentrics is as much a connective tissue workout as one for muscles and joint health. The power of connective tissue has been recognized scientifically only in the last decade or so. Made of collagen, connective tissue supports, binds, or separates every tissue and organ in the body. When it comes to strength, mobility, and how our body moves, healthy connective tissue is as important as healthy muscles and joints. Every time we move, an automatic adjustment of the distribution of effort and tension takes place throughout the connective tissue network, involving peri-fascia, fascia, ligaments, and tendons. This allows the body to withstand tremendous force. When we run, walk, climb stairs, catch a ball, or stumble and fall, the connective tissue of the greater body absorbs much of the tension, not just the knee, hand, or shoulder that takes the direct hit.

Extensive research begun by Dr. Helene M. Langevin when she was at Harvard Medical School and Brigham and Women's Hospital and that she has continued at the NIH has raised awareness of the importance of healthy connective tissue, especially in improving mobility, reducing inflammation, and healing injuries.[8]

The complex, weblike structure of connective tissue that envelops our joints is composed of liquids called lymph and mesh-like fibers designed to absorb the weight and tension of our body as we shift from side to side or up and down, or twist or bend. When muscles contract or extend, the liquid space between the layers of tissue is where the movement happens. When we don't use our full range of motion, these tissues become dehydrated and stiff, constricting our muscles and, in turn, making our joints feel stiff.

This tightness or stiffness is a connective tissue problem, *not* a muscle problem, so it needs

FITNESS MYTHS

Flexibility training weakens muscles.

FALSE. Passive or traditional flexibility programs may weaken muscles, but not Essentrics training! Active dynamic stretching, which combines strengthening with stretching, makes you stronger. For example, male ballet dancers are stronger, pound for pound, than professional boxers.[9]

Targeted training unbalances the joints.

TRUE. Targeted training is just that: working on specific major muscles to either stretch or strengthen them. You'll often see a training program limited to repetitions that work five or six major muscle groups. Targeted muscle training, by definition, unbalances the natural integrity of joints. An unbalanced joint is a weak joint, which increases the chances of injury.

a connective tissue solution. Introducing hydration into dehydrated connective tissue requires slow, gentle movements.

The slowness of Essentrics sequences permits the lymph fluids to enter and hydrate the layers of fascia. This hydration acts as a lubricant that facilitates the fascia's smooth slipping and sliding over our muscles as we move.

Stretching can work only when you balance all the muscles of a joint. Muscle flexibility is the natural by-product of maximum range of motion. The opposite is not true: When an individual muscle is flexible, the full joint may still have limited range of motion. The greater the range of motion, the greater the muscle flexibility and strength. Ballet dancers are trained from childhood to perform hundreds of range-of-motion movements; that's the basis of ballet. This explains why they're some of the strongest and most flexible athletes. Unfortunately, the extreme training of ballet takes them out of the Golden Medium and into the danger zone.

A balanced body is the result of all joints enjoying their full range of motion!

In Aristotle's *Metaphysics*, he suggests that the whole is greater than the sum of its parts. I agree; we need to treat the body as an integrated system, rather than just its individual parts.

The Interdependent Systems of the Human Body

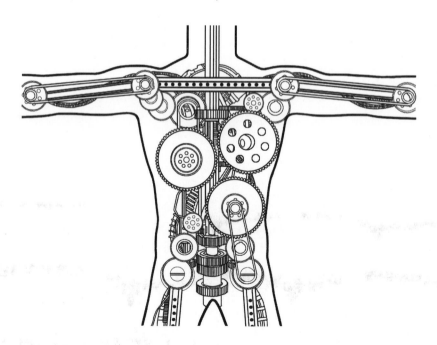

All the moving parts: If one part gets stuck, it affects the whole.

CHAPTER 3
The Musculoskeletal Trifecta

When I started developing a fitness program that would truly heal and energize my clients, I thought that fitness was all about exercising muscles, and that strong, healthy muscles would guarantee people's ability to move. But as I dug deeper, I found that so much of what powers us and keeps us pain-free and mobile is centered in healthy, balanced joints and connective tissue that doesn't tie itself in knots. I leaped into a study of anatomy and the way that joints, connective tissue, and muscles work together to create the miracle of movement that became fundamental to the exercise sequences at the heart of Essentrics. I've found that teaching people about how their musculoskeletal system works transforms the way they think about their bodies and helps them safeguard their all-important joints. So here's a quick anatomy lesson for you.

Our joints work like door hinges. When a door doesn't function properly, the first thing we check is the hinge. If the door doesn't close properly, the hinge could be loose. If the door squeaks, most likely the hinge needs to be lubricated. If one hinge out of three isn't functioning correctly, it will cause a drag on the other hinges, and the door won't swing the way it should.

As with a door's hinge, when a joint is unbalanced, the weight of the attendant limb will make it even more unbalanced. When a hinge is loose, the door pulls on the hinge, causing more damage every time it swings open. We recognize that the problem isn't the door—it's the unbalanced hinge that's making the door difficult to open. When we lift our arms and our shoulders hurt, the problem isn't that we're lifting our arms, it's that the joint is unbalanced. Don't stop lifting the arm; fix the joint and the arm will lift pain-free!

Unbalanced muscles are similar to unbalanced hinges: They pull the limb out of alignment, leading to joint damage and pain. Rebalancing exercises will pull the joint back into alignment.

The key to moving with ease is recognizing that all movement occurs in our joints. There are 360 joints in our skeleton. Each movable joint has a designated range of motion, and the type of joint indicates that range. (The skull joints and some of the spine joints have very little to no ability to move.)

There are three main types of joints:

- Fibrous (immovable), such as the joints of our skull

- Cartilaginous (partially movable), like our vertebrae
- Synovial (freely movable), like our hip or knee joints

Our body adjusts according to the physical demands that are placed on it on a daily basis. The type of those physical demands results in various physiological changes to the muscles, joints, and connective tissue.

The principle of adaptation describes the physiological changes that occur in the muscles, joints, and connective tissue as the body becomes accustomed to a particular sport, fitness regimen, or lifestyle.[1] The body can adapt to the physical demands that are placed on it by growing stronger and more flexible or tighter and weaker.

We are the bosses of our body. We can make our body strong or weak, stiff or fully mobile, elongated or bulky simply by how we train our muscles and connective tissue. Learning to tolerate increased stress or tugging causes adaptive changes to take place in the muscles and connective tissue.[2] If a muscle is stressed beyond its tolerable limits, it will try to adapt its ability to withstand that stress and either lengthen, shorten, or become injured accordingly.

In the study of sports and fitness, a tremendous focus has been placed on muscle strengthening, cardiovascular conditioning, and neuromuscular coordination.[3] Very little attention is paid to connective tissue, which is the part of the musculoskeletal system that is designed to help our body cope with stress and change.

Connective tissue is like a web that reaches from head to toe. It's made of collagenous protein and designed to hold our muscles in their designated shape. When we look in the mirror, we're seeing the shape of our connective tissue, in particular our fascia, which is the glue that holds our body's shape. Ounce for ounce, fascia, ligaments, and tendons are stronger than steel.

Movement and force are generated through the interactions between muscles and fascia. Tendons connect muscles to bones, while ligaments connect bones to bones. If muscles weren't attached to bones or bones attached to each other, humans couldn't move; we would simply be a puddle of flesh and bones on the floor.

Cartilage, a member of the connective tissue family, cushions and prevents wear and tear on the joints, making movement smooth and pain-free. We've all heard how painful joints can be when their cartilage is worn out. Our cartilage is designed to last a lifetime, but we can damage it through poor habits.

Fascia is a subset of the connective tissue system. Fascia gives muscles their shape and rebound tension, which doubles the power of the actual muscle. Our daily movements, lifestyle, and favorite activities are reflected in our fascia, because movement trains the fascia. Someone who spends much of the day sitting has a very different fascial body than an active person.

Healthy connective tissues have a three-dimensional weave that looks like a fishnet pattern. If you looked at that weave through a microscope, you'd see undulations called crimps, which resemble and function like little elastic springs. If you wanted to build a spring that would bounce far, you would make one with many coils smoothly lined up on top of one another. The same concept works for the crimp: a larger degree of crimp will have higher elastic capacity for optimal force production.[4] It was recently found that within the fascia of our legs, humans have a kinetic storage capacity, used when we walk, run, or jump, similar to that of kangaroos and gazelles.[5] It's the crimp pattern that gives fascia, tendons, and ligaments their strength. It's the source of the natural bounce and springiness in a healthy person's movements, the "spring in your step." It makes you feel and look young.

The fascia of inactive or sedentary people loses its crimp formation, so the person has no recoil tension, leading to a constant state of exhaustion every time they try to move. The good news? When lost through injury or inactivity, crimp can be substantially recovered through a proper connective tissue exercise program. Scientific studies have shown that regular exercise, done gently over time, can reorganize connective tissue fibers and lead to the return of a strong crimp formation.[6] Essentrics is full of exercises designed to rebuild the crimp—in particular chair work for the feet and the pliés and lunges.

There is a direct link between our lifestyle and the health of this connective tissue. Unlike muscles, which can strengthen rapidly, fascia is designed to hold the same shape over our entire life span. Fascia is often referred to as a sleeve or a sac surrounding the muscles. The fascia sleeve is made of layers of cellophane-like tissue interspersed with liquid layers of collagenous protein. Muscles are limited in how much they can lengthen and shorten as they stretch or contract by the fascia sleeve. When we move our muscles, the lubrication layer allows the fascia sheets to effortlessly slide over one another. This sliding gives the illusion that the fascia is stretching. Fascia has a limited ability to lengthen or shorten (4 percent to 6 percent) as the muscles contract and relax within the fascia sac. If we're sedentary or we overstretch the fascia, it becomes saggy and loses its powerful web shape.

When our muscles contract and relax, they pull on the fascia sleeve, which showers lubrication into the layers. Imagine the joints of an elevator door receiving a gentle shower of oil every time it opens and closes; that keeps the door sliding smoothly. Now imagine that no one uses the elevator. When this happens, the oil intended to lubricate the elevator door slowly hardens to the point that it prevents the door from opening. That's what happens to our fascia when we don't move our bodies. Moving is the miracle that draws in the lubrication and hydration, which in turn keeps you moving and prevents hardening of the fascia.

The gluing or hardening of fascia occurs over years. Many experts and specialists dismiss it as the result of natural aging, but it's no more natural than a houseplant dying because it wasn't watered. Most houseplants can live for decades if we care for them. Likewise, our fascia can remain healthy and mobile for the full length of our lives if we care for it.

The hardening or gluing of the fascia sheets occurs not only in the large fascia sleeve surrounding the major muscles but also in the fascia sheets surrounding the millions of cells that make up each muscle. This hardening of the fascia can be triggered by different events:

- Scar tissue from injury or surgery
- Glued fascia due to immobility when locked in a brace or cast
- Glued fascia from a sedentary lifestyle
- Wadding of fascia in the upper back due to weak back muscles and poor posture
- Unbalanced joints from habits like always carrying a bag on the same shoulder or always crossing the same leg over the other

In other words, anytime muscle movement is limited or prevented, the fascia will begin the process of hardening. Whether we've experienced that hardening as a result of injury or lifestyle, we can begin to reverse it with awareness and strategic movement designed specifically to rehydrate the fascia. The secret is correct, gentle movement and patience.

The difference between muscle training and fascia training is that muscles strengthen rapidly, while fascia lubricates very slowly. If you begin exercising, within a week of daily sessions you'll notice that you feel stronger and more flexible, but your body may not look that different. That rapid change in strength occurs thanks to our muscles, which can gain (and lose) strength quickly. Fascia, however, takes a long time to change as the layers slowly rehydrate. Once the fascia is rehydrated, however, your shape can change suddenly. When you exercise consistently for six months, your actual body shape will likely change as the muscles reshape the fascia sleeve. If you're weight training, for example, which contracts the muscles, you'll develop shorter muscles; ballet and Essentrics are two types of training that will give you leaner muscles.

Daily movement keeps the layers of fascia hydrated. If you feel stiff when you get up in the morning or after spending hours at your desk, what you're really feeling is the sticking together of the gooey cellophane layers of your fascia. It's why stretching feels so good: You're lubricating and loosening those layers of fascia and liberating your muscles.

Not all movement benefits connective tissue. Repetitive movements and overuse of specific muscles often lead to repetitive strain injuries in the tendons, ligaments, and joint capsules.[7] In many cases, what are considered muscle tears often occur in these structures rather than in the muscle itself.[8] This is an indication that the fascia, tendons, and ligaments were not prepared for the stress that they've had to endure. Training the body for sporting activities should also involve specific training for the connective tissue to ensure that it's well adapted to meet the demands of the sport or exercise.

When any part of the body is immobilized, whether through surgery, injury, or lifestyle, the tissue paper–thin layers of fascia start to stick together and harden, creating general stiffness and an inability to move freely, as well as distorting and weakening the crimp formation. Given the important role connective tissue, especially fascia, plays in movement, it should come as no surprise that healthy, hydrated fascia is critical for developing flexibility and strength. Through Essentrics workouts, we nourish and lubricate the fascia, promoting easy, pain-free movement. We also maintain or restore the fascia's elastic capacity, the rebound tension that gives our movements vitality and ease.

CHAPTER 4

The Poor Posture Epidemic

My mother went to a British boarding school for girls. At the beginning of each new school year, she and the other girls went to see the school doctor, who examined their spine. If their spine wasn't sufficiently straight, they would be given posture exercises to help them achieve the desired result.

All the girls would spend several hours each day balancing books on their heads as they walked around doing other activities. The posture training worked for my mother; she had perfect posture throughout her entire ninety-six years of life. She was very proud of her posture and was instantly admired when she entered a room.

Today, posture like my mother's has gone out of fashion. So little emphasis is put on good posture that we slouch over our desks, when we walk, while we eat, and as we stand. Poor posture is becoming the signature posture of the Western world. My mother regarded her posture as a sign of elegance, but I've come to believe that it was also crucial to her health, allowing her to remain active well into her nineties. The troubling thing is that I now regularly meet children with less mobility and strength than my mother displayed even at an advanced age;

wedded to their devices, they slouch, squishing their organs and weakening their bones, leading to the onset of all kinds of health issues once associated with sedentary old age. And it's not just me who's noticing.

A decade ago, I met with Dr. Mark Tremblay of the Children's Hospital of Eastern Ontario Research Institute in Canada, who predicted that this deterioration would lead to what he had called a posture epidemic—a spiral of health impacts caused by the simple fact that we don't move enough anymore, and neither do our children.[1] "The electronic revolution has fundamentally transformed people's movement patterns by changing where and how they live, learn, work, play, and travel, progressively isolating them indoors, most often in chairs," Dr. Tremblay said. "People sleep less, sit more, walk less frequently, drive more regularly, and do less physical activity than they used to."[2] Judging from the latest health reports,[3] the posture crisis continues to accelerate.

The most frustrating aspect for me is knowing that this epidemic is 100 percent preventable with regular exercise and a healthy diet.

Most people think of an epidemic in relation to a contagious, fast-moving illness like

COVID-19. But the word *epidemic* is not restricted to diseases; it's also used to describe any potentially fatal health condition that affects large populations worldwide. For example, obesity is an accepted health condition that isn't a contagious disease but is classified as an epidemic.

Poor posture destroys the musculoskeletal structure and organs over a long period of time. Most people barely notice the correlation between their changing posture and ill health; even health professionals aren't paying attention. The slow-moving nature of the posture epidemic makes it less frightening than disease epidemics, but its impact on our health can be just as bad.

Poor posture is a condition that depletes our energy and destroys our joints while also interfering with our immune and circulatory systems. It leads to brittle bones and weakens our ability to combat cancer and conditions like diabetes. In addition, poor posture compresses our organs and suppresses hormones, further weakening our ability to fight disease.

THE IMMOBILITY CRISIS

A 2018 study by the US Department of Health and Human Services noted that only 26 percent of American men, 19 percent of women, and 20 percent of adolescents reported being sufficiently active to meet relevant aerobic and muscle-strengthening guidelines. In the introduction to the second edition of the *Physical Activity Guidelines for Americans*, Dr. Alex M. Azar II, secretary of the HHS, wrote:

> The scientific evidence continues to build—physical activity is linked with even more positive health outcomes than we previously thought. And, even better, benefits can start accumulating with small amounts of, and immediately after doing, physical activity.
>
> Today, about half of all American adults—117 million people—have one or more preventable chronic diseases. Seven of the ten most common chronic diseases are favorably influenced by regular physical activity. Yet nearly 80 percent of adults are not meeting the key guidelines for both aerobic and muscle-strengthening activity, while only about half meet the key guidelines for aerobic physical activity. This lack of physical activity is linked to approximately $117 billion in annual health care costs and about 10 percent of premature mortality.[4]

These are facts that we as a society have managed to completely ignore. There's no drumbeat coming from our medical professionals, government, school systems, or the media warning us that we ignore poor posture at our peril.

When people don't move enough, the liquid between the layers of fascia becomes gummy and gluey, and eventually hardens. A vicious cycle sets in where less mobility causes more stiffness and stiffness causes more immobility, which leads to atrophying muscles, less energy, less strength, and less desire to move. This cascade of effects is what causes poor posture.

It seems that as we gain mastery over technology, we lose mastery over our own bodies. Epidemic proportions of the world's population now suffer from once rare diseases like osteoporosis, heart disease, arthritis, type 2 diabetes, cancer, and chronic pain. We pride ourselves on having the most advanced medicine in history, and yet we're confounded by the reality that the children of this generation are destined to die at a younger age than their parents will. It's clear from reports from more than a decade ago that the next generation is destined for a lifetime of chronic sickness in which many will never know what it feels like to be energetic and healthy.

It's a fact that without regular exercise, muscles will atrophy. Let me say that again: *without movement, muscles shrink, atrophy, and die.* What many people don't realize is that atrophy is painful and causes an imbalance in the surrounding joints and tissues. It shows up as a mysterious pain somewhere—hips, knees, or ankles—and seems to migrate around our body. Pain leads to self-protection of the painful area, setting in motion a chain reaction of additional atrophy and even greater pain. We're under the impression that we cannot hurt ourselves by sitting. That assumption couldn't be further from the truth. Nothing can cause more damage, disease, and, ultimately, pain than sitting. As Dr. James Levine,

a professor at the Mayo Clinic, states, "Sitting is the new smoking"—referring to the growing body of research that substantiates the claim that the risk factors associated with time spent sitting pose one of the greatest threats to our health.[5] "Your age does not have to dictate your physical health," points out British physician Sir John Armstrong Muir Gray, former director of the National Knowledge Service for the UK's National Health Service. "The rate at which we lose our fitness is determined not by genes or age but by social factors such as the decisions we make about our lives and the pressures that influence us."[6]

When muscles atrophy, every part of the body is negatively impacted; the cardiovascular and digestive systems slow down, bones weaken, joints become damaged, nerves shrivel, and the brain shrinks from lack of nourishment. Atrophied muscles lead to low energy and unexplained weight gain. Use it or lose it! Atrophy happens when we don't move.

Movement is essential to the development and maintenance of strong muscles and bones. Bones need to be stressed to develop a strong skeleton. When we move, we exert varying degrees of force on our bones, and they strengthen accordingly. Children are especially vulnerable, since their bones are still growing. Bones and bodies develop to match the demands of the activities they perform on a regular basis. For example, tennis players who begin training in childhood develop a dominant arm that's up to 40 percent stronger than their other arm because of the function-dependent adaptability of bones.

Although the most noticeable structural changes take place as the body grows, transformation on the skeletal level can also take place in adulthood. Our bone mass peaks at around age thirty, after which we lose bone density. The less active we are, the faster we'll lose that density. There is no evolutionary benefit to our bones being strong if our environment doesn't require them to be so. When astronauts return to Earth after being in space for an extended period of time, it's not uncommon for them to be carried out of the spacecraft to avoid breaking their weakened bones. Like astronauts, inactive people or patients subjected to extensive bed rest lose significant bone density more quickly than people who are active.[7]

When elderly people's bones are weak due to, for example, osteoporosis, a simple hip fracture can lead to death. This is especially true for women, who represent 80 percent of those affected by the disease.[8] The good news is that studies prove that weight-bearing exercise can reverse bone loss! As with Tai Chi, which has been widely acknowledged for its therapeutic effects in treating osteoporosis, Essentrics workouts involve constant shifting of the weight from side to side to dynamically load the lower body. These weight-bearing exercises, done on various planes of movement, help not only to reduce the rate of bone loss and increase bone mineral density but also to prevent fall-related injuries by improving balance and coordina-

tion.[9] You don't need to lift weights in order to engage in weight-bearing exercise—just get up and move. Carrying around your own body is a sufficiently heavy weight. That being said, we can only develop so much new bone mass in adulthood. The prescription for bone strength at any age could not be simpler or more natural: The activities that children usually engage in at playgrounds—running, jumping, climbing—ensure strong bone development. As adults, we must be equally mindful of our activities in order to ensure that we maintain our strength.

ANATOMY AND POSTURE

Good posture reflects two things: the way we look and the way we feel. Most important, we should feel liberated, weightless, energetic, and pain-free. We tend to dismiss the importance of posture as cosmetic, but that isn't the main reason why we need good posture—good health is. Good posture doesn't threaten our health, but poor posture will.

Let's talk about what good posture is and what's required for us to gain and maintain it.

Good posture refers to the way we hold our full body when we walk, stand, and sit. Good posture should be relaxed, natural, and automatic. Our shoulders should be open and relaxed, our arms should hang easily at our sides, and our upper back and chest should be erect, relaxed, and open. As we walk, our legs should easily swing in the hips.

There should be zero stress or compression anywhere along the spine or in the hips or knees.

Alignment is important for posture. *Clean alignment* refers to the perfect alignment of every joint in our skeleton, from the top of our head to the bottom of our feet. It's essential for good posture. However, clean alignment is not a straight line from our head to our toes; it follows the natural curves in our body. For example, the spine is shaped in two curves. Our shoulders and hips are wide, so our weight gets distributed through the width of our shoulders and hips. The thigh bone (femur) is attached to the outer part of the hip bone and follows a diagonal path inward to the knee. This means that the full weight or load path of an aligned person will flow through many curves as it goes from their head to the magnificent triple arches of their feet. If that person has poor posture, the joints somewhere—or everywhere—along the load path will be poorly aligned. When the load path is interrupted or blocked by poor posture, we are susceptible to back pain and ill health.

It would seem that posture starts at our head, but it actually starts in the soles of our feet. Most people think that in order to improve their posture they simply must straighten their back. That, however, is the end result! It's only achievable if the full body is rebalanced or realigned. The body's musculature must be strong, balanced, and mobile. If any of our muscles are tight, unbalanced, or weak, a chain reaction throughout our entire body will impact our posture. Unbalanced muscles will pull the spine and other bones out of alignment, leading to a cascade of distortion in the body. Every part of our musculoskeletal system participates in good posture; muscles, bones, and connective tissue. This is why good posture requires full-body rebalancing or realigning. To improve posture, Essentrics uses a series of exercises that combine strengthening and stretching sequences that are easy to follow because they mimic everyday movements.

THE SKELETAL SYSTEM: BONES AND JOINTS

The human body is a marvel of engineering. When the bones of our skeleton are aligned, our joints move effortlessly because their designated ranges of motion are unobstructed. When our bones are out of alignment, however, our joints' designated ranges of motion are blocked. I always use the example of a wedge jammed into a door joint, preventing the door from opening or closing easily. Obstruction inevitably leads to pain and structural damage.

The muscles and connective tissue are a mechanical system of levers and pulleys that move the skeleton and are responsible for keeping the bones in alignment. Without the muscles and connective tissue, the skeleton would collapse to the floor in a heap.

LOAD PATH, CURVES, AND ARCHES

When an architect designs a building, whether it be a home, a house of worship, or a skyscraper, they're aware of the load path, or the path the weight of the building will follow from top to bottom. The foundation must be sufficiently solid to support the structure that's being built above it, and each floor has to be able to support the weight of the floors above it. It's not just the physical weight of the building materials that the architect must consider but also the alignment: Is the building straight? The strength of the various building materials also has to be taken into account. The weight of the material at the top of a building multiplies in intensity on the layers below. To prevent a building from collapsing, the supporting structure must be both physically strong enough and correctly aligned.

When we stand upright, our body has a natural load path. It begins at the head (skull) and flows through the spine, hips, and legs, unloading in the feet. Unlike the static structure of a building, the human body is a living, moving structure, so the load path must be able to adjust to movement as well as fluctuating weight. Fortunately, the human body is capable of withstanding stresses that are many times greater than its actual weight.

The study of the human skeleton is a study of the genius of humankind's creation. Our musculoskeletal system is designed to keep us from falling over no matter what kind of awkward position we find ourselves in; yogis balance on one leg for hours, ballerinas pirouette on the tip of one toe, tennis champions successfully reach for a runaway ball.

Centuries ago, architects realized that they could put more weight on an arch than on a square. This gave them the ability to build bigger and higher buildings. You can see this in architectural marvels like the Roman aqueducts, the ruins of the Colosseum, and medieval mosques and cathedrals with their massive arched ceilings, portals, and windows.

Not surprisingly, the arch shape is also found throughout the human skeleton. There are curves and arches in individual bones and in the full skeletal structure. The load path of the body flows downward through the curves of our spine to land on the arches of our feet.

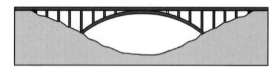

Deck arch bridge.

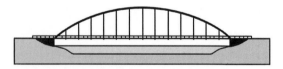

Through arch bridge.

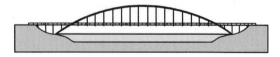

Half-through arch bridge.

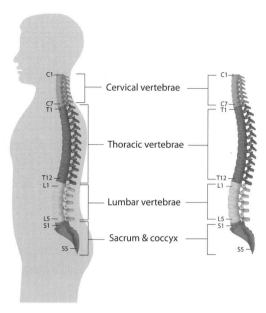

The spine.

SKULL AND SPINE

The skeleton starts at our head with the skull. The skull connects to the spine, which is made up of thirty-three individually pie-shaped vertebrae. The spine's bony structure runs from the nape of the neck to the base of the torso. Shaped in a double *S* curve (arches), the spine consists of five parts: the cervical spine, the thoracic spine, the lumbar spine, the sacrum, and the coccyx. The *S* curve gives the spine the ability to gently spring up and down as we walk, run, climb stairs, and move through our day. Each pie-shaped vertebra is separated from the next by a firm cushion of cartilage called a disc, which is a part of the connective tissue system. The vertebrae are attached to one another by ligaments. Of the thirty-three vertebrae, twenty-four can move and nine are fused together.

The spine is the principal tubular pipeline through which the main conduit of the nervous system runs, but it's equally important as the basic structure that keeps the torso upright. Attached to the spine are three essential bony structures that shape and protect the torso: the clavicle and scapula; the twenty-four ribs; and the ilium, ischium, and pubis, or the hip bones.

CERVICAL SPINE

In humans, cervical vertebrae are the smallest of the true vertebrae, and can be readily distinguished from those of the thoracic or lumbar regions by the presence of a hole in each vertebra,

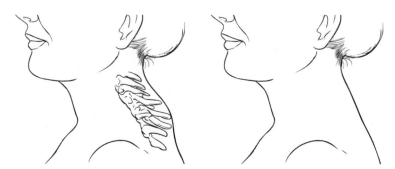

Hyperkyphosis of the upper back.

through which the vertebral artery and veins pass. (Almost every mammal has seven cervical vertebrae—even the giraffe. Their cervical vertebrae are just much longer than those of other mammals. The rare mammal that doesn't have these bones is the sloth.)

The cervical vertebrae are numbered from 1 to 27, with the C1 vertebra closest to the skull. Unlike most vertebrae, the C1 and C2 have been given special names: atlas (C1) and axis (C2). The atlas and axis form the joint connecting the skull to the spine. The axis forms the pivot around which the atlas rotates. When we have poor posture, we tend to lose our ability to turn and lift our head.

The movement of nodding the head is achieved predominantly through flexion and extension at the atlanto-occipital joint between the atlas and the occipital bone of the skull. This joint is often referred to as the *yes joint*. The movement of shaking or rotating the head left and right happens almost entirely at the joint between the atlas and the axis, leading this joint

to often be referred to as the *no joint*. The range of motion of the atlas and axis is inhibited by poor posture.

The last of the cervical vertebrae, the vertebra prominens or C7 vertebra, has a distinctive long bony projection that's palpable from the skin surface.

While poor posture often begins at the C1 and C2 vertebrae when the head bends forward, pulling the rest of the cervical spine with it, the effects are visible in a rounded, immobile upper back. The load path or weight of the head and neck exerts stress on the C7 vertebra. In order to support the load on C7, the fascia in the shoulders and upper back congeals, creating a kind of coat of armor and immobilizing the person's upper back and shoulder area. This wadding of fascia is quite common and is called kyphosis. It's equally common in men and women.

CLAVICLE AND SCAPULA

The bony structures found at our shoulders are the clavicles and scapulae. The clavicles are located at the front of the torso; they're the right and left *S*-shaped bones (more curves!) attached to the top of the cervical spine and ending at the shoulder joint where the arms attach. Clavicle bones come in many shapes and lengths; the variations cause body shapes that are often described as broad, narrow, square, or dropped shoulders. The clavicles perform the role of a coat hanger under which our torso hangs. A rounded upper back will cause the clavicles to drop, pulling the back forward into a rounded position. With good posture, the clavicles should protrude slightly.

The scapulae are located at the back of the shoulders and are often referred to as shoulder blades or wings. The scapulae permit us to lift and lower our arms and use them to pull. Poor posture can cause them to remain in a permanently lifted, overstretched mode, limiting the range of motion of the arms.

When working toward good posture, we must lift the clavicles to a horizontal position and be able to raise and lower the scapulae with ease.

THORACIC SPINE AND RIBS

When we see good posture, what we're seeing is a mobile thoracic spine and rib cage.

The ribs are attached to the thoracic spine at the back and the sternum at the front. There are

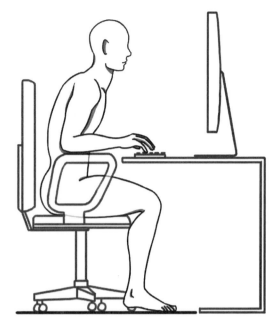

Rounded thoracic spine, or computer posture.

twelve ribs on each side of the spine, making a total of twenty-four. The ribs attach to the twelve thoracic vertebrae, two ribs per vertebra. The rib cage is shaped in a circular or arched formation. It houses and protects most of the vital organs in the body: the lungs, heart, stomach, pancreas, liver, and kidneys. When we slouch, the ribs move close to the spine, reducing the size of the rib cage cavity. This compresses the organs, limiting the ability of the heart and lungs to expand as they pump blood throughout the cardiovascular system. This results in less nourishment being delivered to our cells and fewer toxins removed, causing sickness, exhaustion, slow healing, and premature aging.

HIPS

The bony structure known as our hips is made up of three bones on each side of the spine: the ilium, the ischium, and the pubis. They form what resembles a giant heart shape, and again, we see the arches and curves in the skeleton. Housed inside this massive bony structure is the lower part of our digestive and reproductive systems, including the large intestines and bowels. When the torso rounds with poor posture, these organs are compressed, severely interfering with their efficiency. The health damage caused by compressed organs cannot be overestimated.

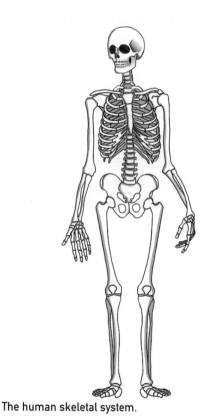

The human skeletal system.

After flowing through the torso, the load path continues downward through the thighs (femur), knees, and shins (tibia) and into the feet. The thigh bone is attached at the outer edge of the top border of the ilium. Rather than going straight down toward the foot, it takes an internal diagonal slope before inserting into the knee joint. There is also a subtle curve in the femur itself. Without that slight curve, the femur would slide off the knee joint, not into it!

Most people incorrectly visualize their legs to be directly below their hips (at a 180-degree angle). That's an optical illusion. They are in fact angled slightly internally at a gentle 170-degree angle. When you place your knees together, a triangle is formed between the hips and the knees.

FEET AND ALIGNMENT

Our ankles and feet are the final landing place of the load path. It's remarkable that our feet, which are relatively small compared to the size of the rest of our body, are capable of withstanding the full weight of the load path as we move through our day. The entire weight of our body goes through the center of the arch of our feet. The way we stand on our feet is where clean alignment and good posture begins. The weight of the body is multiplied to a degree with every step we take. It's extremely important that we learn to walk lightly and not slam our feet into the ground.

Each foot consists of twenty-six bones, thirty-three joints, 107 ligaments, and nineteen mus-

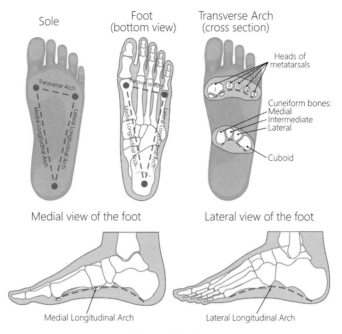

Sole

Foot
(bottom view)

Transverse Arch
(cross section)

Transverse Arch

Medial Longitudinal Arch

Lateral Longitudinal Arch

Transverse Arch

Medial Longitudinal Arch

Lateral Longitudinal Arch

Heads of
metatarsals

Cuneiform bones:
- Medial
- Intermediate
- Lateral

Cuboid

Medial view of the foot

Lateral view of the foot

Medial Longitudinal Arch

Lateral Longitudinal Arch

Arches of the foot.

cles. The twenty-six bones fall into three groups: the tarsal bones, the metatarsal bones, and the phalanges.

Most of us don't realize that we actually have three arches in our feet. The midfoot arch is made of a pyramid-like collection of bones that form one big arch or three individual ones, made of three separate sets of bones. These include the three cuneiform bones, the cuboid bone, and the navicular bone. The lateral and medial arches run the length of the foot. The anterior transverse arch runs horizontally under the pad of the foot from the big toe to the baby toe. The three arches join at the three points of a triangular or pyramidal shape under the foot. Part of the reason the feet can absorb the load path is

this intricate meshing of three arches that make what we know as the arch of the foot.

Incorrect foot alignment leads to structural damage in the knee, the hips, the spine, and even the shoulders. When we evert or invert our ankles, the ripple effect is felt in every other joint in our body, making good posture more difficult. This is one reason that, in Essentrics, we put so much emphasis on how we stand on our feet, as well as their mobility and strength.

Our feet are capable of absorbing a great deal of weight, and of acting like springboards propelling us forward with every step. Their power to absorb and propel is due in part to their pyramid-shaped triple arches and the strength of their ligaments and tendons.

Rebounding power in well-aligned feet comes from two sources: the ligaments and tendons, and the combination of the three arches to make a trampoline-like formation.

Of all the thousands of people I've trained, I can hardly remember anyone having perfectly aligned or well-balanced feet. Weak muscles and poor standing habits cause feet to invert or evert, or roll in or out on the ankles. The poor habits we develop as toddlers we maintain as adults. Even when we're aware that we have dropped or fallen or poor arches, we may be told that it's genetic. Dropped arches lead to knee and hip pain. The common solution for this problem is arch supports or orthotics, which lift the arches, realign the knees, and take the pain away. Orthotics do work, but they don't change the fundamental problem of weak muscles and poor foot alignment. To fix the problem, the entire chain of bones, muscles, fascia, and ligaments needs to be rebalanced.[10] The arch and the skeletal structure need to be rebuilt through exercise; only in the adjustment period are arch supports or orthotics needed.

The easiest way to determine whether you're standing on the full triangular arch or if you're rolling your ankles in or out is to look at the heels of your shoes. Check to see if the heels are worn away in a pie shape or a wedge. If the heels are in perfect shape, it means that you're standing correctly on your full arch. For most people, however, this is not the case.

It's relatively easy to retrain yourself to stand or walk on the full sole of your foot by stretching the overworked side of your leg and strengthening the underworked side. This will remold the fascia and ligaments not just in your feet but all the way up your leg. It becomes a tug-of-war between your attempt to stand correctly and the fascia pulling you back into the original, incorrect shape. For some people it may feel slightly uncomfortable or mildly painful, but once you win the tug-of-war (it takes about three months of a daily five- to ten-minute exercise routine), you'll be amazed at how much stronger, lighter, and better balanced you become. You'll also find that any sports or exercises you do will be easier. I speak from personal experience: I had this problem myself, and had to rebalance my legs. I was in mild discomfort for several weeks, and yes, it was difficult. But the effort and discomfort were well worth it, as I soon stood straighter and moved with greater ease.

When the feet are flat, the knees tend to drop or pull internally. This poor knee alignment strains the knee, hip, and spine joints, which can lead to arthritis and, sometimes, eventual joint replacement. When the knee joint is out of alignment, it creates a ripple effect up the structure of the leg, pulling on the hip and spine and unbalancing the shoulders and arms. Skeletal imbalances leave many different forms of chronic pain in their wake, including hip, back, shoulder, neck, and elbow pain. Reversing flat feet by developing strong arches will indirectly readjust the alignment of your entire body and change your posture.

THE ROLE OF FASCIA IN POSTURE

When it comes to having good posture, healthy fascia is not only essential to establishing it but also plays a major role in maintaining it. Strong, malleable, well-hydrated fascia is as important as strong, flexible muscles. Hardened, dried fascia (sometimes called wadding or scar tissue) impairs the ability of the muscles to move. Hardened fascia behaves like a suit of armor, surrounding muscles and immobilizing them. Brute force is no match for gummed-up, dehydrated fascia. The answer is to melt the buildup of hardened fascia by gentle stretching, which introduces hydration into the fascia layers. Reversing hardened fascia takes time, patience, and gentle movement. Rapid strengthening exercises can actually tear hardened fascia, creating more scar tissue.

If you look at photos of yourself as a child and as an adult, you may notice that the shape of your body has changed over the years. You cannot see those changes on a daily basis, but when you compare a photo of yourself at three years old to one taken ten years later, you can see how your body has changed.

If our muscles remain strong and we maintain roughly the same weight, then our fascia will hold that shape and we'll look approximately the same for decades. However, if we gain a substantial amount of weight or our muscles weaken, or both, our fascia will slowly reshape over time. When the muscles weaken, the fascia surrounding them weakens and deforms. We lose the rebound tension of strong fascia, because the fascia matrix is dependent on strong muscles to push against. Muscles can develop strength rapidly, but it can take months for the fascia to re-form to reflect what the muscles actually should look like. There is an interdependent relationship between the muscular system and the connective tissue system. When one is weak it weakens the other, and when one is strong it strengthens the other.

Over time our fascia remolds based on the way we carry our bodies, reflecting our various habits. For example, people who slouch all the time show signs of a buildup of hardened fascia in their upper back. This posture weakens the muscles of the back; the more this posture becomes a habit, the more difficult it is to hold the spine upright. If this posture is not corrected, it can become almost impossible to straighten the spine.

According to a 2018 study by the market research group Nielsen, American adults spend more than eleven hours per day watching, reading, listening to, or otherwise interacting with media. That's up from nine hours and thirty-two minutes just four years earlier. The time we spend working at a computer or looking at our cell phones causes our neck and upper back muscles to remain relatively still for hours at a

BAD HABITS, BAD POSTURE

Bad habits can imbalance your body and cause stiffness and pain, but a full-body rebalancing program can counteract these habits and keep your body in equilibrium.

If you always carry a bag, or your child, on the same side of your body, over time your fascia will remold around your shoulder and arm, and one shoulder will become visibly lower than the other. This is a shift in your skeleton and could lead to neck pain, back pain, or headaches.

Crossing one leg over the other when sitting stretches the hip muscles of the leg that's crossed. The hip muscles of the crossed leg will slowly lengthen in response to this continuous stretching. Hip muscles are directly connected to both the spine and the legs, which means that any imbalance in the hips will lead to an imbalance in the spine and legs. Unbalanced hips can also pull the femurs out of alignment, which directly pulls on the knee joints, causing knee pain and damage.

Other habits that can cause damage and pain:

- Getting out of bed on the same side every day makes the same hip take the full weight of the body, leading to limping
- Holding the stair rail with the same arm makes one shoulder get stronger and bend sideways, leading to shoulder and neck pain
- Swinging a golf club or a bat in the same direction unbalances the spine muscles, causing pain
- Lifting heavy cooking pots with the same arm creates shoulder and spine imbalance and pain
- Wearing high-heeled shoes causes the shin muscles to lengthen and the calf muscle to shorten, leading to ankle pain and inflammation of the shins
- Wearing poorly fitting shoes that squeeze the toes and feet leads to plantar fasciitis and ankle, knee, and hip pain
- Sitting at a computer for extended periods leads to shortened and weakened full-body muscles
- Brushing your hair with the same arm leads to shoulder imbalance and pain
- Favoring your dominant hand makes that hand and arm get stronger while the other hand and arm get weaker

Many of these daily habits are difficult or impossible to change. If you're left- or right-handed, that's the hand it's easiest to work with; and I know very few golfers or baseball players who swing from both sides. That's why doing a daily rebalancing routine is so important, and such a simple solution to real-life problems.

time. Is it any wonder that the posture of old and young alike suffers?

One immediate solution is to raise your computer screen and hold your cell phone at eye level. This will immediately straighten your neck and upper back. Equally important is taking a three- or four-minute exercise break every hour to stretch your arms, wrists, fingers, and back.

The real issue here is finding the simplest solution to making our lives easy and pain-free. This is why focusing on improving our posture is so important. This book is full of effective routines for sports, daily life, and health, but the most important section in the book is the Posture Routine, which highlights the importance of addressing the flexibility of the hips, spine, and shoulders in one all-encompassing workout. Standing straight doesn't qualify as good posture if your spine and shoulders are locked down from contracted muscles. My definition of good posture is having the fluidity of a cheetah and the ability to twist, turn, reach, and bend effortlessly while sitting, standing, and walking with a straight, relaxed spine.

ESSENTRICS BASIC SPINE MOVEMENTS

In order to improve posture, you will find the following basic movements in every Essentrics workout. These two movements are designed to both improve posture and relieve back pain. They are Neutral C and Neutral Elongation.

Neutral C and Neutral Elongation

The weight of the body should flow uninterrupted from the top of the head down through the spine, hips, and knees and into the feet in what we call a perfect load path. Neutral C is a forward flexion of the upper and lower spine that mimics the letter *C*. The load path of Neutral C shortens the distance between the head and shoulders and the spine as the body bends forward, reducing the load on the lower spine.

Neutral C and Neutral Elongation have two purposes: as a means of stretching and strengthening the spine and as positions to protect the spine from overload and back pain.

Neutral Elongation places the spine in a state of perfect posture as the weight of the body flows through a clean load path. Neutral Elongation reflects the natural double *S*-shaped curves of the spine, helping the vertebrae to hang comfortably from skull to coccyx with no interruption in the flow of the load path at any point.

Almost all Essentrics sequences involve seamless shifting between Neutral C and Neutral Elongation. Sequences such as Shoulder Blasts, Ceiling Reaches, and Embracing a Beach Ball all flow constantly between Neutral C and Neutral Elongation, gently stretching and strengthening the muscles. Full use of the spine in these movements ensures that the lower and upper back are equally strengthened and stretched.

As sequences and exercises shift the spine

constantly between Neutral C and Neutral Elongation, they gently loosen tight vertebrae. The bending and elongating lengthen the many erector spinae muscles, reducing stress and lessening chronic back pain. Shifting between these two positions helps us regain the natural mobility of the spine—and reminds us what good, comfortable posture feels like. Using these positions correctly is vital in achieving good posture.

Neutral C and Correct Posture

We use Neutral C in many of the full-body Essentrics sequences.

Neutral C involves curving the tailbone under while rounding the upper back forward. It's designed to help distribute the weight evenly from the head to the feet when we do forward movements. The forward flexion stretches the vertebrae, and is usually followed by straightening the spine. This pairing of forward movement and straightening the spine safely and gently maintains range of motion of the spine.

Neutral C is often followed by a rotational or diagonal twisting of the spine. When used together, these movements maintain correct range of motion of the vertebrae.

Incorrect positioning involves arching the lower back instead of curving the tailbone under, causing the weight load path to land on the lower back, stressing the lower-back muscles. When shown or indicated in the captions, use Neutral C in forward-flexion sequences.

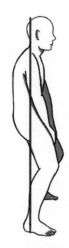

Correct forward flexion in Neutral C.

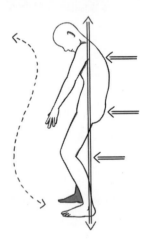

Clean load path through the shoulders and hips into the feet in Neutral C.

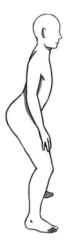

Incorrect forward flexion with the lower back arching.

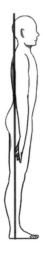

Correct straight spine with load path flowing from the head, down the spine, through the hips, and into the arch of the foot.

Lateral Flexion and Extension

The spine is designed to move in many directions. Lateral flexion of the spine is a movement in which the head and trunk bend toward one side while the spine curves convexly in the opposite direction.[11] In Essentrics it's used to liberate the spine. During lateral flexion, the oblique, intercostal, and rectus abdominis muscles are all eccentrically stretched and strengthened. The strengthening in a lateral extension is achieved by lifting the arms above the head.

Rotation of the Spine

Rotation of the spine is a movement that involves twisting the spine. Each section of the spine has a different degree of flexion, extension, and rotation. The vertebrae of the thoracic T12 and lumbar L4 and L5 rotate the most, while only slight rotation is possible in the thoracic spine above T12. The cervical spine is where the most twisting is possible; it allows for a rotational range of about 90 degrees of head motion.[12]

In Essentrics, spine rotation is frequently combined with diagonal movements. Rotation of the spine allows us to work actively through the muscle chains to increase the range of motion of the spine in each direction, including flexion and extension. Any exercises that include rotation of the spine will stretch, strengthen, and rebalance all the muscles and joints.

ESSENTRICS TECHNIQUES FOR GOOD POSTURE

Alignment

Without good alignment, it's simply impossible to have good posture. Imagine a table with one leg that's shorter than the others. The table will continually wobble until you fix the shorter leg. Likewise, you can work on strengthening your muscles as much as you want, but they will always be unbalanced and incapable of attaining full strength until you focus on your full-body alignment.

Alignment starts with the foundation of the body—the feet—and spirals upward through the entire skeleton. Both inversion and eversion of the soles of the feet will cause torsion of the ankle joints—inversion by rolling the ankle inward, and eversion by rolling it out.

When the feet are positioned correctly—flat on the ground, with the soles neither everted nor inverted—the arches will automatically and naturally lift to their highest comfortable point. Only when the feet are positioned with no eversion or inversion can the rest of the body be correctly aligned to help protect the hips, knees, ankles, and spine from injury and pain. Correct alignment is the most efficient way to strengthen the full-body musculature.

Difficulty in achieving natural alignment may be due to:

- Poor body awareness
- Imbalanced muscles
- Immobility in the ankles from congealed or weakened connective tissue
- Immobility in the ankles from scar tissue caused by injuries
- Immobility in the ankles from tight muscles, dried ligaments, or atrophy
- Weak muscles

Pulling Up and Pulling Out

This technique is derived directly from ballet and offers many benefits, including:

- Improved posture
- Improved alignment
- Joint protection
- Relief and healing of back and knee pain
- Strengthened hip muscles
- Increased energy
- Increased hip flexibility
- Improved circulation

Pulling Up and Pulling Out are fundamental techniques in Essentrics. They provide consistent eccentric tension on the muscles during the entire workout. When you use them, you're lifting your bones, which takes strength. Lifting the weight of the body up and out of the joints gives the sensation of becoming lighter. Strengthening in the elongated position relieves tightness and immobility of the joints, including the spine, hips, knees, and ankles.

Pulling Up the Arms

The action of lifting the arms above the head stretches and strengthens all the muscles of the spine. Lifting the arms above the head helps reverse shrinking as people age, improves posture, slenderizes the waist, and reverses muscle atrophy.

CHAPTER 5

Neuromuscular Techniques

Eccentric, Concentric, Isotonic, and Isometric

There are several ways in which muscles change length while moving. Anytime a muscle moves, it immediately contracts. The word *contraction* implies a "shortening" when referring to muscles, but this is not true. Contractions can shorten muscles, lengthen them, or maintain the same length. When muscles shorten, it's called a *concentric contraction*. When the muscle stays the same length, it's called an *isometric contraction*. When the muscle lengthens, it's called an *eccentric contraction*. *Isotonic contractions* do both as they flow through a movement. Essentrics uses traditional neuromuscular techniques to consciously stimulate the brain to contract or relax the muscles for flexibility and strength.

ECCENTRIC CONTRACTIONS

In literal terms, *eccentric* means proceeding from the center. Imagine that you're holding a ten-pound weight and doing a biceps curl. As you do the curl, you bend your elbow while pulling the weight toward your shoulder. Your biceps muscle will shorten. That's a concentric contrac-

tion. Now straighten your elbow, keeping your arm at shoulder height. The biceps muscle will lengthen and look longer, even though you're still holding the ten-pound weight. This is an eccentric contraction; the muscles are contracting (getting stronger) *and* lengthening at the same time. This sends a conflicting message to the protein filaments: One message says to contract or slide together, and the other says to lengthen or pull apart, creating a tug-of-war.

Here are other examples of concentric and eccentric contractions:

When you're putting a heavy pile of dishes into a kitchen cupboard, your elbows bend as you lift the dishes off the counter and straighten as you lift the dishes into the cupboard. As the elbow bends, the biceps muscle contracts concentrically, and as the arm extends, the biceps muscle contracts eccentrically.

When you're painting a wall with a roller, your elbow bends and straightens as you move the roller up and down the wall. As you straighten your elbow to reach upward, your biceps and latissimus dorsi contract eccentrically.

Eccentric contractions are actually more

efficient builders of strength than concentric contractions, and eccentric training has been scientifically proven over and over again to develop stronger muscles than concentric strengthening.[1] The ability to produce greater force in the lengthening phase of muscle contraction is largely attributed to the passive elements of the muscle fibers—the structural protein titin and the collagen-based connective tissues, which act like little elastic bands within the muscle. As a contracted muscle is elongated, these structures gradually unravel and resist the lengthening movement, leading to greater strengthening adaptation than concentric contractions provide. Furthermore, when the muscles are targeted through their full range of motion, as with eccentric contractions, it can help the muscle produce maximum force through greater lengths.[2]

Due to the enhanced strengthening potential associated with eccentric contractions, many bodybuilding and strength programs have adapted eccentric training principles to include the use of external weights. The pitfall of this is that eccentric training with weights is also known to cause more damage to the connective tissue and requires a longer recovery time. The adverse effects of this damage can interfere with performance, increase the risk of injury, and potentially decrease range of motion if adequate recovery time isn't allotted.[3] Eccentric training with weights is a completely different type of eccentric training than that used in Essentrics, where we never use external weights. We use only the weight of the person's body.

Ballet dancers, who eccentrically strengthen their muscles throughout maximum ranges of movement, are well known for their strong physiques, seemingly effortless posture, excellent balance, and powerful jumping capabilities. Eccentric training is the principal technique used by classical ballet dancers. They straighten their limbs and joints in large, elegant, controlled full-body movements. It takes a lot of strength to hold your legs straight and high above your shoulders with pointed toes.

CONCENTRIC CONTRACTIONS

In a concentric contraction, the muscle being strengthened is pulled toward the body. This brings the attachment points of the muscle closer together, shortening it. When you lift a weight by bending your elbow, pulling the weight toward your body, your biceps flexes as it shortens. Concentric training is referred to as positive training.

Most sports, fitness, and dance (with the exception of ballet) training programs focus primarily on concentric training; little attention is paid to eccentric training. This makes the muscles grow tighter and tighter, leading to unnecessary injuries and pain.

Muscles are designed to shorten *and* lengthen. When they're trained only to shorten, they compress the joints, reduce the range of motion, and become unbalanced and injury prone.

ISOTONIC CONTRACTIONS

Isotonic means equal resistance. Isotonic movement replicates the movements we perform in everyday life. In exercise science, an isotonic contraction is one in which the resistance or weight remains constant as the muscle changes length, shortening or lengthening during the movement. In the isotonic contraction of lifting and lowering a limb, the muscles of that limb change length as the limb lifts and lowers. At every stage of isotonic movement, the weight remains constant while the muscle length changes.

Examples of isotonic contractions are the actions we take when putting on our clothes in the morning. We might bend forward to put on our socks and shoes and reach over our head to pull on a T-shirt or sweater. The twists and turns we make when drying our legs, backs, arms, and hair after a shower are other classic examples of isotonic contractions.

ISOMETRIC CONTRACTIONS

Isometric means equal length. An isometric movement is one in which no change in muscle length occurs. Pushing against an immovable object like a door frame or the floor is an example of an isometric movement.

Isometric contractions are used mainly in physical therapy; they're the safest way to strengthen a weak or injured muscle. An isometric contraction is held in a static position and does not move through the range of motion of a joint.

In Essentrics, we use isometrics in standing leg lifts by pressing the standing leg into the floor or contracting the hips to stabilize the joints while balancing. In arm exercises, we isometrically contract the torso to liberate blocked range of motion in the shoulders.

RELAXATION

Muscular relaxation is the release of a contraction. Relaxation is a powerful technique in helping to fully stretch and strengthen muscles. The muscles surrounding any joint must be able to flow rapidly between tension and relaxation in order to permit the full range of motion of the joint.

Many people have trouble releasing tension from their muscles. If muscles cannot relax, they cannot stretch. Ironically, releasing tension from muscles on command is as tiring and challenging as strengthening them.

AGONIST/ANTAGONIST

In the skeletal structure, muscles are arranged in opposing pairs. When one muscle group (the agonist) contracts and shortens, the opposing muscle group (the antagonist) relaxes and lengthens. The degree of strength or tension in the working (agonist) muscle is equally matched by the degree of flexibility in the opposing (antagonist) muscle; they work harmoniously to permit full range of motion of the joints.

If a joint isn't able to achieve its maximum potential range of motion, then you know that either the agonist group or the antagonist group is too tight, holding back the movement.

CHAPTER 6

Getting Started

This chapter explains how to get started doing an Essentrics routine. You'll learn what equipment is needed, why you need it, and how to use it correctly. You'll also learn the difference between good and bad posture, as well as common mistakes people make when doing Essentrics. As a beginner, you may find that you have trouble standing straight or doing the exercises correctly or comfortably; however, by using the equipment and correct alignment, you will see rapid changes to your flexibility and strength.

EQUIPMENT

Most equipment used in Essentrics, like a chair or a towel, can easily be found in your home. The following is a list of what you may need to support you in your workouts.

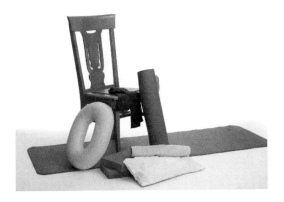

Basic Essentrics Equipment:

1. Chair, ballet barre, or banister.
2. Blocks or risers.
3. Small rolled-up towel.
4. TheraBand or other resistance band.
5. Hemorrhoid "donut" cushion.
6. Cushion for the head.
7. A solid mat (not a squishy one).

1. CHAIR, BALLET BARRE, OR BANISTER

A chair (or a barre or banister) is needed for balancing and stretching. Make sure your chair is sturdy and stable and has a relatively high back.

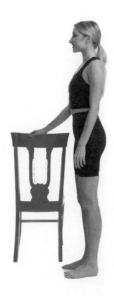

Correct: Stand about five inches away from the chair. Hold the chair with a bent elbow well in front of your body.

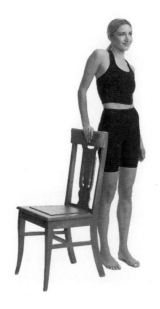

Incorrect: Do not lift your shoulder or elbow while holding the chair.

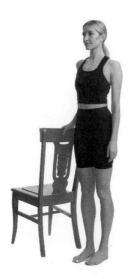

Incorrect: Do not stand directly beside the chair.

It's extremely important to hold the chair or barre slightly in front of your shoulders. Stand about five inches away from the chair and bend your elbow, dropping it toward your waist. Never lift your elbow, as that will lift your shoulder.

2. BLOCKS OR RISERS

During the seated floor sequences, people with tight back, hip, and leg muscles should sit on blocks or foam risers to lift their hips off the ground. Elevating the hips makes it easier to keep the back and knees straight while sitting. Some people need to sit on as many as three or four risers in order to straighten their spine. The recommended size is 30.5 cm x 20 cm x 5 cm (12 in x 8 in x 2 in).

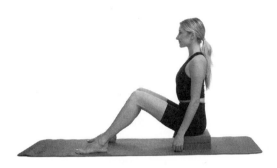

Use blocks, risers, or a wide book to elevate the hips off the floor when the legs are extended in front (with knees bent or straight).

3. SMALL ROLLED-UP TOWEL

If your ankles feel uncomfortable during leg-on-the-barre or seated stretches, place a small towel under your heels or ankles. The towel acts as a barrier to alleviate discomfort caused by pressure from the hard surface.

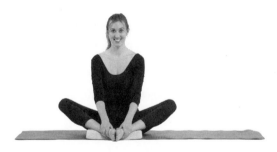

Place a small towel under the heels or ankles to relieve any pressure.

4. THERABAND OR OTHER RESISTANCE BAND

A TheraBand or other resistance band is a tool for people with tight muscles to make it easier for them to reach their feet or ankles.

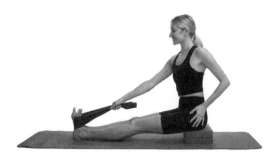

Use a TheraBand or other resistance band when it's difficult to reach your feet while keeping your back straight at the same time.

5. HEMORRHOID "DONUT" CUSHION

A hemorrhoid cushion is used in Side Leg Lifts to correctly position the hips. For some people, getting into the correct position for leg lifts requires lying directly on their hip bone, which is painful. To prevent your hip bone from digging into the floor, you can rest it in the hole of a donut cushion. Without the cushion, people tend to roll their hips backward, therefore losing many of the benefits of this powerful exercise.

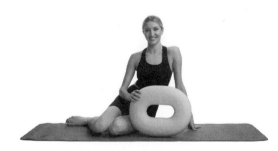

A hemorrhoid "donut" cushion can be used in Side Leg Lifts sequences.

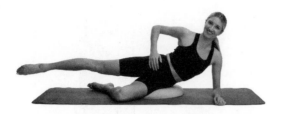

Placing your hip in the donut hole takes the weight off your hip bone, making it easy to target the gluteus medius without pain.

6. CUSHION FOR THE HEAD

A small cushion is used to stop the chin from protruding forward and the head from falling backward. Placing a cushion under your head will help you straighten your neck and release tension.

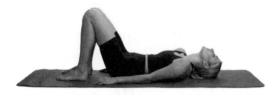

Incorrect: Chin protrudes upward and the head falls backward.

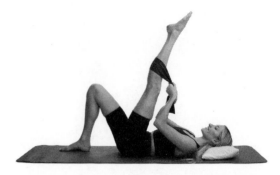

Correct: Find the correct thickness of cushion to raise the head off the floor so that the neck is straight and the head doesn't fall backward.

7. MAT

Using a thin mat (3 mm thick) is optional during the standing sequences to support your feet and provide a non-slippery surface. For floor work, some people prefer a thicker mat (8 mm thick) for added comfort.

CORRECT/INCORRECT POSITIONS

In this section, you'll learn common mistakes people make and how to safely do these exercises.

Correct/Incorrect Positions:

1. Neck and Head Positioning
2. Neutral Elongation (Standing Straight)
3. Neutral C (Curving the Spine)
4. Foot Positioning
5. Ankle Positioning
6. Foot and Knee Positioning in Pliés
7. Spine Positioning in Pliés
8. Hip Isolation

1. NECK AND HEAD POSITIONING

Many people develop tight, rounded upper backs by overbuilding the trapezius (upper back) muscles, which causes the chin to protrude. Forward drooping of the head and chin causes compression of the cervical spine.

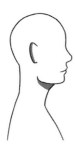

Correct positioning of the neck and chin. This prevents the upper back from rounding and creates a well-aligned load path to distribute the weight of the head in an unimpeded flow through the spine and into the feet.

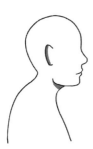

Incorrect positioning of the neck and chin. When the chin protrudes, the weight of the skull pulls the spine forward and causes the upper back to round.

A dropped head and rounded upper back are clear visual evidence of poor posture. When the chin protrudes, it pulls the weight of the upper spine forward, and, over time, the cervical spine will assume this rounded position. Forward head posture is often caused by sitting at a desk, leading to a rounded upper back (called kyphosis).

2. NEUTRAL ELONGATION (STANDING STRAIGHT)

Good posture permits the load path to flow unobstructed from head to toe, leaving the joints fully mobile and stress-free. A poor load path puts stress and strain on the joints from head to toe.

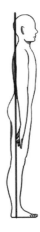

Correct alignment and distribution of weight through a clean load path flowing from the head, down the spine, through the hips, and into the arch of the foot.

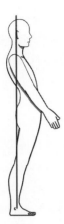

Incorrect alignment and distribution of weight through a poor load path.

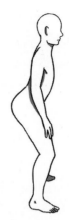

Incorrect forward flexion with the lower back arching.

3. NEUTRAL C (CURVING THE SPINE)

Neutral C is designed to increase the flexion of the spine by curving the tailbone under while rounding the upper back forward. The forward flexion stretches the vertebrae. Neutral C is usually followed by straightening the spine. This pairing of forward flexion and straightening safely and gently maintains the range of motion of the spine. Neutral C and spine straightening are often followed by a side, rotational, or diagonal twisting of the spine.

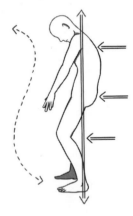

Clean load path through the shoulders and hips and into the feet in Neutral C.

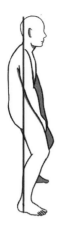

Correct forward flexion in Neutral C.

Neutral C is meant to help distribute weight evenly from the head through to the feet when we do forward movements. Incorrect positioning involves arching the lower back instead of curving the tailbone under, causing the weight load path to land on the lower back, stressing the lower back muscles. When indicated in the captions, always use Neutral C in forward flexion sequences.

4. FOOT POSITIONING

Always stand with your weight distributed over the entire soles of your feet. Do not roll your feet in or out (eversion or inversion). Doing so weakens the muscles and joints of your entire leg: as one side of the leg overworks, the other weakens. This leads to a chain reaction of joint damage, starting at the ankle and spiraling through the knee, hip, and spine. Rolling your feet is a common cause of knee, hip, and back pain, as well as of arthritis.

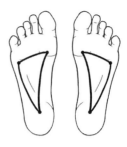

The arches of the feet form a triangle on the sole of each foot.

Between the toes and heel of each foot is the arch, which consists of three separate arches that form a triangle on the sole of the foot. These three arches are designed to absorb the weight of the body with every step we take.

Practice standing on the full triangles of your feet. This will require standing with your weight distributed from the heel to the full pad of the foot, where the toes join the sole. You want to spread the weight of your body evenly from the front pad of each foot to the heel pad, with the center point being the middle of the arch of each foot (the center of the triangle).

It takes two or three months to retrain your feet to stand correctly. This may not feel natural for the first few weeks, but slowly the connective tissue and muscles will reshape. Until you have finished training your feet and legs, they will continuously try to pull you back into the rolling position. It's exhausting but worth the effort—standing fully on the soles of your feet will instantly improve your balance and relieve knee and ankle pain.

5. ANKLE POSITIONING

It's important to avoid twisting or rolling the ankles. Ankles have a limited side-to-side range of motion, which is controlled by ligaments that act as stabilizers. Weak ankles are often caused by eversion or inversion. This is one of the most common reasons for sprained ankles, shin splints, plantar fasciitis, and most chronic ankle pain.

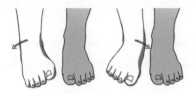

Eversion or inversion of the ankles.

When we spend our lives either everting or inverting our ankles, our ligament stabilizers get overstretched. When that happens, the ligaments become limp and are no longer capable of supporting the ankle. It doesn't matter how strong an athlete or dancer may be—if their ankles are everted or inverted, their feet will be prone to injury and pain. Sequences in this program are designed to rebuild and strengthen overstretched ligaments.

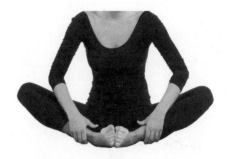

Correct positioning of shins: When doing the butterfly stretch, it's important not to overstretch your ankles. Hold your legs above your ankles and not your toes, as seen in the next photo.

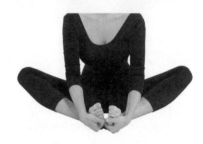

Incorrect positioning of feet: Holding your feet during this stretch will cause overstretching of your ankle ligaments.

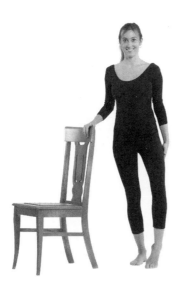

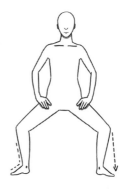

Correct positioning: In a wide plié, the knees should be over the arches or toes and should feel no stress.

Incorrect rolling of ankles: When pointing your foot, don't let your ankle and foot roll inward or outward as your heel lifts; keeping a clean line through your shin to the center of your arch will properly align your ankles.

6. FOOT AND KNEE POSITIONING IN PLIÉS

Take the time to set up your knee positioning for lunges and pliés. Turn your feet comfortably outward; never force the turnout position beyond proper alignment and what feels comfortable for your knees. Keep in mind that these are not ballet pliés or squats.

Pliés are used to strengthen the quadriceps and liberate the knees. If your feet are placed correctly, there should be zero stress on your knees. When your feet are either too wide apart or too close, it will put pressure on your kneecaps, possibly leading to pain.

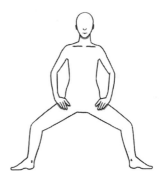

Incorrect positioning: Too wide. The feet are too far apart.

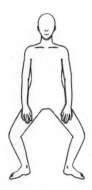

Incorrect positioning: Too narrow. The feet are too close together.

Stabilize your knees by keeping them in line with your feet and pushing your thighs outward; this will stretch your groin. Stand flat on your feet, without everting or inverting them. This will protect your knees.

7. SPINE POSITIONING IN PLIÉS

The purpose of pliés in Essentrics is to eccentrically strengthen and stretch the quadriceps and gluteus muscles. Pliés are not the same as squats. Pliés use Neutral Elongation; your spine should remain straight. Do not round your lower back. Your shoulders should remain in line with your hips.

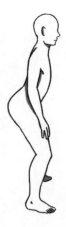

Incorrect: Forward flexion with the lower back arching.

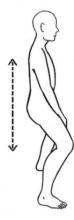

Correct: Keep the spine straight and the knees over the arches of the feet. Keeping the back straight liberates the hip flexors and increases the range of motion of the lower spine.

8. HIP ISOLATION

Legs are designed to swing freely at the hip joint. The torso should not move when we walk, run, or kick. However, a common mistake many people make is to tilt their body sideways when they lift their leg to the side or curl their buttocks under as they lift their legs to the front. In time the quadriceps, psoas, and hamstring muscles weaken from disuse. This is where isolating the torso and the hip joint is important. The correct way to lift the legs is to isolate the legs from the hips. This leaves the legs free to swing in the hip sockets while the torso remains upright.

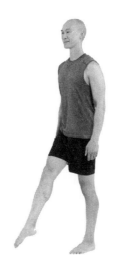

Correct: Isolate the leg from the hip when lifting the leg to the front.

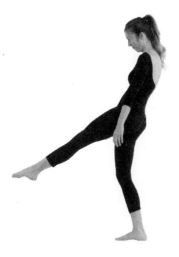

Incorrect: Do not lean back as you lift your leg. This will compress your spine and strain your back, as well as prevent your leg muscles from strengthening.

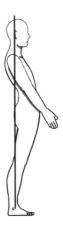

Incorrect: Leaning backward to lift your leg will stress your lower spine.

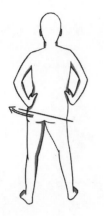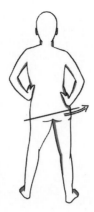

Lifted hips are incorrect.

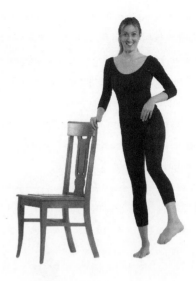

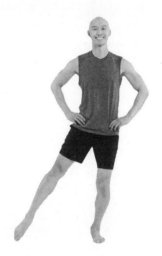

Incorrect: When kicking or lifting your leg to the side, don't let your buttocks or hips do the lifting. This is referred to as "lifting the leg with the hips." To liberate your hips and legs, keep both hips parallel to the ground as you lift your leg. Isolating your leg in the hip socket helps strengthen the leg muscles, increase hip flexibility, and rebalance your spine. It also helps to relieve and prevent back pain.

Correct: When lifting your leg to the side, try to isolate your leg from your torso. Lift your leg using only the gluteus and other leg muscles. This liberates the range of motion of both the hips and the spine.

CHAPTER 7
The Warm-Up

In this chapter you'll find eleven sequences that make up a fully balanced warm-up routine. Once you become familiar with these eleven sequences, it should take between four and five minutes to execute them.

Raising the body temperature is the basic principle behind doing a warm-up. The primary objective is to make the muscles warmer so that all movements are easier and more comfortable. To do that, we focus on relaxing the muscles and pumping blood into the extremities, which transports nutrients and oxygen while flushing toxins. As in every Essentrics routine, the full body is involved in the warm-up, which means we move through the range of motion of all the joints—for example, Simple Side-to-Side Steps for the hips or Swinging Both Arms Forward and Back for the spine and shoulders.

Never skip the warm-up and jump straight into stretching—it is an essential component to prepare your body for every Essentrics routine.

SIMPLE SIDE-TO-SIDE STEPS

JOINTS: hips, knees, shoulders, elbows.

Condyloid.   Hinge.   Saddle.

Plane.   Ball and socket.

MUSCLES: quadriceps, hamstrings, hip flexors, gluteus group, hip adductors, soleus, gastrocnemius, pectorals, deltoids, trapezius, rhomboids, latissimus dorsi, triceps, biceps.

Neutral spine.   Knees bent.   Side hip hinge.

Plantar flexion.   Elbow rotation.   Elbow hinge.   Fist open/close flexion.

1

Start with your feet together, arms bent at shoulder height, and knees bent.

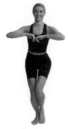

2

Open your arms and take as wide a step as possible. Timing: 1 second.

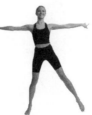

3

Land with control, not heavily, bringing your arms and legs together. Timing: 1 second. Repeat from side to side eight times. Timing: 8–9 seconds. Sixteen times takes 16 to 18 seconds.

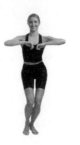

4

Start with your feet together, arms bent at shoulder height, knees bent. Timing: 1 second.

5

Lift your arms above your head while taking as wide a step as possible. Timing: 1 second.

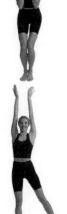

6

Land with control, not heavily, bringing your arms and legs together. Timing: 1 second. Repeat from side to side eight times. Timing: 8–9 seconds. Sixteen times takes 16 to 18 seconds.

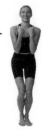

SWINGING BOTH ARMS FORWARD AND BACK

JOINTS: spine, shoulders, hips, knees, ankles.

Condyloid.

Hinge.

Saddle.

Plane.

Ball and socket.

MUSCLES: erector spinae, quadratus lumborum, abdominals, latissimus dorsi, trapezius, triceps, rhomboids, pectorals, deltoids, triceps, biceps, quadriceps, gluteus group, hip flexors, soleus, gastrocnemius.

Neutral spine.

Spine curved.

Knees bent.

180° arm rotation.

Elbow hinge.

1

You should be completely relaxed when doing all warm-up exercises to encourage maximum blood flow and to release tension in your muscles. Start with your arms above your head.

2

Bend your elbows and knees while rounding your upper back and tucking your tailbone under.

3

Gently swing your arms down and finish behind your hips. Timing: 2 seconds.

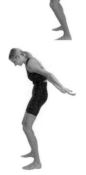

4

Swing your arms up to the start position. Timing: 2 seconds.

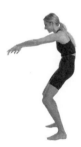

5

Repeat eight double-arm swings in a row. Timing: 30 seconds.

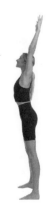

CEILING REACH WITH WAIST ROTATION

JOINTS: spine, shoulders.

Condyloid.

Saddle

Plane.

Ball and socket.

MUSCLES: obliques, abdominals, latissimus dorsi, intercostals, erector spinae, quadratus lumborum, trapezius, rhomboids, deltoids, triceps, biceps, pectorals.

Spine circle.

Shoulder lift.

1

Reach one arm toward the ceiling. Keep your body relaxed and let your shoulders lift as your arm reaches higher. Timing: 4 seconds.

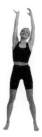

2

Alternate arms eight times, reaching upward. Timing: 30 seconds.

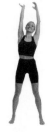

3

When performing a ceiling waist rotation, imagine that your fingers are following a small circle drawn on the ceiling.

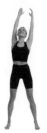

4

Stay relaxed.

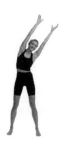

5

When bending forward, let your knees bend slightly.

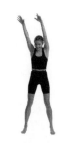

6

Finish the circle and then reverse, going in the opposite direction. Timing: 10 seconds per ceiling rotation.

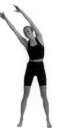

DOUBLE-ARM SWINGS, SIDE TO SIDE

JOINTS: spine, shoulders, knees.

Condyloid.

Hinge.

Saddle.

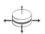
Plane.

Ball and socket.

MUSCLES: obliques, abdominals, latissimus dorsi, intercostals, erector spinae, quadratus lumborum, trapezius, rhomboids, pectorals, deltoids, quadriceps, hamstrings, gluteus group, soleus, gastrocnemius.

Neutral spine.   Spine curved.

Knees bent.   180° arm rotation.

1

With feet comfortably apart, swing both arms upward. Throughout this sequence your arms, elbows, fingers, and shoulders should be very relaxed.

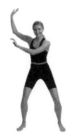

2

Swing your arms downward, bending your knees.

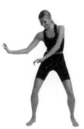

3

Lowering your head slightly, let your arms graze the tops of your thighs.

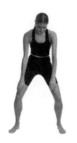

4

Swing your arms to the other side, following your arms with your head.

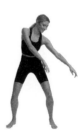

5

Slightly shift your weight over your leg.

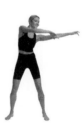

6

Finish with your arms above shoulder height, elbows relaxed and bent, eyes looking upward. The swing should feel like the pendulum of a clock. Timing: 2½ seconds. Eight swings should take roughly 15 seconds.

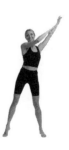

SINGLE-ARM ROTATIONS

JOINTS: spine, shoulders, hips. knees.

Condyloid.

Hinge.

Saddle.

Plane.

Ball and socket.

MUSCLES: latissimus dorsi, obliques, abdominals, erector spinae, quadratus lumborum, trapezius, rhomboids, deltoids, pectorals, quadriceps, hamstrings, hip flexors, gluteus group, soleus, gastrocnemius.

Neutral spine.

Spine curved.

Knees bent.

Spinal rotation.

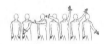

360° arm rotation.

1

Stand with your feet apart. Lift your arm toward the back of the room, rotating your spine as much as possible. Keep your shoulders down and your feet in place.

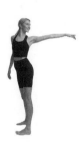

2

Sweep your arm downward, close to your thigh, while rounding your back. Your knees should be bent, your spine facing the front.

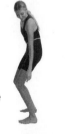

3

Continue the windmill motion, sweeping your arm forward. Let your spine begin to rotate.

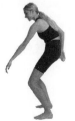

4

Finish the full rotation of your spine as you lift your arm in a windmill motion.

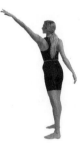

5

Continue the windmill motion by lifting your arm over your head and rotating your spine in the other direction.

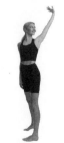

6

Start a new windmill from the beginning. Timing: 8 to 10 seconds. Repeat three times per arm. Timing: 25 to 30 seconds per arm.

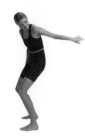

DIAGONAL TWISTS

JOINTS: spine, shoulders, elbows, hips, knees.

Condyloid.

Hinge.

Saddle.

Plane.

Ball and socket.

MUSCLES: latissimus dorsi, obliques, abdominals, intercostals, erector spinae, quadratus lumborum, trapezius, rhomboids, deltoids, pectorals, triceps, biceps, quadriceps, hamstrings, hip flexors, gluteus group, soleus, gastrocnemius.

Neutral spine.

Spinal rotation.

Plantar flexion.

Knees bent.

Elbow hinge.

1

Bend both knees and elbows.

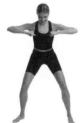

2

Shift your weight into a forward lunge and extend one arm in front and the other upward and behind. Rotate your torso to its maximum.

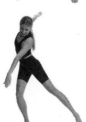

3

Take 5 seconds to go from the starting position to the diagonal lunge and back to the starting position. Repeat the diagonal lunge to the floor four times.

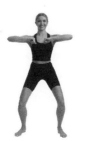

4

Repeat the diagonal lunge shoulder height four times.

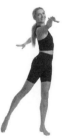

5

Always return to the neutral stance.

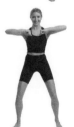

6

Repeat the diagonal lunge ceiling height four times. Repeat the sequence on the opposite side.

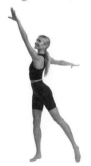

KNEE KICKS WITH SPINE TWISTS

JOINTS: spine, hips, knees, shoulders.

Condyloid.   Hinge.   Saddle.

Plane.   Ball and socket.

MUSCLES: latissimus dorsi, obliques, erector spinae, quadriceps, hamstrings, hip flexors, gluteus group, hip adductors, trapezius, rhomboids, deltoids, pectorals, triceps, biceps.

 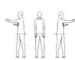

Neutral spine.   Spinal rotation.   Knees bent.   Hip hinge.

Hip joint rotation.   Shoulder lift.   Elbow hinge.

1

A. Bend your supporting leg, lift your other knee across the midline, and twist your spine. Hit your hips with both hands.

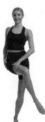

2

B. Open your arms and step sideways onto your other leg.

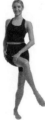

3

Repeat A and B eight times. Timing: 10 seconds to complete eight stepping-into-knee-lifts.

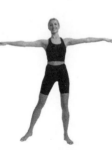

4

Continue the same side-to-side knee lifts with a spine twist.

5

In this series, lift both your arms to the ceiling instead of to the side when stepping sideways.

6

Repeat eight times. Timing: 10 seconds to complete eight kicks. Repeat the sequence on the opposite side.

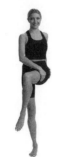

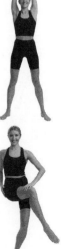

THROW A FRISBEE

JOINTS: spine, shoulders, hips, knees.

Condyloid.

Hinge.

Saddle.

Plane.

Ball and socket.

MUSCLES: erector spinae, quadratus lumborum, latissimus dorsi, obliques, abdominals, trapezius, rhomboids, deltoids, pectorals, triceps, biceps, quadriceps, hamstrings, hip flexors, gluteus group, soleus, gastrocnemius.

Neutral spine.

Spine curved.

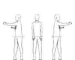
Spinal rotation.

Knees bent.

Hip hinge.

Elbow hinge.

1

Bend both knees, feet apart. Imagine you're about to throw a Frisbee.

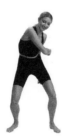

3

Toss the Frisbee to the other side. Repeat four times. Timing: 15 seconds to throw four Frisbees.

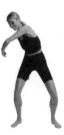

2

Toss the Frisbee to the side.

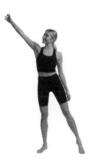

TAI CHI SPINE ROTATIONS

JOINTS: spine, shoulders, hips, knees.

Condyloid.　Hinge.　Saddle.

Plane.　Ball and socket.

MUSCLES: erector spinae, quadratus lumborum, latissimus dorsi, obliques, abdominals, trapezius, rhomboids, deltoids, pectorals, triceps, biceps, quadriceps, hamstrings, hip flexors, gluteus group, soleus, gastrocnemius.

Neutral spine.　Spine curved.　360° arm rotation.

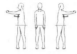

Spinal rotation.　Knees bent.　Heel lift.

1

Wrap your arms around your body. Bend both knees, tuck your tailbone under, and round your upper body in a crunch.

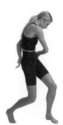

2

Windmill your front arm toward the ceiling.

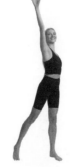

3

Start your body rotation by opening both arms as you shift your weight onto the opposite leg.

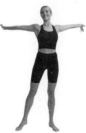

4

Windmill your other arm above your head as you continue the rotation.

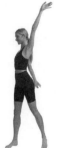

5

Lower your top arm as you wrap both arms around your body, one arm in front, the other behind. Timing: 7 seconds for one wraparound sequence.

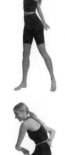

6

Repeat on the other side.

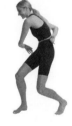

FAST PLIÉS WITH FULL ARM CIRCLE

JOINTS: shoulders, hips, knees.

Condyloid.

Hinge.

Saddle.

Plane.

Ball and socket.

MUSCLES: latissimus dorsi, trapezius, rhomboids, deltoids, pectorals, triceps, biceps, quadriceps, hip adductors, hamstrings, hip flexors, gluteus group, soleus, gastrocnemius.

Neutral spine.

Knees bent.

Plantar flexion.

1

Raise your arms above your head. Keep your knees straight and your feet comfortably apart.

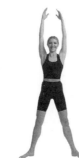

2

Lower your arms and bend your knees, contracting your quadriceps as you do so. Timing: 1 second.

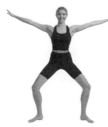

3

This is not a squat! As you bend your knees, keep your back straight and make sure that your feet are always flat on the ground, never everting or inverting. Timing: 1 second.

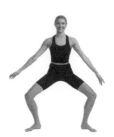

4

At the depth of the plié, finish the arm circle and cross your arms in a relaxed mode in front. Timing: 1 second.

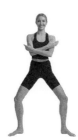

5

Reverse the movement by opening your arms and slowly straightening your knees. Timing: 1 second.

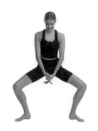

6

Finish with your arms above your head, as you started. Timing: 5 seconds for the entire plié sequence. Repeat four times.

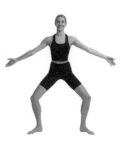

ARCHES, TOES, AND ANKLES

JOINTS: ankles, toes.

Hinge.

Plane.

MUSCLES: soleus, gastrocnemius, tibialis anterior and posterior, flexors and extensors of the toes.

Neutral spine.

Knees bent.

Heel lift.

Toe flexion.

Ankle flexion/extension.

1

Start by putting your weight on your front foot.

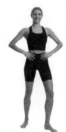

2

Keep your heel on the floor while raising the rest of your foot. This will stretch and strengthen the tibialis and gastrocnemius. Repeat the flat-to-flex movement four times. Timing: 10 seconds.

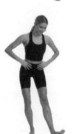

3

Raise your heel as much as possible while keeping all your toes flexed and flat on the floor. Push against the floor to help raise your heel farther.

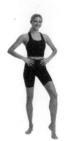

4

Point your toes, keeping your ankle extended.

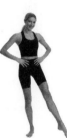

5

Keep your ankle extended and flex your toes. This will increase the power in your toes, enhancing the rebound action when you walk or run.

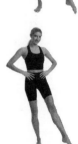

6

Flex your ankle. Take 10 seconds to repeat the point and flex four times. Repeat on the opposite side.

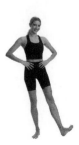

THE ESSENTRICS WARM-UP ROUTINE

TIME: Three to four minutes

FOCUS: Range of motion of every joint in all three planes

TECHNIQUES: Relaxation, mobility, deep breathing

OBJECTIVE: Increased blood flow, hydrated fascia, relaxed muscles, loose joints, decreased risk of injury, increased ability to adapt to the intensity of training

1. Simple Side-to-Side Steps, page 58.

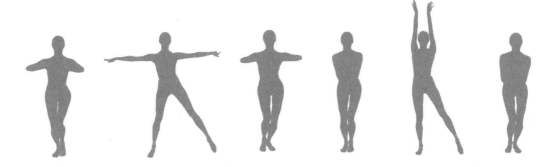

2. Swinging Both Arms Forward and Back, page 59.

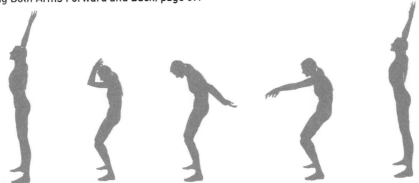

3. Ceiling Reach with Waist Rotation, page 60.

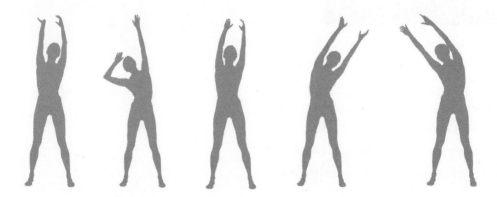

4. Double-Arm Swings, Side to Side, page 61.

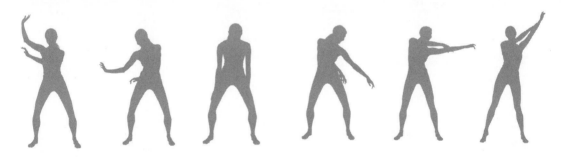

5. Single-Arm Rotations, page 62.

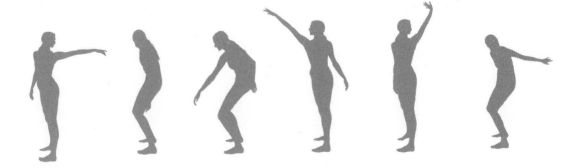

6. Diagonal Twists, page 63.

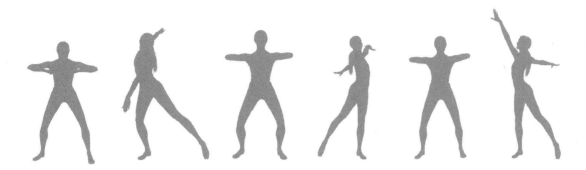

7. Knee Kicks with Spine Twists, page 64.

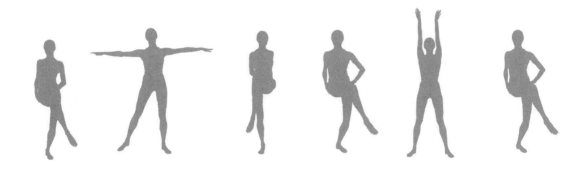

8. Throw a Frisbee, page 65.

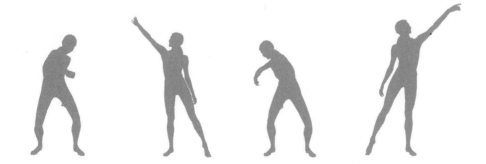

9. Tai Chi Spine Rotations, page 66.

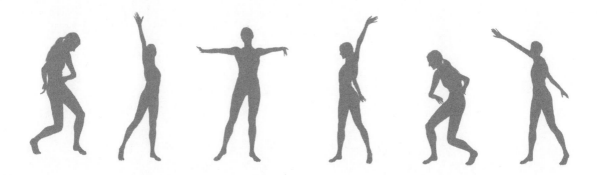

10. Fast Pliés with Full Arm Circle, page 67.

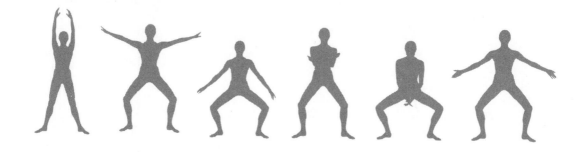

11. Arches, Toes, and Ankles, page 68.

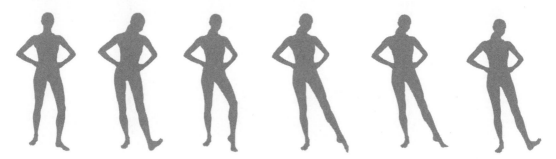

DANCE OUT YOUR STIFFNESS

Try these simple dance sequences to shake out stiffness and release tension. They're great for releasing the joints after long periods of sitting at your desk or traveling.

SEQUENCE 1

MUSCLES: gluteus group, quadriceps, hamstrings, soleus, gastrocnemius, quadratus lumborum, latissimus dorsi, obliques, abdominals.

Knees bent.   Elbow hinge.

Hip sway.   Pelvic tuck.

1

Dancing relaxes your hip and spinal muscles and hydrates and liberates the surrounding fascia, ligaments, and tendons.

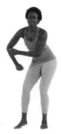

2

Put on music and dance, swinging your hips in every direction.

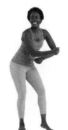

3

Relax and let your body move fluidly.

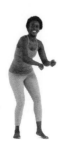

4

Keep dancing and moving!

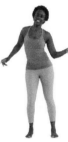

5

Enjoy yourself! Smile!

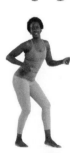

6

Exaggerate your moves to loosen your hips and spine as much as possible. Dance for 3 to 5 minutes until you're relaxed and warmed up.

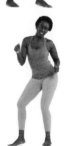

SEQUENCE 2

MUSCLES: gluteus group, hamstrings, quadriceps, hip flexors, quadratus lumborum, erector spinae, abdominals, obliques.

Knees bent.

Pelvic tuck.

Hip sway.

1

The rumba is a dance that relaxes your hip and spinal muscles. It hydrates and liberates the surrounding fascia, ligaments, and tendons.

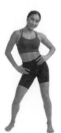

2

Put on dance music and dance a rumba, swinging your hips in every direction.

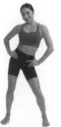

3

Relax and let your body move fluidly.

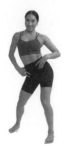

4

Keep dancing and moving until your body moves fluidly, like a well-oiled machine.

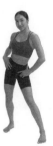

5

Take 2 to 3 seconds to focus on tucking your tailbone under.

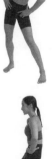

6

Take 2 to 3 seconds to focus on arching your back or sticking out your buttocks.

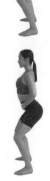

SEQUENCE 1

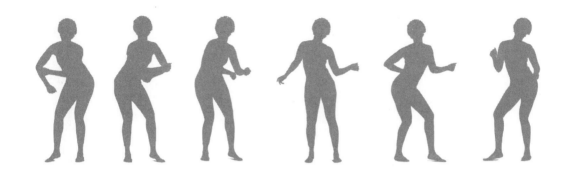

SEQUENCE 2

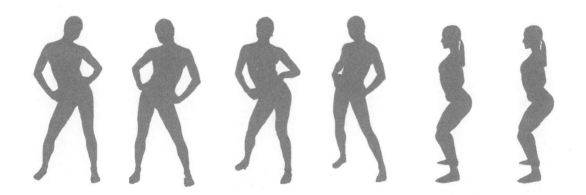

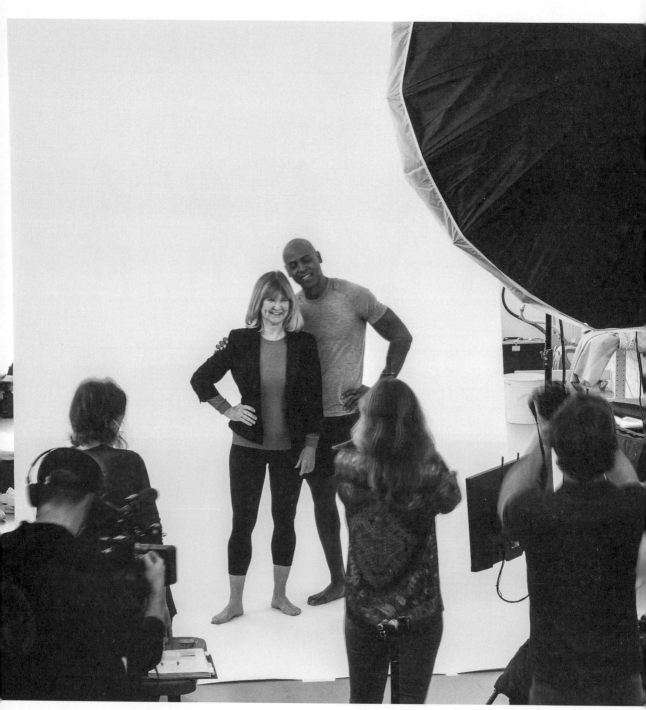

Behind the scenes: Miranda Esmonde-White guiding the photo shoot for this book.

CHAPTER 8
The Essentrics Sequences

In this chapter, you'll find more than a hundred different range-of-motion exercises, or sequences, as we call them in Essentrics.

Each Essentrics sequence focuses on different joints and muscles, moving through the range of motion of each given joint. The sequences consist of flowing movements based on imagery, such as washing a table. In Essentrics, the body is in constant motion, so there are no static, standing-still exercises. Keep moving throughout a sequence, trying to gently wiggle your joints into an even deeper stretch.

There is one sequence per page, and each page provides an overview of the primary muscles and joints that are being targeted for strengthening or flexibility and what equipment, if any, will be needed. The line drawings at the top of the page indicate the direction of every movement.

This chapter will tell you how to perform each sequence properly. The captions are as important as the pictures, as they indicate the speed at which the sequence should be performed. The Essentrics routines in later chapters are all made up of Essentrics sequences, and you should choose the routine or routines that best fit your needs. The sequences themselves are not stand-alone exercises; they're to be used only in the routines, and in the order specified.

CATEGORY 1: FORWARD FLEXION

ZOMBIE

JOINTS: spine, shoulders, knees.

MUSCLES: latissimus dorsi, erector spinae, quadratus lumborum, trapezius, rhomboids, deltoids, triceps, biceps, quadriceps, gluteus group.

1

Round your entire spine. Lower your head and bend your knees with your feet slightly apart. Repeat three times.

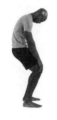

2

Slowly roll down your spine (5 seconds), hands following your thighs. Once you've finished your downward roll, relax your arms, shoulders, and upper back and sway for 5 seconds.

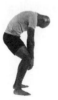

3

Slowly straighten your spine by rolling upward, one vertebra at a time.

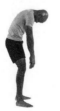

4

Slowly roll up. Timing: 5 seconds. Keep following your body with your hands, and keep your head lowered.

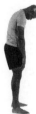

5

Fully straighten your spine and bring your arms to shoulder height, elbows bent.

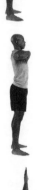

6

Take 5 seconds to finish by raising your arms above your head, relaxing your torso and shoulder muscles while pulling up as far as you can toward the ceiling. Timing: 20 seconds from start to finish.

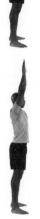

ROCK THE BABY

JOINTS: spine, shoulders, elbows, hips, knees.

Hinge.

Ball and socket.

MUSCLES: latissimus dorsi, obliques, intercostals, rhomboids, trapezius, deltoids, triceps, biceps, quadriceps, hamstrings, gluteus group.

Knees bent.

Bent elbows.

Spine curved.

Spine side to side.

1

Start with both knees bent. Imagine you're holding a baby in your arms and rocking it gently from side to side. Shift your weight slightly over one knee.

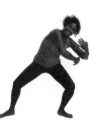

2

Shift your weight to the opposite knee, keeping your spine slightly rounded.

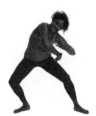

3

Rock the baby to the other side of your body and go into a lunge with your back knee straight.

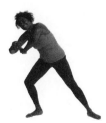

4

Start shifting your weight back over both knees.

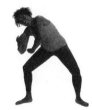

5

Now move your torso in a gently rocking motion.

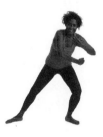

6

Bend slightly forward, cuddling the baby. Timing: 10 seconds for the full sequence. Repeat three times.

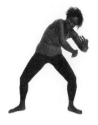

LULLABY AND LOWER A BLANKET

JOINTS: spine, shoulders, elbows, hips, knees.

Ball and socket.   Hinge.

MUSCLES: latissimus dorsi, quadratus lumborum, erector spinae, obliques, intercostals, rhomboids, trapezius, triceps, biceps, deltoids, pectorals, hamstrings, quadriceps, gluteus group.

Spine curved.   Bent elbows.   Knees bent.

Spine side to side.   Spine toe touch.   Straight spine.

1

From a side lunge, bend your spine toward the straighter leg, rounding your spine (ribs) and raising your arms to chest height, holding your elbows and hands together.

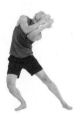

2

Sway side to side eight times, taking 3 seconds to change sides. Timing: 30 seconds total for eight sways.

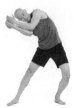

3

Finish with your body aligned, facing forward.

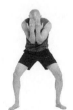

4

Imagine you have a precious blanket in your arms; lower the blanket to the floor. Roll down the spine one vertebra at a time. Timing: 7 seconds.

5

Roll up your spine one vertebra at a time. Timing: 7 seconds.

6

Finish with your arms outstretched, ready to repeat the sequence on the other side.

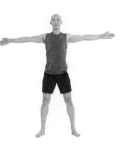

EMBRACE YOURSELF WITH SINGLE-ARM EXTENSIONS

JOINTS: spine, ribs, shoulders, elbows, hips, knees.

Ball and socket.

Hinge.

Saddle.

MUSCLES: latissimus dorsi, erector spinae, obliques, intercostals, trapezius, rhomboids, deltoids, pectorals, quadriceps, gluteus group.

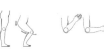

Knees bent.   Bent elbows.   Spine curved.

Spine side to side.   Straight spine.

1

Stand in a comfortably wide stance with your knees bent. Rounding only your upper spine/back, wrap your arms tightly around your chest or ribs.

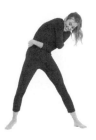

2

Move side to side in a slow swaying motion. Timing: 5 seconds.

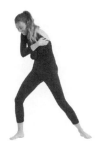

3

Make sure you engage your ribs and spine, feeling the individual ribs and upper vertebrae being stretched. Timing: 20 seconds for four sways.

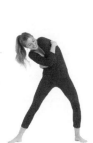

4

Keep your body bending sideways and reach one arm diagonally across.

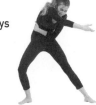

5

Sweep your arm across your body, opening it into a full side extension.

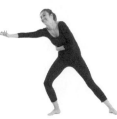

6

Repeat the same large sweep with your other arm, then stretch both arms open as wide as possible, raising your head and straightening your spine. Timing: 15 seconds for the two arm extensions. Repeat on the opposite side.

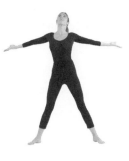

EMBRACE YOURSELF WITH CEILING REACHES

JOINTS: spine, shoulders, elbows, hips, knees.

Ball and socket.

Hinge.

Saddle.

MUSCLES: intercostals, obliques, latissimus dorsi, erector spinae, quadratus lumborum, trapezius, rhomboids, deltoids, pectorals, hamstrings, quadriceps. Connective tissue: deep fascia stretch.

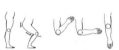

Knees bent.   Bent elbows.   Spine curved.   Spine side to side.

Spine leaning forward.   Straight spine.   Elbow hinge.   Arms up above head.

1

Start in a side lunge. Embrace yourself, holding your shoulders. Bend sideways toward your straight leg.

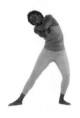

2

In a slow, gentle swaying movement, bend toward your bent knee. Timing: 5 seconds.

3

In the same fluid movement, shift your side lunge onto your other leg while continuing to sway your spine. Timing: 3 seconds.

4

Shift your spine to the front and then over your other knee. Keep your spine moving the entire time. Timing: 3 seconds.

5

To release the stretch on your spine, raise one arm at a time toward the ceiling. Timing: 3 seconds.

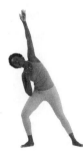

6

Finish with both arms stretched toward the ceiling and legs straight. Timing: 3 seconds. Total timing for one sequence: 17 seconds.

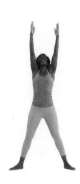

SHOULDER BLAST

JOINTS: shoulders, elbows, spine, ribs, knees.

Ball and socket.

Hinge.

Saddle.

MUSCLES: trapezius, rhomboids, deltoids, triceps, biceps, latissimus dorsi, erector spinae, quadratus lumborum, intercostals, hamstrings, quadriceps.

Spine curved.

Bent elbows.

Knees bent.

Spine toe touch.

Straight spine.

Shoulder arm rotation.

Shoulders up.

1

Create an *S* shape from the top of your head to your heels. Keep your elbows close to your waist and pull them as far behind your body as possible. Timing: 3 seconds.

2

Take 3 seconds to internally rotate your arms in their sockets while lifting your shoulders and straightening your elbows. Be careful not to bend forward.

3

Take 3 seconds to slowly sweep your arms in front at chest height. Timing: about 45 seconds for the full sequence.

4

Clasp your fingers together while pressing your hands toward the front of the room and pushing your upper back (rhomboid muscles) toward the back wall. Tip your shoulders very slowly up and down to feel a stretch in the muscles between your ribs. Timing: 5 seconds for each tip movement.

5

Bring your clasped hands up until they're almost touching your collarbone. Tip slowly sideways, alternating sides, four times. Timing: 3 seconds for each movement. Try to pull your fingers apart but don't let it happen. Timing: 12 seconds for the cycle of four.

6

Release your fingers and, in a relaxed mode, raise your arms above your head. Timing: 5 seconds.

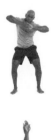

ARMS FOLLOWING THE CIRCUMFERENCE OF A BEACH BALL—CEILING TO WAIST

JOINTS: spine, shoulders, hips, knees.

Ball and socket.

Hinge.

Bent elbows.

Bent knee.

Curved spine.

1

Imagine that you're embracing a large, lightweight beach ball. You'll be holding or following the circumference of this beach ball throughout this sequence.

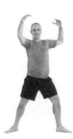

2

Stand facing forward with your feet in a wide stance. Twist slightly to face one knee and begin to follow the circumference of the ball.

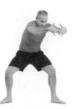

3

Bring your hands in to touch your body as the ball would be touching your body. Round your body to follow the circumference of the ball.

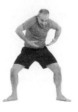

4

Keep circling the invisible ball.

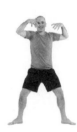

5

Repeat twice on the same side. Timing: 10 seconds.

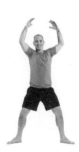

6

Repeat twice on the other side. Timing: 40 seconds total for both sides.

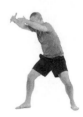

ARMS FOLLOWING THE CIRCUMFERENCE OF A BEACH BALL—CEILING TO FLOOR

JOINTS: spine, shoulders, hips, knees.

Ball and socket.

Hinge.

MUSCLES: abdominals, obliques, intercostals, latissimus dorsi, quadratus lumborum, triceps, biceps, deltoids, rhomboids, pectorals, trapezius, hamstrings, quadriceps, hip flexors, soleus, gastrocnemius.

Bent elbows.   Bent knee.   Spine leaning forward.

1

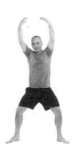

Imagine that you're embracing a large, lightweight beach ball. You'll be holding or following the circumference of this beach ball throughout this sequence.

2

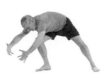

Follow the circumference of the ball to the floor, shifting your weight onto your front leg as you bend forward.

3

As you begin to straighten, shift your weight onto your back leg.

4

Follow your body with your hands, keeping your back rounded. Keep your feet flat so that your knee stays over your foot.

5

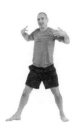

Slowly straighten up as you complete one sequence. Repeat twice on each side. Timing: 12 seconds for one sequence. Total timing for entire sequence: 50 seconds.

EMBRACE A BALL OVERHEAD— SWAYING SIDE TO SIDE

JOINTS: spine, shoulders, hips, knees.

Ball and socket.

Hinge.

MUSCLES: abdominals, obliques, intercostals, latissimus dorsi, quadratus lumborum, triceps, biceps, deltoids, rhomboids, pectorals, trapezius, hamstrings, quadriceps, hip flexors, soleus, gastrocnemius.

Bent elbows.

Bent knee.

Spine curved.

Spine side to side.

1

Imagine that you're embracing a large, lightweight beach ball. Bend sideways and hold the ball above your head.

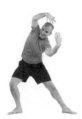

2

Continue holding the ball while moving it from one side of your body to the other.

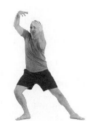

3

Keep holding the ball in the same position while bending your torso.

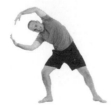

4

Hold the ball above your head as you shift your lunges and torso side to side. Shift side to side four times.

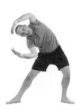

5

Timing: 8 seconds for one side.
Total timing: 40 seconds.

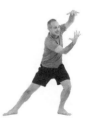

EMBRACE A BALL WITH DIAGONAL MOVEMENTS

JOINTS: spine, shoulders, hips, knees.

Ball and socket.   Hinge.

MUSCLES: abdominals, obliques, intercostals, latissimus dorsi, quadratus lumborum, triceps, biceps, deltoids, rhomboids, pectorals, trapezius, hamstrings, quadriceps, hip flexors, soleus, gastrocnemius.

Knees bent.   Spine curved.   Bent elbows.

Spine side to side.   Spine leaning forward.

1

Imagine you're holding a giant beach ball in your arms. Hold the beach ball in your embrace throughout this sequence. Stand in a wide stance with both knees bent.

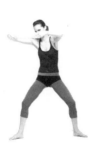

2

Bend forward, rounding your spine. Timing: 4 seconds.

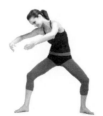

3

Bend diagonally sideways. Lift the beach ball to the opposite corner. Timing: 5 seconds.

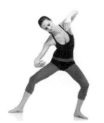

4

Once you've bent as far as you can, lifting the beach ball to the top corner, bend in the opposite direction. Timing: 5 seconds.

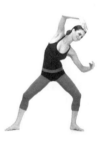

5

Turn your torso to face the corner and lift the beach ball above your head. Timing: 4 seconds.

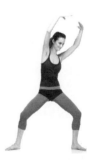

6

Repeat on the other side. Timing: 18 seconds.

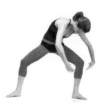

CATEGORY 2: DIAGONAL ROTATION

WAIST ROTATIONS

JOINTS: spine, shoulders, hips, knees.

MUSCLES: abdominals, obliques, latissimus dorsi, quadratus lumborum, rhomboids, trapezius, triceps, biceps, deltoids, pectorals, quadriceps, hamstrings, soleus, gastrocnemius.

1

Waist rotations liberate the upper torso from the lower torso. Lock your hips and don't let them move throughout this sequence.

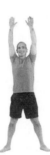

2

Reach above your head with both arms. Your shoulders should be relaxed. Bend from the waist. Timing: 5 seconds.

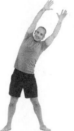

3

Reach forward, bending your knees while rounding your back. This will protect your back muscles from being stressed.

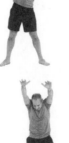

4

Side view of the forward portion of the waist rotation.

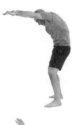

5

Rotate to the other side, pulling as much as possible toward the ceiling.

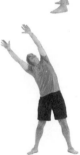

6

Rotate until you have a small arch in your upper back. Start the sequence from the beginning, rotating in the opposite direction this time. Timing: 20 seconds. Timing for both sides: 40 seconds.

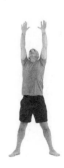

WASHING A SMALL ROUND TABLE

JOINTS: spine, shoulders, hands, hips, knees, ankles.

Hinge.

Ball and socket.

Plane.

MUSCLES: obliques, abdominals, erector spinae, trapezius, rhomboids, triceps, quadriceps, gluteus group, tibialis posterior, soleus, gastrocnemius.

Knees bent.

Body twist.

Bent elbows.

Rotation in the hip joint.

Heel lift with toe flexion.

Hands open.

1

Imagine that you're standing in the middle of a round table and washing it. Bend both legs and place both hands flat on the imaginary tabletop.

2

Start to wash the top of the table behind you, lifting your back heel and twisting your spine.

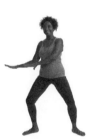

3

Twist around as far as your spine and hips will permit. Timing: 8 seconds.

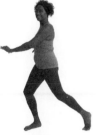

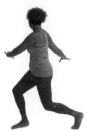

4

Return to the front, but keep washing the table with your hands flat and your fingers spread out.

5

Continue to wash the table in the opposite direction.

6

Try to bend your back knee to get a quad stretch as you twist back as far as you can. Timing: 18 seconds for the full sequence. Repeat two or three times in a row.

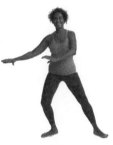

SIMPLE WINDMILL—FEET PARALLEL

JOINTS: spine, shoulders.

Saddle.

Ball and socket.

MUSCLES: erector spinae, obliques, latissimus dorsi, abdominals, trapezius, rhomboids, triceps, biceps, pectorals, deltoids.

Straight spine.

Shoulder arm rotation.

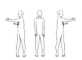

Torso rotation.

1

Start with your feet apart, one arm in front of your body and the other behind, shoulders and shoulder blades pulled down. Rotate as far to one side as possible. Keep your muscles relaxed to facilitate the rotation.

2

Slowly raise your back arm while lowering your front arm.

3

Bring your back arm to the ceiling and your other arm beside your body while rotating your spine to face the front.

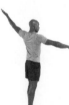

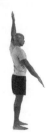

4

Keep the windmill action going by bringing your lower arm behind and your top arm to the front. Rotate your spine as far as you can. Timing: 7 seconds.

5

Complete the windmill by taking the arm that's behind and bringing it over your shoulder and back to the starting position.

6

It should take 15 seconds to complete a full windmill. Do three windmills in a row.

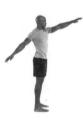

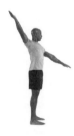

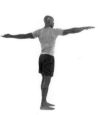

WRAPAROUND ARMS

JOINTS: shoulders, elbows, spine, hips, knees.

Ball and socket. Hinge.

MUSCLES: triceps, biceps, deltoids, rhomboids, pectorals, trapezius, obliques, latissimus dorsi, abdominals, quadriceps, hamstrings, soleus, gastrocnemius.

Bent elbows. Knees bent.

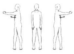

Torso rotation. Spine leaning forward.

1

Bend both your knees slightly and open both arms to the side.

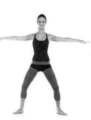

2

Wrap one arm around your waist in the front and the other arm around the back of your waist. Timing: 4 seconds.

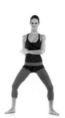

3

Rotate on your spine and turn your torso toward your front knee. Timing: 4 seconds.

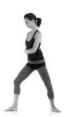

4

Lie on your front knee, lowering your forehead to touch your knee. Timing: 8 seconds.

5

Slowly straighten your spine. Timing: 4 seconds.

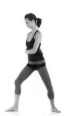

6

Face front and open your arms to prepare to do the exercise in the opposite direction. Timing: 4 seconds. Total timing of sequence: 26 seconds. Repeat on the opposite side.

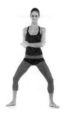

SINGLE-ARM PULLING A ROPE

JOINTS: shoulders, elbows, spine, hips, knees.

Saddle.

Ball and socket.

Hinge.

MUSCLES: triceps, biceps, deltoids, rhomboids, pectorals, trapezius, abdominals, obliques, latissimus dorsi, quadriceps, hip flexors, hamstrings, soleus, gastrocnemius.

Hip hinge side for wide stance.

Knees bent.

Shoulder arm rotation.

Bent elbows.

Spine curved.

Cross-body rotation.

Hands open and closed.

1

Start in a side lunge, reaching your arm toward the corner in a deep side bend.

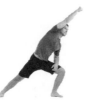

2

Grab a stiff invisible rope, rounding your back slightly, and contract your muscles as you pull the rope. Timing: 3 seconds.

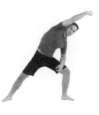

3

Keep pulling toward the opposite corner, shifting your weight to the opposite side in a lunge. Timing: 3 seconds.

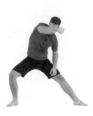

4

Continue moving. Timing: 3 seconds.

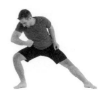

5

Reach as far away as possible before releasing the rope and the muscle tension. Timing: 3 seconds.

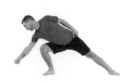

6

Slowly straighten your back and rotate your torso while lifting your arm to shoulder height. This will stretch your chest muscles. Timing: 3 seconds. Timing for one sequence: 15 seconds. Repeat two or three times per side.

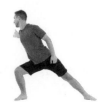

DIAGONAL PRESSES AT VARIOUS HEIGHTS

JOINTS: shoulders, elbows, spine, hips, knees.

Ball and socket.

Hinge.

MUSCLES: triceps, biceps, deltoids, rhomboids, pectorals, trapezius, abdominals, obliques, latissimus dorsi, quadriceps, hamstrings, soleus, gastrocnemius.

Hip hinge side for wide stance.   Knees bent.   Bent elbows.

Spine curved.   Spine leaning forward.

1

Imagine that you're pressing or pushing away a heavy weight at different heights: above the shoulders and to the floor. Play with the imagery to press or push at various heights. Timing: 2 seconds for preparation.

2

Start in a deep front lunge and bend your elbow, preparing to push or press the weight. Contract all your muscles and slowly press or push the weight until your elbows straighten. Timing: 6 to 8 seconds.

3

Change your arm position to press or push another weight. Timing: 2 seconds for preparation.

4

Push or press the weight, deepening your lunge and bending farther forward. Timing: 6 to 8 seconds.

5

When aiming toward the floor, start in a standing position and prepare the bent elbow. Timing: 2 seconds for preparation.

6

Slowly press or push as heavy a weight as you can imagine to the floor. Repeat three times per side. Timing: 6 to 8 seconds. Total time per side: 30 seconds.

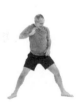

DOUBLE-ARM PULLING ROPES TO THE FLOOR

JOINTS: shoulders, elbows, spine, hips, knees.

Ball and socket.   Hinge.

MUSCLES: triceps, biceps, deltoids, rhomboids, pectorals, trapezius, abdominals, obliques, latissimus dorsi, quadriceps, hamstrings, soleus, gastrocnemius.

Hip hinge side for wide stance.   Knees bent.   Shoulder arm rotation up.

Shoulders up.   Bent elbows.   Spine circle.   Hands open and closed.

1

Start in a side lunge, reaching both arms toward the corner in a deep side bend.

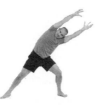

2

Grab a stiff invisible rope and pull toward the opposite corner on the floor. Timing: 3 seconds.

3

Attach the rope to the floor. Timing: 3 seconds.

4

Continue moving in a half circle upward. Timing: 3 seconds.

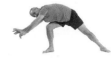

5

When you reach the halfway point, face forward with both arms beside your ears and slowly finish the movement. Timing: 3 seconds. Total timing for one sequence: 12 seconds.

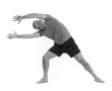

6

You should be in the starting position to begin pulling the rope toward the other foot. Repeat the rope pulls four times, alternating sides each time. Timing: 48 seconds for four sequences.

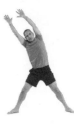

DEEP DIAGONAL REACHES AT THREE HEIGHTS

JOINTS: spine, ribs, shoulders, hips, knees, ankles

Ball and socket.

Saddle.

Hinge.

Plane.

MUSCLES: latissimus dorsi, erector spinae, obliques, abdominals, intercostals, quadratus lumborum, trapezius, pectorals, hamstrings, quadriceps, hip flexors, gluteus group, hip adductors, soleus, gastrocnemius.

Straight spine.   Hip hinge.   Knees bent.   Bent elbows.

Torso rotation.   Shoulder arm rotation up.   Shoulders up.

1

This is a relatively quick exercise. It should take 10 seconds to go through the entire sequence. It's designed to develop dynamic flexibility and rapid agility. Start with your feet apart and your arms facing front.

2

Twist into a diagonal lunge toward the floor. Timing: 2.5 seconds.

3

Return to the starting position. Timing: 2.5 seconds.

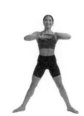

4

Twist into a diagonal lunge, reaching your arm toward the wall. Timing: 2.5 seconds.

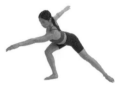

5

Return to the starting position. Timing: 2.5 seconds.

6

Twist into a diagonal lunge, reaching your arm above your shoulder. Timing: 2.5 seconds. Repeat the lunge sequence of low, medium, and high arms three times, then change sides. Timing: 12.5 seconds for all repetitions.

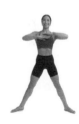

WINDMILL WITH SPINE FLEXION

JOINTS: spine, shoulders, hips, knees.

Saddle.

Ball and socket.

Hinge.

MUSCLES: abdominals, obliques, erector spinae, latissimus dorsi, triceps, biceps, deltoids, rhomboids, pectorals, trapezius, quadriceps, hamstrings, hip flexors, hip adductors, soleus, gastrocnemius.

Shoulder arm rotation.

Hip hinge side for wide stance.

Knees bent.

Bent elbows.

Spine leaning forward.

Body rotation.

Hands: fists, open, closed.

1

Stand with your feet comfortably apart and your arms as wide as possible on a diagonal.

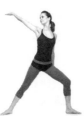

2

Bending your front knee, windmill your top arm toward the opposite knee, using your arms to open your chest.

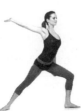

3

Continue to windmill your arms as you bend your body deeper into a front lunge.

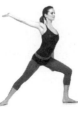

4

Grab an imaginary rope, bend both knees, and round your back as you pull the rope in toward your navel.

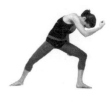

5

Timing: 12 seconds.

6

Open your arms as wide as possible to transition to the other side. Repeat four times. Total time: 50 seconds.

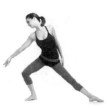

TRICEPS STRETCH INTO WINDMILLS

JOINTS: shoulders, spine, ribs, hips, knees.

Ball and socket.

Saddle.

Hinge.

MUSCLES: obliques, triceps, deltoids, rhomboids, pectorals, trapezius, abdominals, latissimus dorsi, gluteus group, hamstrings, gracilis, quadriceps, sartorius.

Straight spine.

Spine side to side.

Bent elbows.

Shoulder arm rotation.

Knees bent.

1

Stand with your feet comfortably apart. Try to touch your shoulder blade with one hand while bending toward the arm hanging at your side.

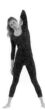

2

Bend farther sideways while walking your fingers down your leg. Timing: 5 seconds.

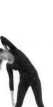

3

Stay in the deep side bend while extending your other arm toward the ceiling, turning your head to look at your hand and the ceiling. Timing: 5 seconds.

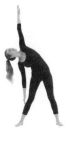

4

Slowly straighten your back and begin a windmill arm sequence.

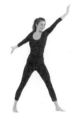

5

Shift your legs into a deep front lunge as you perform the windmill arms. Timing: 5 seconds.

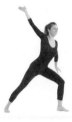

6

Finish the windmill arms in a deep lunge, twisting your spine to deepen the reach of your front arm. Timing of the full sequence: 20 seconds. Repeat on the opposite side.

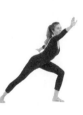

DEEP LUNGES WASHING A LARGE ROUND TABLE

JOINTS: spine, shoulders, hips, knees, ankles.

Ball and socket.

Hinge.

Plane.

MUSCLES: abdominals, obliques, latissimus dorsi, triceps, biceps, deltoids, rhomboids, pectorals, trapezius, hip flexors, quadriceps, hamstrings, soleus, gastrocnemius.

Knees bent.

Body twist.

Bent elbows.

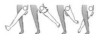

Hip ball joint rotation.

Heel lift with toe flexion.

1

Imagine that you're standing in the middle of a round table, washing the circumference of the table. You'll make a 360° rotation on your spine. With your spine straight, start in a deep lunge, rotating your spine as fully as possible toward the back of the room. Bend your back knee and lift your back heel to enable a greater rotation.

2

Unwind the twist on your spine but keep washing the circumference of the table.

3

As you come toward the front, bend both knees in a deep plié. Bend forward to try to reach the outer edges of the table.

4

As you continue following the edge of the table, shift your weight into a deep lunge.

5

Finish washing the circumference of the table by fully rotating toward the back of the room. Bend your back knee and lift your back heel to enable a greater rotation. Repeat on the opposite side.

PUSH A PIANO AND PULL A DONKEY

JOINTS: shoulders, spine, hips, knees.

Hinge.

Ball and socket.

MUSCLES: triceps, biceps, deltoids, trapezius, rhomboids, latissimus dorsi, quadratus lumborum, gluteus group, quadriceps, hamstrings, sartorius, soleus, gastrocnemius.

Knees bent.   Bent elbows.   Spine curved.

Hands: fists, open, closed.   Wrist extension.   Full-body lunge, push, pull.

1

Imagine that you're pushing a heavy piano. Prepare your legs to push in a lunge, bending your knees. Prepare your arms and hands to push a heavy weight, rounding your back.

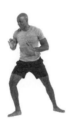

2

Start to push the invisible piano using all the muscles you would need to move a real piano.

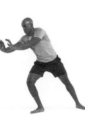

3

Take 8 seconds to complete the pushing of the piano. Your spine will straighten slightly by the end of the push.

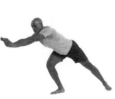

4

Now imagine you have a stubborn donkey at the end of a rope. Lift your upper back and shoulders to get all your arm and back muscles involved.

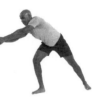

5

Pull the donkey with all your strength, taking 8 seconds to shift your weight onto your back leg in the lunge. Timing:16 seconds for the full sequence. Repeat on the opposite side.

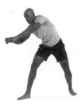

ADVANCED PULLING SACKS OF RICE

JOINTS: shoulders, spine, hips, knees.

Ball and socket.   Hinge.

MUSCLES: triceps, biceps, deltoids, rhomboids, pectorals, trapezius, abdominals, obliques, latissimus dorsi, quadriceps, sartorius, gluteus group, hamstrings, hip adductors, soleus, gastrocnemius.

Hip hinge side for wide stance.   Knees bent.

Elbows bent.   Fist open/close flexion.

1

Imagine that you're dragging a heavy sack of rice. You'll be shifting from a deep front lunge through a side lunge to an opposite-side front lunge. Reach as far away as possible to grab the sack.

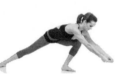

2

Start pulling the sack slowly across your body, keeping as low to the floor as possible.

3

Shift into a side lunge as you keep dragging the sack of rice.

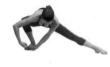

4

Finish in a deep side lunge facing the other way. Extend your arms and prepare to repeat the motion in the other direction. Timing: 10 seconds. Repeat on the other side.

ADVANCED AIRPLANE HAMSTRING STRETCH

JOINTS: spine, shoulders, ribs, hips.

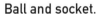

Ball and socket.   Saddle.

MUSCLES: latissimus dorsi, erector spinae, quadratus lumborum, obliques, trapezius, rhomboids, deltoids, pectorals, hamstrings, hip adductors, quadriceps, gluteus group.

Straight spine.   Hip hinge.   Shoulder: up, down.

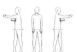

Torso rotation.   Spine leaning forward.

1

Stand with your legs wide apart, but not too wide. Lift your arms to the side.

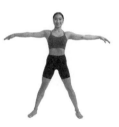

2

Keeping your arms in line with your shoulders, slowly bend forward with your back straight. Modification: Bend your knees if your hamstrings or back are too tight. Timing: 5 seconds.

3

Imagine your arms are attached at your sides like airplane wings. Rotate your spine, keeping it straight and maintaining a straight alignment between the fingers of both hands. Timing: 5 seconds.

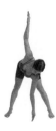

4

Grab your shin and pull your body toward your leg. Timing: 8 seconds.

5

Reach your arm diagonally forward as far as possible to pull on the spine muscles. Timing: 5 seconds.

6

Return to center, bend both knees, and totally relax your entire body. Swinging gently to remove tension from your body, roll up one vertebra at a time. Timing: 10 seconds. Timing of the full sequence: 33 seconds. Repeat on the other side.

CATEGORY 3: SIDE TO SIDE

SINGLE-ARM SWEEPS INTO CELEBRATION ARMS

JOINTS: shoulders, spine, knees.

MUSCLES: pectorals, triceps, deltoids, trapezius, obliques, abdominals, latissimus dorsi, quadratus lumborum, quadriceps, gluteus group, gracilis.

1

Start with your legs apart and both knees bent. Wrap one arm around your ribs and reach your opposite arm across your body.

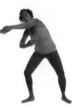

2

Slowly sweep your arm across your body, shifting your weight in the direction of your open arm. Timing: 7 seconds.

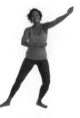

3

Repeat with the other arm.

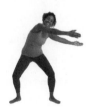

4

Feel a pectoral stretch as you fully open your arm.

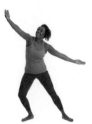

5

Stand with your weight equally spread over both feet, knees bent.

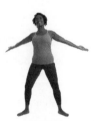

6

Slowly lift your arms, stretching your elbows, wrists, and fingers while raising your head. This should feel like a celebration. Timing: 20 seconds for the full sequence.

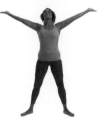

BOW AND ARROW

JOINTS: shoulders, elbows, spine, hips, knees.

Ball and socket.

Hinge.

Saddle.

MUSCLES: pectorals, triceps, biceps, deltoids, rhomboids, trapezius, abdominals, obliques, latissimus dorsi, quadratus lumborum, erector spinae, quadriceps, hip flexors, gluteus group, hamstrings, soleus, gastrocnemius.

Hip hinge side for wide stance.   Knees bent.   Bent elbows.

Spine curved.   Shoulder arm rotation.   Fist open/closed.

1

Imagine you're shooting a bow and arrow. Mimic the action required to pull an arrow on a tight bow string. This will build tension between your arms. Timing: 3 seconds.

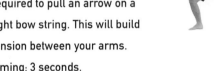

2

Stand in a wide lunge with both knees bent. Slowly pull the arrow back. Round your back to create the tension needed to pull the arrow back. Timing: 3 seconds.

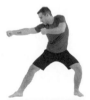

3

Release the arrow, relaxing your shoulders as you do so. Timing: 3 seconds.

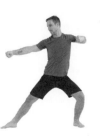

4

Extend your arm behind your shoulders, keeping your torso facing forward. Relax your shoulder joint as much as possible. This will stretch your chest muscles. Timing: 3 seconds.

5

Lift your arm above your head and prepare to start again from the beginning. Timing: 3 seconds. Timing for one sequence: 15 seconds. Repeat on the opposite side.

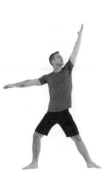

SWEEPING BEHIND HEAD INTO CUTTING THE AIR

JOINTS: shoulders, elbows, spine, hips, knees.

Ball and socket.

Hinge.

Saddle.

MUSCLES: triceps, deltoids, pectorals, trapezius, rhomboids, intercostals, obliques, abdominals, latissimus dorsi, erector spinae, quadratus lumborum, quadriceps, gluteus group, hamstrings, soleus, gastrocnemius.

Spine side to side.   Shoulder arm rotation.   Knees bent.

1

Stand in a wide side lunge. Bend sideways and raise one arm to shoulder height. Raise your other arm and bend it over your head, trying to touch your other arm with your fingers.

2

Drag your fingers along your arm and behind your neck. As your elbow bends while you're dragging it back, pull it backward and down. Shift your weight from one leg to the other. Timing: 5 seconds.

3

Turn your hand to face the side wall, preparing to push an invisible weight.

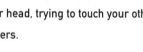
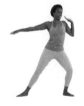

4

Push the invisible weight toward the wall, lunging as deeply as possible. Timing: 5 seconds.

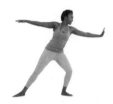

5

Shift your weight equally as you pretend to cut the air with the underside of your arm. Bend your body against the cutting direction.

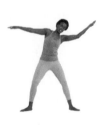

6

Finish cutting the air and prepare to start the sequence again on the same side. Timing: 5 seconds. Timing for total sequence: 15 seconds. Repeat on the opposite side.

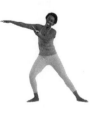

WASHING WINDOWS ABOVE THE SHOULDERS

JOINTS: shoulders, elbows, spine, hips, knees.

Ball and socket.

Hinge.

MUSCLES: triceps, biceps, pectorals, deltoids, trapezius, rhomboids, obliques, abdominals, intercostals, latissimus dorsi, erector spinae, quadratus lumborum, gluteus group, quadriceps, soleus, gastrocnemius.

Shoulder rotation arms up.   Spine side to side.   Shoulders: up, down.

Knees bent.   Bent elbows.   Spine curved.

1

Extend both arms while in a deep side lunge. Bend sideways until you feel your ribs being stretched.

2

Start the sequence by shifting your weight from one lunge to the other. Sweep your arms across your body at head height. Take 7 seconds to go from one side to the other.

3

Keep your elbows wide open and close to your head throughout the wash.

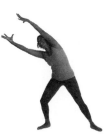
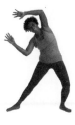
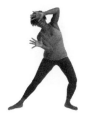

4

Finish the first half of the sequence by extending your arms while reaching toward the side wall. Timing: 10 seconds.

5

Start the second half of the sequence by bending your elbows to frame your face and shifting the weight of your torso sideways.

6

Continue the wash until you finish with your arms extended sideways. Timing: 20 seconds for the complete sequence. Repeat three times.

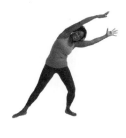
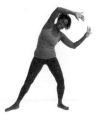
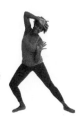

DEEP SIDE LUNGE WASHES

JOINTS: shoulders, elbows, spine, hips, knees.

Ball and socket.

Hinge.

MUSCLES: triceps, biceps, deltoids, rhomboids, pectorals, trapezius, obliques, abdominals, intercostals, latissimus dorsi, quadratus lumborum, erector spinae, quadriceps, gluteus group, hamstrings, soleus, gastrocnemius.

Hip hinge side for wide stance.

Shoulder rotation arms up.

Shoulders up.

Spine side to side.

Spine curved.

Bent elbows.

Knees bent.

1

Start in a wide side lunge. Your knee should be over your foot. Bend sideways and reach toward the side wall. Imagine that you're pinned between two glass walls as you shift from side to side.

2

Shift the lunge and side bends from one side to the other. Bend deeper sideways, framing your head with your bent elbows.

3

Imagine that you're washing the upper part of a wall as you continue to shift the lunge.

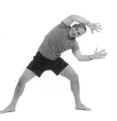

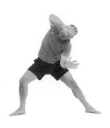

4

Slowly continue the wash, trying to feel the stretch in every rib, shoulder, and glute muscle.

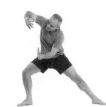

5

Finish the wash in as deep a lunge as you started in, making sure you're reaching as far as possible toward the opposite wall. Timing: 15 seconds for the full sequence.

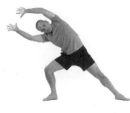

6

Repeat on the other side.

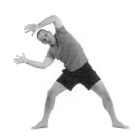

FINGERS WALKING DOWN THE ARM

JOINTS: shoulders, spine, hips, knees.

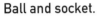

Ball and socket.   Hinge.

Saddle.

MUSCLES: deltoids, triceps, pectorals, trapezius, rhomboids, intercostals, obliques, abdominals, latissimus dorsi, erector spinae, quadratus lumborum, gluteus group, quadriceps, hamstrings, soleus, gastrocnemius.

Spine standing.   Shoulder rotation arm up.   Spine side to side.

Knees bent.   Shoulders up.   Bent elbows.

1

Stand with your arms stretched out to the sides and your feet comfortably apart.

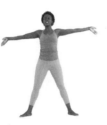

2

Go into a side lunge while wrapping one arm over your head and trying to touch your shoulder. Timing: 4 seconds.

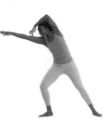

3

Start to walk your fingers down your extended arm.

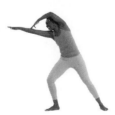

4

Timing: 5 seconds.

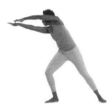

5

Stretch both arms, reaching in a deeper side bend. Timing: 3 seconds.

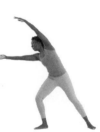

6

Finish with both arms above your head while reaching as far as possible toward the ceiling. Timing: 15 seconds for the full sequence. Repeat on the other side.

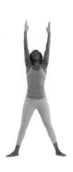

DOUBLE-ARM HALF-BODY ROTATION

JOINTS: spine, shoulders, hips, knees.

Ball and socket.

Hinge.

MUSCLES: abdominals, obliques, latissimus dorsi, erector spinae, quadratus lumborum, trapezius, triceps, rhomboids, biceps, deltoids, pectorals, quadriceps, hamstrings, gluteus group, soleus, gastrocnemius.

Hip hinge side for wide stance. Knees bent. Shoulder rotation arm up.

Shoulders up.   Spine circle.

1

Stand with your legs comfortably apart. Start with both arms above your head, letting your shoulders lift as you reach upward.

2

Imagine that you're following the circumference of your full body. Keeping your arms beside your ears, bend sideways while deeply bending your knees. Timing: 3 seconds.

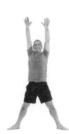

3

When you get to waist height, start the half circle. Timing: 3 seconds.

4

Keep moving to complete the half circle.

5

When you reach the side, turn your torso and adjust your arms so that they're beside your ears. Timing: 3 seconds.

6

Keeping your arms beside your ears, bend sideways while deeply bending your knees. Timing: 3 seconds. Repeat on the opposite side.

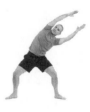

ADVANCED SIDE STRENGTHENING WITH SCISSOR ARMS

JOINTS: spine, shoulders, hips, knees, ankles.

Plane.

Ball and socket.

Hinge.

Saddle.

MUSCLES: latissimus dorsi, obliques, abdominals, erector spinae, quadratus lumborum, trapezius, rhomboids, triceps, biceps, deltoids, pectorals, gluteus group, quadriceps, soleus, gastrocnemius.

Straight spine.

Spine side to side.

Knees bent.

Shoulder rotation arms up.   Shoulders up.   Wrist extension.

1

Stand with your feet and arms wide apart.

2

Lunge deeply, bending sideways. Take your top arm and try to touch both hands together. Timing: 5 seconds.

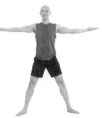

3

Maintain your deep side bend and open both arms as widely as possible, flexing your wrists. Timing: 5 seconds.

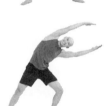

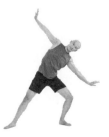

4

Bring both hands together. Timing: 5 seconds. Repeat the opening and closing of your arms three times, as if your arms are the blades of scissors cutting the air.

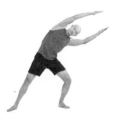

5

Return to center and repeat on the other side.

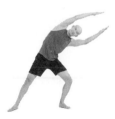

ADVANCED SIDE STRENGTHENING WITH SIDE PRESSES

JOINTS: ribs, spine, shoulders, wrists, hips, knees.

Ball and socket.

Hinge.

Saddle.

Condyloid.

MUSCLES: intercostals, latissimus dorsi, obliques, abdominals, erector spinae, quadratus lumborum, pectorals, trapezius, rhomboids, triceps, biceps, flexors and extensors of the hands and wrists, quadriceps, hamstrings, gluteus group, gracilis, soleus, gastrocnemius.

Spine side to side.

Bent elbows.

Knees bent.

Shoulders up.

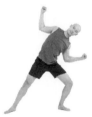

Hands: fists, open, closed.

Wrist extension.

1

Stand in a side lunge. (Do not attempt an extremely deep lunge.) Lock your hips down and bend sideways from your ribs. Imagine you're pulling a stiff rope hanging from the ceiling. Timing: 5 seconds.

2

Start to shift to the other side, keeping both knees bent. Now imagine you're lifting a heavy weight.

3

Keep lifting the heavy weight above your head as you bend to the opposite side. Timing: 5 seconds.

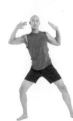

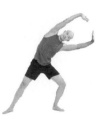

4

Remain in the deep side bend and imagine that you're pulling stiff ropes from the ceiling. Timing: 3 seconds.

5

Still in the side bend, flip your hands and imagine again that you're lifting a heavy weight, pushing toward the corner. Timing: 3 seconds.

6

Stretch your hands and try to bring your arms as close to your ears as possible. Timing: 3 seconds. Repeat immediately on the other side.

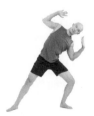

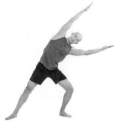

ADVANCED CLOCK SEQUENCE

JOINTS: spine, ribs, shoulders.

Ball and socket.

MUSCLES: latissimus dorsi, erector spinae, inter-costals, quadratus lumborum, obliques, abdominals, triceps, biceps, deltoids, trapezius, pectorals, quadratus lumborum, gluteus group.

Spine standing.　　Shoulder arm rotation up.

Shoulders up.　　　Spine circle.

1

Imagine that you are the hands of a clock. Go through both the clockwise and counterclockwise directions of the clock, taking 20 seconds for each.

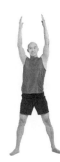

2

As you bend, support your spine with your abdominal muscles. Do not move your hips. Keep your arms straight and held beside your ears

3

Bend your knees and turn your torso to face toward the floor.

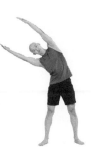

4

Drop your head at the bottom.

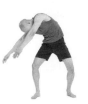

5

Start to rotate your spine and shoulders as you leave the six o'clock position.

6

Straighten your knees and turn your body flat sideways as you continue to the twelve o'clock position. Timing: 20 seconds per rotation.

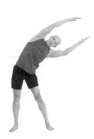

CATEGORY 4:
UPPER-BODY EXTENSION

OPEN CHEST SWAN

JOINTS: spine, shoulders, elbows.

MUSCLES: abdominals, latissimus dorsi, trapezius, quadratus lumborum, triceps, biceps, deltoids, pectorals.

1

Open Chest Swan is a signature Essentrics sequence used in floor work, chair work, and standing. It's a basic movement for improving posture.

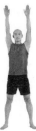

2

Stand with your arms above your head and beside your ears. Keep your arms and elbows straight.

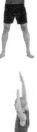

3

Slowly bend your elbows, pulling them behind your shoulders as much as possible. Flip your hands outward. Don't lean backward or change the position of your spine. Timing: 5 seconds.

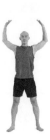

4

Make very tight fists with your hands, pulling backward with your arms and elbows. Timing: 5 seconds.

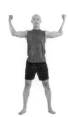

5

Release your fists and turn your hands toward the wall, opening your chest even farther. Lifting your chest, slowly pull your arms down behind you. Timing: 5 seconds.

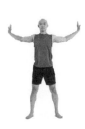

6

Release your spine, rounding it while relaxing all your muscles. Drop your arms and relax them in front. Timing: 5 seconds.

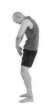

FLUID SPINE

JOINTS: spine, shoulders, elbows, hips, knees.

Ball and socket.

Hinge.

MUSCLES: obliques, latissimus dorsi, abdominals, trapezius, rhomboids, triceps, biceps, deltoids, pectorals, quadriceps, hamstrings, soleus, gastrocnemius.

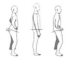

Hips forward and back.

Knees bent.   Bent elbows.

Reach up and back.   Shoulders up.

1

Starting position: Stand with one foot in front of the other, feet flat on the floor, with no eversion or inversion. Make a *C* curve with your spine, tailbone tucked under and shoulders rounded. Bend your elbows and lift them in line with your shoulders. Make your hands into fists.

2

Reverse the *C* curve of your spine, push your buttocks out, and arch your spine. Twist your elbows toward your waist, keeping them bent. Slowly return to the starting position. Timing: 6 to 8 seconds for the full sequence. Repeat three times.

3

Resume your starting position. Reverse the *C* curve of your spine, push your buttocks out, and arch your spine. Stretch and straighten your arms behind your spine

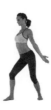

and downward, pulling your shoulder blades down, palms of your hands facing upward. Slowly return to the starting position. Timing: 6 to 8 seconds for the full sequence. Repeat three times.

4

Stretch your arms at shoulder height, turning the palms of your hands toward the ceiling. Slowly return to the starting position. Timing: 6 to 8 seconds for the full sequence. Repeat three times.

5

Resume your starting position. Reverse the *C* curve of your spine, push your buttocks out, and arch your spine. Straighten your arms above your head, stretching them toward the ceiling. Slowly return to the starting position. Timing: 6 to 8 seconds for the full sequence. Repeat three times.

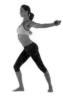

CEILING REACH AND OPEN CHEST SWAN

JOINTS: spine, shoulders, elbows.

Ball and socket.

Hinge.

MUSCLES: latissimus dorsi, erector spinae, quadratus lumborum, abdominals, deltoids, triceps, biceps, trapezius, rhomboids, pectorals.

Straight spine.

Shoulders: up, down.

Bent elbows.   Reach up and back.

1

Stand with your feet comfortably apart. Raise your arms above your head, keeping your spine completely straight. Try to keep your elbows straight. Timing: 4 seconds.

2

Pull one arm at a time toward the ceiling, relaxing your shoulder and permitting it to rise along with the arm. When you reach your maximum upward stretch, pull your arm behind your ear, stretching the chest muscles. Timing: 4 seconds.

3

Repeat with your other arm, alternating sides two times.

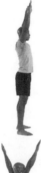

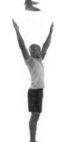

4

Stretch both arms directly above your head. Timing: 2 seconds.

5

Rotate your arms in their sockets while bending your elbows. Pull your elbows behind your shoulders, but do not lean your spine backward.

6

As you pull your elbows back, rotate your shoulders to sink or depress your shoulder blades. This will stretch the chest muscles. Timing: 6 to 8 seconds. Total time for the full sequence: 30 to 35 seconds.

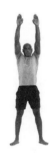

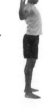

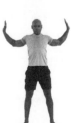

REMOVE A SWEATER

JOINTS: spine, shoulders, elbows, hips, knees.

Ball and socket.

Hinge.

MUSCLES: abdominals, obliques, latissimus dorsi, triceps, biceps, deltoids, rhomboids, pectorals, trapezius, quadriceps, hamstrings, soleus, gastrocnemius.

Knees bent.

Hips forward and back.

Bent elbows.

Reach up and back.

Shoulders: up, down.

1

Stand with your legs apart in a comfortable stance. Bend your knees and round your spine while crossing your arms in front of your thighs. Imagine that you're taking off a large, baggy sweater.

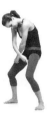

2

Slowly straighten your knees and lift your arms.

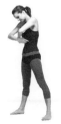

3

Move slowly, keeping your elbows crossed until your spine is completely straight.

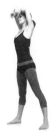

4

Reach to the ceiling, straightening your elbows. Timing: 9 seconds for the full sequence.

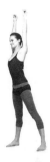

5

Without leaning backward, bend your elbows and pull them behind you in an Open Chest Swan move. Timing: 6 seconds. Total timing of sequence: 15 seconds. Repeat two times.

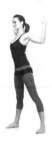

LIFT IMAGINARY WEIGHTS ABOVE YOUR HEAD

JOINTS: shoulders, elbows, wrists, hips, knees.

Ball and socket.

Hinge.

Condyloid.

MUSCLES: abdominals, latissimus dorsi, triceps, biceps, trapezius, deltoids, pectorals, hamstrings, gluteus group, quadriceps.

Spine standing.

Knees bent.

Shoulders: up, down.

Bent elbows.

Reach up and back.

Wrist extension.

1

Imagine that you're lifting a very heavy weight. Hold the weight for 5 seconds.

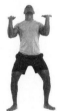

2

Slowly lift the weight above your head, taking 5 to 7 seconds to straighten your elbows above your head.

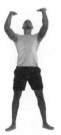

3

When your arms are completely above your head, relax your arms and shoulders and let your arms lift even higher. Timing: 5 to 7 seconds.

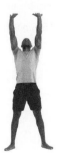

4

Take 5 seconds to slowly open your arms, pushing your chest upward to stretch your chest muscles.

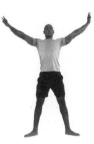

5

Relax your arms as you lower them and get ready to start again. Repeat two times.

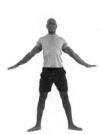

CATEGORY 5:
FULL-BODY FIGURE EIGHTS

SMALL SINGLE-ARM FIGURE EIGHTS

JOINTS: shoulders, spine, hips, knees.

MUSCLES: trapezius, rhomboids, triceps, biceps, deltoids, pectorals, latissimus dorsi, abdominals, quadratus lumborum, hamstrings, quadriceps, gluteus group.

1

Stand with your feet apart, one arm extended with your elbow bent.

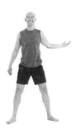

2

Round your spine and slowly rotate your arm inside the shoulder joint. Timing: 4 seconds.

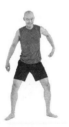

3

Twist your arm more as you slowly draw it toward the front. Do not move your shoulders; keep them square to the front and only move your arm. Timing: 4 seconds.

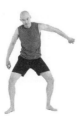

4

Bend your knees and round your spine more as you sweep your arm directly in front of your breastbone. Timing: 3 seconds.

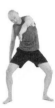

5

Bending slightly sideways, slowly sweep your arm around your head, straightening your spine. Timing: 3 seconds.

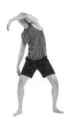

6

Completely straighten your spine and legs as you finish sweeping your arm upward. Timing: 4 seconds. Total timing of sequence: 18 seconds. Repeat on the opposite side.

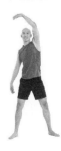

LARGE SINGLE-ARM FIGURE EIGHTS

JOINTS: shoulders, spine, hips, knees.

Saddle.

Ball and socket.

Hinge.

MUSCLES: triceps, biceps, deltoids, rhomboids, pectorals, trapezius, obliques, latissimus dorsi, abdominals, quadriceps, hamstrings, soleus, gastrocnemius.

Spine standing.

Spine curved.

Knees bent.

Elbows bent.

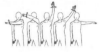

Shoulder arm rotation.

1

Start in a deep side lunge with your arm held diagonally behind your body. Imagine that you're drawing a large figure eight with your hand as you sweep your arm across your body.

2

Twist your arm inside the socket until it forces your shoulders and upper back to round. Bend both legs equally. Timing: 5 seconds.

3

Shift your weight into an opposite-side lunge and bend your torso toward the lunge.

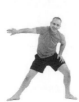

4

Slowly draw your arm in front of your shoulders. Timing: 5 seconds.

5

Shift your weight back between both bent legs while lifting your arm above your head. Timing: 3 seconds.

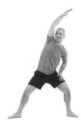

6

Shift your weight back into the original lunge while opening your arm and pulling it behind your shoulders with the palm of your hand facing the ceiling.

Timing: 4 seconds. Timing of full sequence: 16 to 20 seconds. Repeat twice on each side.

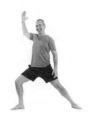

DOUBLE-ARM FIGURE EIGHTS

JOINTS: spine, shoulders, elbows, hips, knees.

Ball and socket.

Hinge.

MUSCLES: quadratus lumborum, latissimus dorsi, abdominals, trapezius, rhomboids, deltoids, triceps, biceps, pectorals, gluteus group, quadriceps, hip flexors, hamstrings.

Hips forward and back.

Bent elbows.

Arms up and open.

1

Stand straight with your arms above your head.

2

Arch your upper back and stick your tailbone out behind. Bend your knees while pulling your bent elbows behind your shoulders. Timing: 6 seconds.

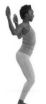

3

Reverse the position by tucking your tailbone under and rounding your upper back. Lift your elbows toward the ceiling while lowering your hands to touch your waist.

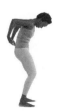

4

Keep lifting your elbows up and over your shoulders with your arms bent. Timing: 6 seconds.

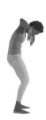

5

Stretch your arms out so that they're in line with your shoulders. Try to round your spine more as you stretch your arms in front. Bend your knees more deeply. Timing: 4 seconds.

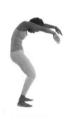

6

Raise your arms above your head, pulling them toward the ceiling and completely straightening your spine and knees. Lift your chin. Timing: 3 seconds. Total timing for the sequence: 19 seconds.

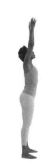

LARGE FULL-BODY FIGURE EIGHTS WITH ROTATION

JOINTS: shoulders, spine, hips, knees, ankles, toes.

Plane.

Ball and socket.

Hinge.

Saddle.

MUSCLES: trapezius, rhomboids, biceps, triceps, deltoids, pectorals, abdominals, latissimus dorsi, quadratus lumborum, hamstrings, quadriceps, gluteus group, soleus, gastrocnemius.

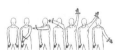

Shoulder arm rotation.

Spine curved.

Full-body twist.

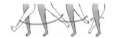

Rotation in the hip joint.

Heel lift with toe flexion.

1

Take a wide stance and bend both knees equally. Lift one arm to shoulder height, twisting it in the shoulder socket. Round your spine, bending forward slightly. Timing: 4 seconds.

2

Sweep your arm to the floor as you shift your weight into a wide side lunge. Timing: 3 seconds.

3

Keep sweeping your arm in a circular motion, pulling it toward the ceiling to stretch your ribs. Timing: 3 seconds.

4

Shift your weight to the other side. Rotate your arm within your shoulder joint as you rotate your spine to face the back of the room. Timing: 3 seconds.

5

As you twist to face the back of the room, bend your back knee while lifting your heel. Turn your head to look at the back of the room. Timing: 3 seconds.

6

Finish in as deep a lunge as possible and with maximum rotation of your spine while gently lowering your arm. Repeat the sequence two or three times before changing sides. Timing: 16 seconds per rotation.

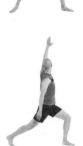

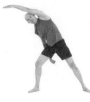

CATEGORY 6: PLIÉS

PLIÉS WITH QUADRICEPS STRENGTHENING

JOINTS: hips, knees, ankles.

MUSCLES: gluteus group, hamstrings, quadriceps, sartorius, hip adductors, soleus, gastrocnemius, tibialis posterior.

1

Stand in a comfortably wide stance, feet turned out, knees over the arch of your feet. Do not evert or invert your ankles. This will stabilize and prevent strain on your knees.

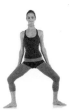

2

Bend and straighten your legs eight times. Timing: 5 seconds to bend and 5 seconds to straighten your legs.

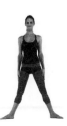

3

Stand with your heels touching, feet comfortably turned out. Squeeze your buttocks while rotating your inner thighs open.

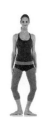

4

Straighten your legs, fighting against an imaginary steel coil between your knees. Timing: 5 seconds to bend and 5 seconds to straighten your legs. Repeat eight times.

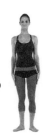

5

Stand with your feet parallel and slightly apart. Slowly bend and straighten your knees. As you bend and straighten your knees, contract your quads, pushing against the floor. Squeeze your buttocks as tightly as possible and contract your stomach muscles throughout this sequence.

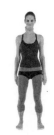

6

Straighten your legs. Timing: 3 seconds to bend and 3 seconds to straighten your legs. Repeat eight times.

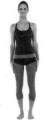

PLIÉS WITH SQUEEZE AN ORANGE UNDER YOUR HEEL

JOINTS: spine, hips, knees, ankles.

Ball and socket.

Hinge.

Plane.

MUSCLES: erector spinae, quadriceps, sartorius, hamstrings, hip adductors, gluteus group, tibialis posterior and anterior, soleus, gastrocnemius.

Knees bent.

Wide legs rotated in the hip joint.

Heel lift with toe flexion.

1

Stand in a wide plié, feet flat on the floor, knees over your feet. This is not a squat! Keep your back upright. Take 3 seconds to bend your knees.

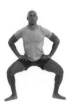

2

Take 3 seconds to lift one heel as high as possible while keeping your toes flat on the floor. Repeat three times.

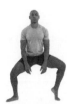

3

Imagine that there's an orange under your heel and you're squeezing all the juice out of it as you lower your heel. Time: 4 seconds per heel squeeze. Repeat three times, raising and lowering your heel.

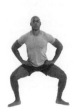

4

Shift your weight onto the opposite leg and bend forward. Timing: 3 seconds.

5

Pull your buttocks farther back as you flex your foot. Timing: 6 seconds.

6

Return to center and repeat with your other heel. Timing: 30 seconds for the full sequence.

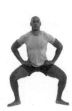

PLIÉS WITH SINGLE-ARM FULL-BODY ROTATION

JOINTS: spine, hips, knees, shoulders.

Ball and socket.

Hinge.

Plane.

Saddle.

Condyloid.

MUSCLES: pectorals, rhomboids, trapezius, latissimus dorsi, abdominals, obliques, gluteus group, quadriceps, sartorius, hip adductors, hamstrings, soleus, gastrocnemius.

Spinal circle.

Knees bent.

360° shoulder rotation.

1

Stand with both feet apart and both arms fully extended to the side. You'll be following the circumference of a large imaginary circle with one arm. Throughout the entire sequence, hold your stationary arm in line with your shoulder.

2

Move into a deep plié while simultaneously beginning to draw a full circle with your arm. Round your spine diagonally forward, making sure your tailbone is tucked under during any forward bend.

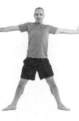

3

While drawing the circle, try to sweep the floor with your fingertips.

4

As your body shifts from forward bend to side bend, straighten and elongate your spine. When you're in a side bend, do *not* tuck your tailbone under.

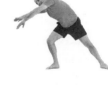

5

When you reach the point in the arm circle where your two arms are parallel to each other, your entire torso should be facing front.

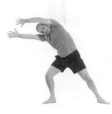

6

Finish drawing the full arm circle, ending with your arm straight above your head and pulling as much as possible toward the ceiling. Timing: 25 to 30 seconds for the full sequence. Repeat with the other arm.

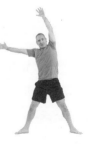

PLIÉS WITH SINGLE-ARM FIGURE EIGHTS

JOINTS: shoulders, elbows, spine, hips, knees.

Hinge.

Saddle.

Ball and socket.

MUSCLES: pectorals, rhomboids, trapezius, latissimus dorsi, abdominals, obliques, gluteus group, quadriceps, sartorius, hip adductors, hamstrings, soleus, gastrocnemius.

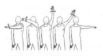

Shoulder arm rotation.

Bent elbows.

Knees bent.

Wide legs rotated in the hip joint.

1

Bend your knees in a wide stance, with your arms open to the side and your back straight. Do not bend forward.

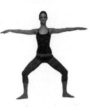

2

Hold one arm at shoulder height throughout the sequence. Bend the other elbow and pull it toward your waist as you rotate toward the back of the room. Timing: 4 seconds.

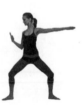

3

Straighten one arm behind your back and rotate the arm inside the shoulder joint. Timing: 4 seconds.

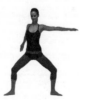

4

Slowly twist your arm forward while keeping your opposite arm extended and your torso facing front. Timing: 4 seconds.

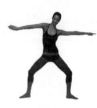

5

Keep your torso facing forward and your spine straight, isolating your arm from your shoulder. Slowly sweep your arm across the front of your body to join the other arm that's extended to the side. Timing 4 seconds.

6

Slowly pull your arm upward, finishing in line with your ear. Reach toward the ceiling, while keeping your other arm at your side. Timing: 4 seconds. Repeat twice with each arm.

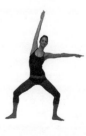

PLIÉS WITH DEEP SIDE BENDS

JOINTS: spine, shoulders, elbows, hips, knees.

Saddle.

Ball and socket.

Hinge.

MUSCLES: abdominals, obliques, latissimus dorsi, erector spinae, quadratus lumborum, trapezius, rhomboids, pectorals, biceps, triceps, quadriceps, sartorius, hamstrings, hip adductors, gluteus group.

Straight spine.   Knees bent.   Wide legs rotated in the hip joint.

Shoulder arm rotation up.   Spine side to side.   Elbows bent.

1

Starting position. Arms straight above the head, legs wide apart.

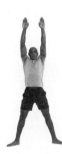

2

Stand on the entire soles of your feet and bend your knees. Bend your torso sideways, pulling an invisible elastic from the ceiling while touching your knee with your elbow.

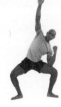

3

Straighten your elbow and touch the floor in front of your heel. Timing: 5 seconds.

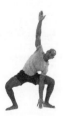

4

While reaching toward the ceiling, move your arm from in front of your leg to behind your leg. Timing: 5 seconds.

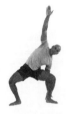

5

Straighten your knees and bring your arms together beside your ears, pulling them toward the ceiling. Relax your shoulders, raising them as you pull toward the ceiling. Timing: 15 seconds for the full sequence. Repeat three times on each side. Total time: 120 seconds.

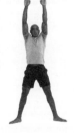

PLIÉS WITH SINGLE-ARM HALF-BODY ROTATION

JOINTS: shoulders, spine, hips, knees.

Saddle.

Ball and socket.

Hinge.

MUSCLES: triceps, biceps, deltoids, rhomboids, pectorals, trapezius, abdominals, obliques, latissimus dorsi, quadratus lumborum, erector spinae, hip adductors, quadriceps, sartorius, gluteus group, hamstrings, soleus, gastrocnemius.

Straight spine.

Knees bent.

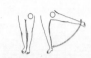

Wide legs rotated in the hip joint.

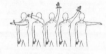

Shoulder arm rotation.

Spine side to side.

1

Stand with your feet apart, knees bent, arms extended to the side.

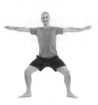

2

Rotate one arm within the socket while moving it directly in front of your shoulders. Keep your torso facing front; do not rotate it. Timing: 5 seconds.

3

Continue slowly moving your arm across your body until it joins the other arm. Bend to the side, stretching your rib cage.

Don't let your hips lift as you bend sideways, and keep your knees in the deep plié. Timing: 5 seconds.

4

Slowly lift your arm over your head, partially straightening your knees.

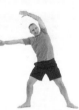

5

Keep your arm moving until it finishes in line with your shoulder. Timing: 5 seconds.

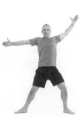

6

Straighten your knees at the end of one single-arm half rotation. Repeat twice with both arms.

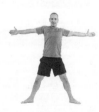

PLIÉS WITH HIP AND GROIN STRETCH

JOINTS: hips, knees.

Ball and socket.

Hinge.

MUSCLES: quadratus lumborum, obliques, hip adductors, gluteus group, quadriceps, sartorius, hamstrings, soleus, gastrocnemius.

Wide legs rotated in the hip joint.

Knees bent.

Hips side to side.

1

Stand with your feet apart in a comfortable stance, arms at your side.

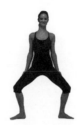

2

Bend forward, sticking out your buttocks, hands on your thighs above your knees. Put the weight of your body into your arms as you try to push your knees open, slowly shifting your hips left and right.

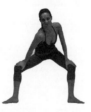

3

Try to dig into the hip socket to loosen it. Repeat four to eight times. Go at your own speed!

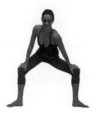

4

Straighten your spine and slowly shift your hips left to right.

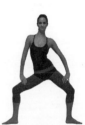

5

This will loosen up a different part of your hips. Go slowly and at your own pace. Repeat four to eight times.

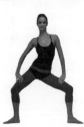

6

Finish with your legs straight and relaxed.

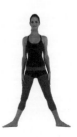

PLIÉS WITH SIDE-BEND ARM REACHES

JOINTS: shoulders, spine, hips, knees.

Saddle.

Ball and socket.

Hinge.

MUSCLES: trapezius, rhomboids, pectorals, biceps, triceps, abdominals, obliques, latissimus dorsi, quadratus lumborum, erector spinae, hip adductors, quadriceps, sartorius, hamstrings, gluteus group.

Straight spine.

Knees bent.

Wide legs rotated in the hip joint.

Shoulder arm rotation up.

Spine side to side.

1

Take a wide stance, feet comfortably turned out, knees bent, spine straight. Lift both arms above your head, elbows straight. If you have knee pain, stop before the pain begins.

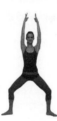

2

Remain in the deep plié throughout this sequence. Lower one arm. Timing: 4 seconds.

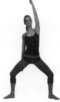

3

Bend sideways as much as possible. Timing: 4 seconds.

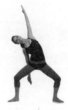

4

Remain in the deep side bend and raise your arm slowly to shoulder height. Timing: 4 seconds.

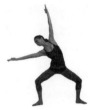

5

Straighten your spine and return your arm above your head. Timing: 3 seconds. Timing for one full sequence: 15 seconds. Repeat four times, alternating sides.

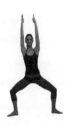

CATEGORY 7: HANDS, ARMS, AND SHOULDERS

HANDS, FINGERS, AND WRISTS MOBILITY SEQUENCE #1

JOINTS: wrists, fingers.

MUSCLES: flexors and extensors of the hands and fingers.

1

Open the fingers of both hands as wide as possible. Hold for 3 seconds, then open farther. Repeat eight times.

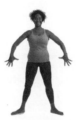

2

With your hands facing the back of the room, close and open your fingers. Repeat eight times.

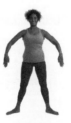

3

With your hands facing the floor, close and open your fingers. Repeat eight times.

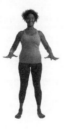

4

Make tight fists with both hands. Open and close your fists. Repeat eight times.

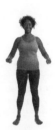

5

Move one finger at a time. Start with the thumb and finish with the pinkie. Repeat eight times on each hand.

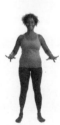

6

Make a claw. Starting with the thumb, move each finger one at a time. Repeat with each hand eight times.

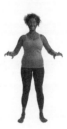

HANDS, FINGERS, AND WRISTS MOBILITY SEQUENCE #2

JOINTS: wrists, fingers.

Condyloid.

Hinge.

Ball and socket.

MUSCLES: extensors of the wrist, flexors and extensors of the hands and fingers.

Fingers: open, closed.　　Fists: open, closed.

Fingers: up, down.　　Wrist extension.

1

Position A. Use this as your starting position. Squeeze your fingers and thumbs together, keeping your knuckles straight.

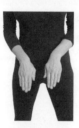

2

Open your fingers as wide as possible. Hold them open for 2 seconds, then close them and hold for 2 seconds. Repeat eight times. Timing: 32 seconds for the full sequence.

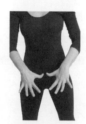

3

Using A as your starting position, open and close your fists. Hold them open for 2 seconds, then close them and hold for 2 seconds. Repeat eight times. Timing: 32 seconds for the full sequence.

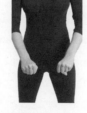

4

Using A as your starting position, move your fingers as fast as possible for 6 seconds.

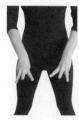

5

Return to position A. Imagine that you're hitting a piano key one finger at a time, over and over again. Repeat ten times.

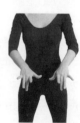

6

Put your hands together in a prayer position and try to keep your palms and fingers glued together while you lift your hands toward your chin and lower them toward your belly button. Repeat slowly for 10 seconds.

DOUBLE-ARM SHOULDER ROTATIONS

JOINTS: shoulders.

Ball and socket.

Saddle.

MUSCLES: trapezius, rhomboids, deltoids, triceps, biceps, pectorals, latissimus dorsi, obliques, abdominals, hip flexors.

Straight spine.

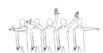

Shoulder arm rotation.

1

Stand with your feet comfortably apart and both arms above your head, elbows straight.

2

Do not lean backward. Keep your spine completely straight throughout the arm rotations.

3

Start the rotation, imagining that you're pulling your arms out of their sockets.

4

Continue the rotation, imagining that you're dropping your shoulder blades into a back pocket.

5

Pass by your hips and continue the rotation upward.

6

Continue the rotation until you reach the ceiling. Repeat three times. Timing: 12 seconds for each complete rotation.

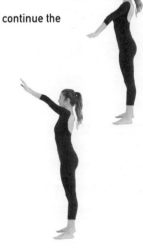

ARM PUMPS FOR SHOULDER JOINT LIBERATION

JOINTS: shoulders, elbows, wrists.

Ball and socket.

Saddle.

Condyloid.

Hinge.

MUSCLES: trapezius, rhomboids, deltoids, pectorals, triceps, biceps, extensors of the wrist, flexors and extensors of the hands and fingers, abdominals.

Straight spine.

Bent elbows.

Fists: open, closed.

Wrist extension.

1

Stand with your legs comfortably apart, elbows bent and raised in line with your shoulders, hands in fists.

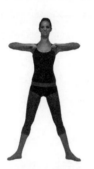

2

Lock your spine straight and your deltoids down throughout these arm exercises. Open your arms to the side, hands facing the floor. Timing: 3 seconds.

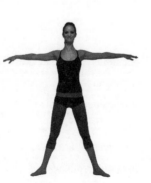

3

Flex your wrists, fingers together. Pump your arms down, pushing against an invisible force by contracting your deltoids. Don't let your deltoids move as you pump up and down; the size of each pump should be no greater than six inches. Timing: 3 seconds per pump. Repeat thirty-two times.

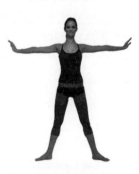

ARM PUMPS FOR PECTORAL STRETCH

JOINTS: shoulders, elbows, wrists.

Ball and socket.

Saddle.

Condyloid.

Hinge.

MUSCLES: trapezius, rhomboids, deltoids, pectorals, triceps, biceps, extensors of the wrist, flexors and extensors of the hands and fingers, abdominals.

Straight spine.

Bent elbows.

Fists: open, closed.   Wrist extension.

1

Open your arms to the side, straighten your elbows, and flex your wrists.

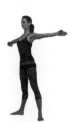

2

Pump your arms backward, pushing against an invisible force by contracting your deltoids. Don't let your spine arch or move as you pump your arms behind. The size of each pump should be no greater than six inches. Timing: 3 seconds per pump. Repeat sixteen times.

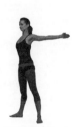

3

Rotate your shoulders in their sockets while imagining that you're dropping your shoulder blades into a back pocket. Do not lean back. Lower your arms to hip height with your wrists flexed. Slowly try to touch your

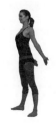

fingertips together behind you in a gentle pump. Timing: 3 seconds per pump. Repeat eight times.

4

Bring your arms in front, elbows bent at shoulder height. Contract your fists, shoulders, and arm muscles as much as possible.

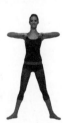

5

Keep your arms and shoulders tight and contracted. Open and close your arms, returning to the bent-elbow position each time. Timing: 4 seconds. After completing these arm pumps, shake out your arms and completely relax your arms and shoulders. Repeat eight times.

ARM PUMPS FOR TRICEPS

JOINTS: shoulders, elbows, wrists.

Ball and socket.

Saddle.

Condyloid.

MUSCLES: trapezius, rhomboids, deltoids, pectorals, triceps, biceps, extensors of the wrist, flexors and extensors of the hands and fingers, abdominals.

Straight spine.   Bent elbows.   Wrist extension.

1

Stand with your feet comfortably apart, elbows bent at the sides at waist height, hands in fists.

2

Straighten your elbows, pushing an invisible force toward the floor. Keep your shoulders still.

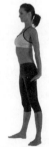

3

With flexed wrists, pump your arms backward, isolating your arms within your shoulders. Timing: 3 seconds per pump. Repeat eight to sixteen times.

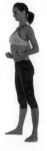

4

Rotate your arms outward to turn the palms of your hands to face opposite walls. Flex your wrists.

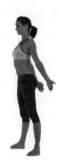

5

Try to touch your fingers together in a gentle pumping action. Timing: 3 seconds per pump. Repeat eight to sixteen times.

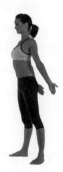

ARM PUMPS FOR POSTURE

JOINTS: shoulders, elbows, wrists.

Ball and socket.

Saddle.

Condyloid.

Hinge.

MUSCLES: trapezius, rhomboids, deltoids, pectorals, triceps, biceps, extensors of the wrist, flexors and extensors of the hands and fingers, abdominals.

Straight spine.

Bent elbows.

Hands open.

Wrist extension.

1

Stand with your legs comfortably apart, elbows bent and raised in line with your shoulders, hands in fists.

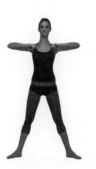

2

Open your arms to the side, straighten your elbows, and flex your wrists.

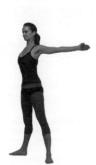

3

Pump your arms backward, pushing against an invisible force by contracting your deltoids. Don't let your spine arch or move as you pump your arms behind. The size of each pump should be no greater than six inches.

Timing: 3 seconds per pump. Repeat sixteen times.

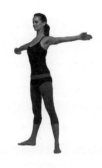

CATEGORY 8: LEGS AND HIPS

LOW RAPID KICKS

JOINTS: hips, ankles.

MUSCLES: abdominals, latissimus dorsi, quadratus lumborum, hamstrings, quadriceps, gluteus group, soleus, gastrocnemius, tibialis posterior and anterior.

1

These rapid low kicks will strengthen your glutes, improve your balance, and loosen your hip joints. As your leg strengthens and your hips loosen, your leg will feel as light as a feather. Kick behind and only move your leg, not your buttocks. Timing: 1 second. Repeat eight times.

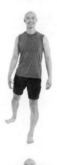

2

Perform eight kicks in a row behind with your knee bent and turned out.

3

Perform eight kicks in a row diagonally across the front of your body.

4

Perform sixteen kicks in a row forward with your front foot pointed.

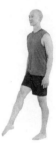

5

Perform sixteen kicks in a row forward with your front foot flexed.

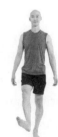

6

Perform eight kicks in a row to the side with your knee facing front and your foot pointed, then eight more kicks with your foot flexed. Timing: 60 seconds for all seventy-two kicks. Repeat the entire sequence on the opposite side.

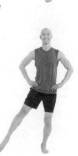

KARATE KICKS TO THE FRONT—CHAIR

JOINTS: spine, hips, knees.

Ball and socket.

Hinge.

MUSCLES: abdominals, obliques, quadratus lumborum, latissimus dorsi, quadriceps, hamstrings, gluteus group, hip flexors, soleus, gastrocnemius.

Straight spine.

Knees bent.

Hip hinge.

1

Hold the back of the chair with one hand. Bend both knees.

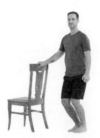

2

Lift one knee as high as possible while flexing your foot. Bend your arm in front, making a fist. Timing: 1 second.

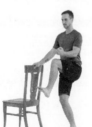

3

Leading with your heel, kick as fast as possible while simultaneously pulling your bent elbow backward. Timing: 1 second.

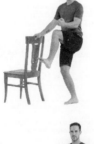

4

Return your knee and arm to their bent positions. Timing: ½ second.

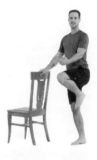

5

Put your feet together, straighten your knees, and relax your arm. Timing: ½ second. Timing for the total sequence: 3 seconds. Repeat eight times per leg.

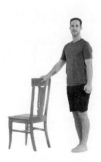

KARATE KICKS TO THE SIDE—CHAIR

JOINTS: spine, hips, knees.

Ball and socket.

Hinge.

MUSCLES: abdominals, obliques, quadratus lumborum, latissimus dorsi, quadriceps, hip flexors, hamstrings, gluteus group, soleus, gastrocnemius.

Straight spine.

Knees bent.

Hip hinge.

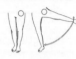

Hip hinge side.

1

Hold the back of the chair with one hand and bend both knees.

2

Lift one knee as high as possible while flexing your foot. Bend your elbow and make a fist. Timing: ½ second.

3

Bend sideways, lifting your hip. Timing: ½ second.

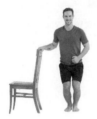

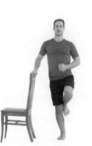

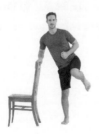

4

Kick to the side as fast as possible, leading with your heel. Timing: 1 second.

5

Return your body to an upright position while bringing your knee back beside your leg. Timing: ½ second.

6

Put your feet together. Timing: ½ second. Timing for the total sequence: 3 seconds. Repeat eight times per leg.

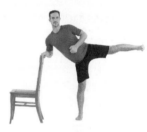

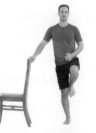

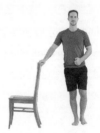

FAN KICKS WITH LUNGES

JOINTS: spine, hips, knees.

Ball and socket.

Hinge.

MUSCLES: abdominals, obliques, quadratus lumborum, latissimus dorsi, quadriceps, hip flexors, hamstrings, hip adductors, gluteus group, soleus, gastrocnemius.

Straight spine.

Rotation in the hip joint.

1

Bend your standing leg and kick your opposite leg across your body. Your arms should stay relaxed. Timing: ½ second.

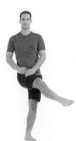

2

Rapidly swing your leg in a fan shape across your body. Timing: ½ second.

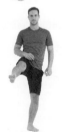

3

When your leg arrives at your side, try to hold it for one or two seconds at its maximum height. Timing: 1 second.

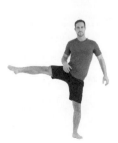

4

Land softly in a lunge; contract your quadriceps and abdominals and pull your weight upward as you land. Timing: 1 second.

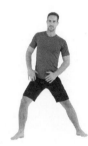

5

Shift your weight to the other side in a deep side lunge. Start again by rapidly standing and kicking your leg across your body again. Timing: 1 second. Repeat three fan kicks in a row. Timing: 9 to 12 seconds for three fan kicks.

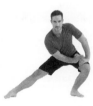

6

Start again by rapidly standing and kicking your other leg across your body. Timing: 1 second. Repeat three fan kicks in a row. Timing: 9 to 12 seconds for three fan kicks.

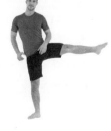

SQUASH LUNGES

JOINTS: spine, hips, knees, ankles.

Ball and socket.

Hinge.

Plane.

MUSCLES: abdominals, latissimus dorsi, quadratus lumborum, hamstrings, hip flexors, quadriceps, gluteus group, tibialis posterior and anterior, soleus, gastrocnemius.

Straight spine.

Knees bent.

Hip hinge.

Ankle flexion and extension.

1

This sequence is quite fast. Start with both knees bent and together, spine straight.

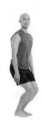

2

Lift one knee and straighten your standing leg. Timing: 1 second.

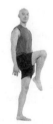

3

Extend your leg straight in front; do not lean backward. Isolate your leg in the joint. Do not use your buttocks to lift your leg. Timing: 4 seconds.

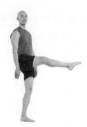

4

Slowly lower your body into a front lunge with both knees bent and your back straight. Timing: 4 seconds.

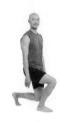

5

Return to the starting position, keeping your spine straight and your leg isolated in the joint. Timing: 3 seconds.

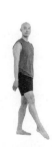

6

Finish standing on both legs, knees straight. Repeat the squash lunges three times. Timing: 12 seconds for one sequence. Timing for three sequences: 36 seconds. Repeat on the opposite side.

LUNGE HIP MOBILITY SEQUENCE

JOINTS: hips, knees, ankles.

Ball and socket.

Hinge.

Plane.

MUSCLES: quadriceps, hamstrings, hip adductors, sartorius, gluteus group, tibialis posterior and anterior, soleus, gastrocnemius.

Knees bent.

Hip hinge to the side.

Ankle flexion and extension.

1

Start in a front lunge, bending your front knee and making sure your back leg is straight and your heel is on the floor. Hold for 5 seconds to feel your knees being strengthened and the back of your leg being stretched.

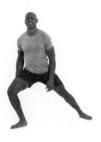

2

Shift your weight into a side lunge, keeping both feet on the ground and your back as straight as possible. Hold for 5 seconds to feel your inner hips being stretched.

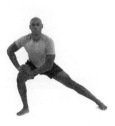

3

Flex your foot for 5 seconds. Place your foot flat on the ground and hold for 5 seconds. Change legs.

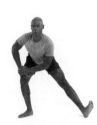

4

Shift your weight onto your back leg, bending your knee and making sure your foot is flat on the floor and your knee is over the arch of your foot. Hold for 5 seconds to feel the front of your leg being stretched. Repeat on the opposite side.

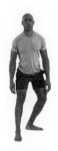

STANDING QUAD STRETCH

JOINTS: hips, knees, ankles.

Ball and socket.

Hinge.

Plane.

MUSCLES: abdominals, quadriceps, hip flexors, hamstrings, gluteus group, tibialis posterior and anterior, soleus, gastrocnemius.

Knees bent.

Heel lift with toe flexion.

1

Stand straight and extend one leg straight behind you, lifting your back heel as high as possible while leaving your toes flexed on the floor. Bend your standing leg.

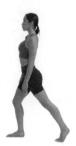

2

Tuck your buttocks under while lowering your back knee toward the floor. Return to your starting position. Do not hold at the bottom of the stretch. Timing: 4 seconds to lower your knee and 3 seconds to return to your starting position.

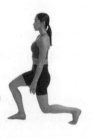

3

As soon as you're upright, lift your back foot, grabbing it with your hand or with a TheraBand. Let your knee swing slightly in front of your thigh, then pull it back in line with your thigh. Timing: 5 seconds.

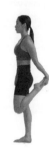

4

Pull your heel toward your buttocks. Do not let your lower back arch. Continuously pull and release the tension on your quad in a pulsing motion. Timing: 6 seconds. Repeat on the other leg.

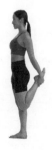

MUSKETEERS BOW—IT BAND AND LONG ADDUCTOR STRETCH

JOINTS: spine, hips, ankles.

Ball and socket.

Hinge.

MUSCLES: latissimus dorsi, abdominals, obliques, hip adductors, gluteus group, hamstrings, hip flexors, sartorius, tibialis anterior, soleus, gastrocnemius.

Hip hinge.   Hip hinge side.   Ankle flexion and extension.

1

Bend one knee and extend the other leg in front, flexing your foot. Bend forward slightly, hinging from your hips while keeping your spine straight.

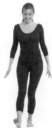

2

Shift your hips as far as possible, rotating your extended leg in the hip joint while trying to touch the floor with the outside of your ankle. Timing: 5 seconds.

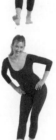

3

Shift your hips in the other direction, rotating your leg inward. Timing: 4 seconds. Repeat two times.

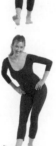

4

Balance on one leg and lift the stretching leg into a bent position at hip height. Ensure that your hips are level and your knee is in front of your hip.

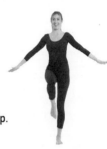

5

Transfer into a deep side lunge. Place your hands on your bent knee and keep your hips in line with the heel of your bent leg.

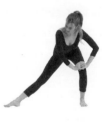

6

Flex your foot while swaying your hips toward the back of the room. Timing: 6 seconds for three sways. Repeat on the opposite side.

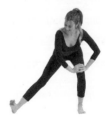

CATEGORY 9: FEET, ANKLES, AND CALVES

ANKLE, CALF, AND SHIN STRETCH

JOINTS: knees, ankles, toes.

MUSCLES: hamstrings, soleus, gastrocnemius, tibialis anterior and posterior, muscles of the foot.

1

Stand with one foot in front of the other. Bend both knees, keeping your spine straight. Shift your weight onto your back leg.

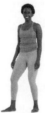

2

Lift your front heel as high as possible without poor alignment in the ankle. Timing: 3 seconds.

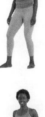

3

Lift your front leg off the floor, pointing your foot. Straighten both your back and front legs. Timing: 3 seconds. Repeat on the other side.

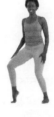

4

Place your toes back on the floor, keeping your heel lifted. Bend your knee and carefully push the weight of your body forward into the arch of your foot. Timing: 3 seconds.

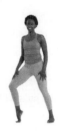

5

Place your heel flat on the floor, bending your front knee as much as possible. Timing: 3 seconds.

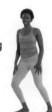

6

Shift your weight onto your back leg while bending your back knee and straightening your front leg. Flex your front foot as you pull your buttocks backward. Keep your spine straight as you bend forward. Timing: 3 seconds. Total timing for full sequence: 18 seconds. Repeat two times, then repeat on the opposite side.

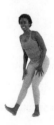

CALF STRETCH SEQUENCE

JOINTS: hips, knees, ankles, toes.

Ball and socket.

Hinge.

Plane.

MUSCLES: hip flexors, gluteus group, tibialis anterior and posterior, soleus, gastrocnemius.

Straight spine.

Knees bent.

Hip hinge.

Heel lift with toe flexion.

Elbows bent.

1

Stand with one leg in front of the other, feet comfortably parallel. Keeping your back straight, bend both knees and shift your weight onto your back leg. Dig your back heel into the floor and keep bending your knee. Timing: 6 to 8 seconds.

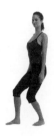

2

Shift your weight onto your front leg, lift your back heel, and straighten your back knee. Keep your back straight. Timing: 2 seconds.

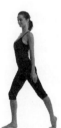

3

Slowly lower your back heel, digging it into the floor. Keep your weight and buttocks forward. Timing: 6 to 8 seconds.

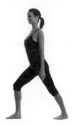

4

Shift your weight onto your back heel, keeping it glued flat to the floor and bending your back knee. Timing: 6 to 8 seconds.

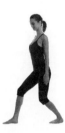

5

Straighten your back knee, bend slightly forward, and lift your buttocks. Glue your back heel to the floor and gently shift your weight forward. Timing: 6 to 8 seconds.

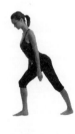

6

Lift your elbows to shoulder height and straighten your arms in front. Timing: 4 to 6 seconds. Change legs and repeat the sequence.

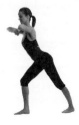

ANKLE MOBILITY WITH HIP ROTATION—FLOOR

JOINTS: hips, ankles.

Hinge.

Ball and socket.

Plane.

MUSCLES: gluteus group, soleus, gastrocnemius, tibialis anterior and posterior.

Straight spine.

Hip hinge.

Ankle flexion and extension.

1

Use a riser if necessary. Sit comfortably on the floor and point your feet. Hold for 3 seconds.

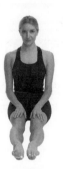

2

Flex your feet and keep trying to increase the degree of flexion. Timing: 3 seconds.

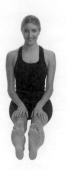

3

Rotate your hips and feet to one side, trying to put the outside of your foot on the floor. Timing: 3 seconds.

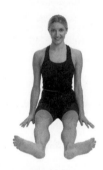

4

Rotate your ankles and hips internally to stretch the range of motion of your ankles. Timing: 3 seconds. Repeat three times.

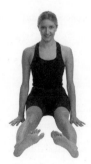

SHIN STRETCHING AND STRENGTHENING—CHAIR

JOINTS: knees, ankles, toes.

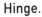

Hinge.

Plane.

MUSCLES: abdominals, quadriceps, hip flexors, hamstrings, sartorius, soleus, gastrocnemius, muscles of the foot, tibialis anterior.

Straight spine.   Knees bent.   Ankle flexion and extension.

1

A: Hold the back of a chair with both hands. Your feet should be slightly apart and parallel. Bend your knees. Timing: 2 seconds.

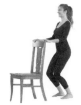

2

B: Lift your heels as high as possible. Timing: 2 seconds.

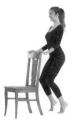

3

C: Imagine that you're pushing the full weight of your body away from the floor as you slowly straighten your knees. Timing: 2 seconds.

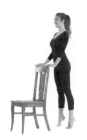

4

D: Slowly lower your heels. Timing: 2 seconds. Total time to complete steps A to D: 8 seconds. Repeat four times.

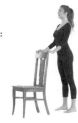

5

Variation 1: Repeat steps A to D four times with your knees turned out.

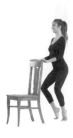

6

Variation 2: Repeat steps A to D four times in a wider stance, also with your knees turned out.

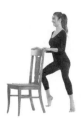

ADVANCED ANKLE STRENGTHENING— CHAIR

JOINTS: knees, ankles, toes.

Hinge.

Plane.

MUSCLES: abdominals, gluteus group, quadriceps, soleus, gastrocnemius, tibialis anterior, muscles of the foot.

Straight spine.

Knees bent.

Hip hinge.

Heel lift with toe flexion.

1

Hold a chair at waist level. Your feet should be together and your knees bent.

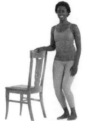

2

Preparation position: Lift the leg farthest from the chair and touch your toes to the ankle of your standing leg. Timing 2 seconds.

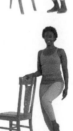

3

Slowly lift the heel of your standing leg while keeping your opposite knee bent. Timing: 3 seconds.

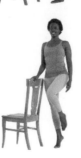

4

Extend your leg to the front, straightening your knee and keeping the heel of the standing leg raised. Timing: 4 seconds.

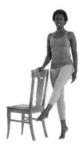

5

Return to the preparation position. Timing: 3 seconds. Total timing of one sequence: 15 seconds. Repeat the sequence four times per foot.

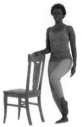

CALF STRETCH SEQUENCE FOR BALANCE

JOINTS: spine, shoulders, hips, knees.

Ball and socket.

Hinge.

MUSCLES: abdominals, obliques, intercostals, latissimus dorsi, quadratus lumborum, deltoids, triceps, quadriceps, hamstrings, sartorius, hip flexors, tibialis posterior, soleus, gastrocnemius.

Shoulder arm rotation up.

Spine circle.

1

Stand in a deep front lunge. Raise one arm above your head and the other sideways to shoulder height.

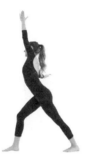

2

Bend sideways to start a body rotation.

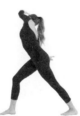

3

When you can bend to the side no farther, start to bend forward.

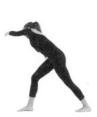

4

Continue the forward bend until you can touch your torso to your front thigh, lowering your head until your forehead touches your knee.

5

Continue the side rotation using your abdominal muscles to maintain your balance as your body moves upward in the rotation.

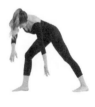

6

Continue the full side rotation until you return to the starting position. Timing: 15 seconds for one full side rotation. Repeat in the opposite direction.

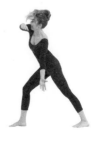

CATEGORY 10:
CHAIR/BARRE STRETCHING

HIP CLEANERS—CHAIR

JOINTS: hips, knees.

MUSCLES: abdominals, gluteus group, hamstrings, quadriceps, hip flexors, gracilis.

1

The purpose of the Hip Cleaner is to loosen any congealed debris that's restricting movement within the hip socket. Hold a chair for balance and stand on the leg close to the chair. Bend your other knee while touching both knees together. Swing the foot of the bent leg behind and across the standing leg.

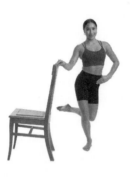

2

Keep your knees touching and swing your leg toward the other wall. Timing: 2 seconds.

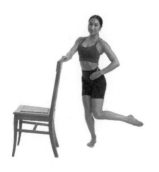

3

Lift your knee across your body. Timing: 2 seconds.

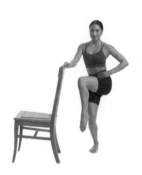

4

Open your leg, lifting it to the side. Repeat three times per leg. Timing: 6 seconds for one Hip Cleaner. Total timing for three Hip Cleaners: 18 to 20 seconds.

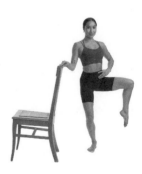

FOUR-DIRECTIONAL HIP STRETCH— CHAIR

JOINTS: spine, hips, knees.

Hinge.

Ball and socket.

MUSCLES: abdominals, obliques, quadratus lumborum, erector spinae, latissimus dorsi, gluteus group, hip adductors, quadriceps, hamstrings, soleus, gastrocnemius.

Hips forward and back.   Hip hinge in front.   Knees bent.

1

Stand relatively close to the seat of the chair and place one flexed foot on the seat. Bend your supporting leg, place your hand on your knee, and lightly press downward to stretch your hip. Keep your back straight and your buttocks protruding slightly backward. Timing: 4 to 6 seconds.

2

Lift your hip as high as possible to loosen the ball and socket of the hip hinge. Place your hand lightly on your knee and keep your standing leg bent. Let your spine bend sideways during this movement. Timing: 4 to 6 seconds.

3

Drop your hip, rocking it as far in the opposite direction as possible. Use the hand on your knee to stretch your hip farther. Let your back relax into a curve to permit the hip to move through its maximum range of motion. Timing: 4 to 6 seconds.

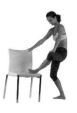

4

Keep your standing knee bent and straighten your spine, keeping your buttocks protruding. Shift your weight toward the seat of the chair to stretch the inside of your hip. Timing: 4 to 6 seconds.

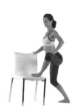

5

Shift your weight back onto your standing leg, pulling your buttocks back and straightening your spine. Timing: 4 to 6 seconds.

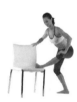

6

Straighten your spine, keeping your knee bent, and twist or rotate your spine toward the leg of the chair. Timing: 4 to 6 seconds. Repeat on the opposite side.

PREPARATION: HIP FLEXOR AND HAMSTRING STRETCH—CHAIR

JOINTS: spine, hips, knees, ankles.

Ball and socket.

Hinge.

Plane.

MUSCLES: abdominals, latissimus dorsi, erector spinae, quadratus lumborum, gluteus group, quadriceps, hamstrings, gracilis, tibialis anterior and posterior, soleus, gastrocnemius.

Straight spine.

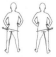

Hip hinge.

Ankle flexion and extension.

Hips: left, right.

Spine curved.

Knees bent.

1

Stand with one foot placed flat on the seat of a chair. Shift your full weight forward onto the foot on the chair. Lift your standing heel if needed.

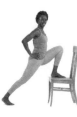

2

Slowly shift your weight completely onto your standing leg while trying to straighten the leg on the chair and pointing that foot. Wiggle gently as you're stretching. Keep your spine straight. Timing: 6 seconds.

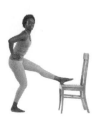

3

To release the stretch, bend the knee on the chair. Timing: 3 seconds.

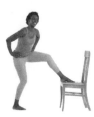

4

Move your hips as much as possible toward your standing leg. Timing: 3 seconds.

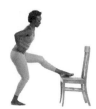

5

Shift your hips, lifting your buttocks as much as possible. Timing: 3 seconds.

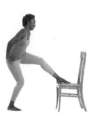

6

Face the chair with both hips and tuck your tailbone under, rounding your spine. Timing: 3 seconds. Repeat the entire sequence two times. Total timing of one sequence: 18 seconds. Repeat with the opposite leg.

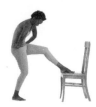

INNER AND OUTER THIGH ROTATIONS: IT BAND AND LONG ADDUCTOR STRETCH—CHAIR

JOINTS: spine, hips, knees.

Ball and socket.   Hinge.

MUSCLES: abdominals, latissimus dorsi, erector spinae, gluteus group, hip adductors, hip flexors, quadriceps, hamstrings, tibialis anterior, soleus, gastrocnemius.

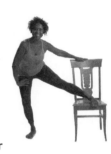

Hip hinge.   Hip hinge to the side and rotation in the hip joint.

1

Place one foot on the seat of the chair, flexing it. Bend slightly forward with your spine completely straight. Bend your standing leg.

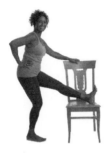

2

Hold the back of the chair and twist your hips toward the back of the room, keeping your spine straight while bending forward. Adjust your standing foot to face the back of the room. Rotate your leg externally on the chair, trying to touch the seat of the chair with the outside of your foot. This will stretch the outside of your leg, or the IT band. Timing: 6 to 8 seconds.

3

Rotate your standing leg to face the front of the room, adjusting the placement of your foot and knee to face forward. Turn your hips and torso to face front. Keep your back straight while bending forward. Rotate the leg on the seat of the chair internally, trying to touch the seat of the chair with the inside of your foot. This will stretch the inside of your leg, or the long adductor. Timing: 6 to 8 seconds. Repeat, turning back to front three times before changing legs and repeating the exercise.

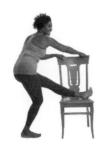

DEEP HAMSTRING AND SPINE STRETCH WITH RELEASE—CHAIR

JOINTS: spine, shoulders, hips, knees, ankles.

Ball and socket.

Hinge.

Plane.

MUSCLES: rhomboids, deltoids, triceps, hamstrings, gluteus group, tibialis anterior, soleus, gastrocnemius.

Straight spine.

Hip hinge.

Ankle flexion and extension.

Spine curved.

Hips side to side.

1

Place your foot on the seat of a chair and point your toes. Raise the arm on the same side as the leg on the chair and reach as far forward as possible. Bend your standing leg while bending slightly forward. Keep your spine as straight as possible. Reach forward for 5 seconds.

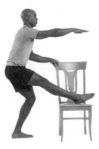

2

Flex your foot and keep reaching over it. This will stretch the hamstrings. Remain flexed for 5 seconds. Repeat the pointing and flexing movement three times.

Timing: 30 seconds for the full sequence.

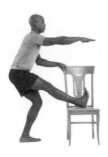

3

Round your back and hold the back of the chair with both hands. Move your hips up and down to engage different parts of your glutes and hamstrings.

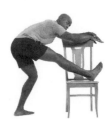

4

Move slowly and continuously for 10 seconds. Change legs and repeat the sequence.

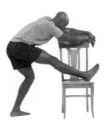

PULL A ROPE IT BAND AND HAMSTRING STRETCH—CHAIR

JOINTS: spine, shoulders, elbows, hips, knees.

Ball and socket.

Hinge.

Plane.

MUSCLES: abdominals, obliques, erector spinae, latissimus dorsi, quadratus lumborum, trapezius, biceps, triceps, deltoids, pectorals, gluteus group, hamstrings, quadriceps, hip flexors, soleus, gastrocnemius.

Straight spine.　　Hip hinge.　　Bent elbows.

Hands open and closed.　　Body twist.

1

Stand straight, holding the chair.

2

Lift the leg nearest the front onto the seat of the chair. Bend the knee of your supporting leg, keeping your spine as straight as possible. Reach over your leg and imagine you're grabbing a rope.

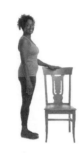

3

Round your back and imagine you're pulling a really tight rope toward your chest.

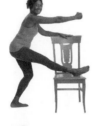

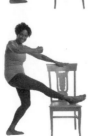

4

Straighten your spine as you pull the rope behind you. Timing: 10 seconds for the full sequence. Repeat three times.

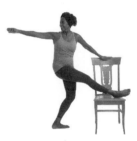

5

Once you get to your maximum twist, breathe slowly and try to rotate a little farther. Change legs and repeat the sequence.

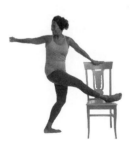

HIP FLEXOR AND HAMSTRING STRETCH—CHAIR

JOINTS: spine, hips, knees, ankles, toes.

Ball and socket.

Hinge.

Plane.

MUSCLES: latissimus dorsi, quadratus lumborum, erector spinae, hip flexors, iliopsoas, hamstrings, gluteus group, tibialis anterior and posterior, gastrocnemius.

Straight spine.

Knees bent.

Heel lift with toe flexion.

Spine curved.

1

Stand near the chair with one foot on the seat.

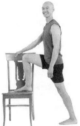

2

Raise the heel of your standing leg and shift your hips toward the seat of the chair. Timing: 3 seconds.

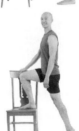

3

Bend the knee of your supporting leg and shift your hips forward while simultaneously tucking your tailbone under and pushing your heel flat onto the floor. This is the iliopsoas stretch. Timing: 5 seconds.

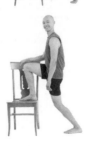

4

Slowly bend your standing knee while shifting your weight closer to the chair. Timing: 6 seconds. Do not hold at the bottom of the movement.

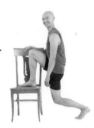

5

To relax the tension on your quads, shift your weight onto your back bent leg and round your spine. Timing: 4 seconds. Switch legs and repeat the sequence.

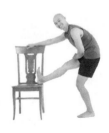

HAMSTRING STRETCH—CHAIR

JOINTS: spine, hips, knees, ankles.

Ball and socket.

Hinge.

MUSCLES: abdominals, latissimus dorsi, erector spinae, quadratus lumborum, hamstrings, gluteus group, quadriceps, tibialis anterior and posterior, soleus, gastrocnemius.

Straight spine.

Hip hinge.

Ankle flexion and extension.

Spine curved.

Knees bent.

1

A: Place one heel on the seat of the chair with your foot flexed and your knee straight, if possible. Bend your standing leg and keep your spine straight.

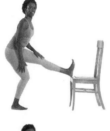

2

B: Point and flex your foot. Timing: 3 seconds to flex and 3 seconds to point. Repeat four times. Total time: 24 seconds.

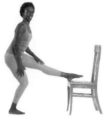

3

Bend forward and try to touch the back of the chair, keeping your spine as straight as possible. Timing: 5 seconds.

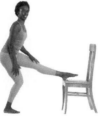

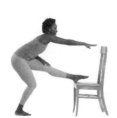

4

Switch arms and reach again. Timing: 5 seconds per reach. Repeat the sequence two times. Total timing for four reaches, alternating arms: 20 seconds.

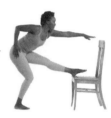

5

To release the tension on your spine and hamstrings, stand upright, round your spine, and tuck your tailbone under while bending the leg on the chair. Slowly wiggle around in this position. Timing: 5 seconds. Total timing of the sequence: 25 seconds. Change legs and repeat the sequence.

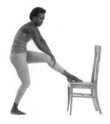

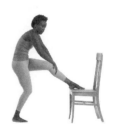

WINDMILL HAMSTRING AND SPINE STRETCH—CHAIR

JOINTS: spine, shoulders, hips.

Ball and socket.

Saddle.

MUSCLES: latissimus dorsi, erector spinae, quadratus lumborum, abdominals, obliques, trapezius, rhomboids, pectorals, hamstrings, quadriceps, hip flexors, gluteus group.

Hip hinge.   Straight spine.   Spine leaning forward.

Upper body twist.   Shoulder arm rotation.   Knees bent.

1

Move your arm in a windmill motion throughout this sequence. Turn the chair to the side. Bend your standing leg and place your other foot on the chair. Keep the foot on the chair pointed as you raise the arm on the same side as your raised leg, relax your shoulder, and lift your arm as high as you can, feeling the stretch through your spine.

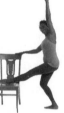

2

Take 5 to 7 seconds to windmill your right arm, keeping your spine straight as you reach as far as possible over your extended leg.

3

Take another 5 to 7 seconds to slowly windmill your arm toward the floor, breathing deeply as you do.

4

Take another 5 to 7 seconds to windmill your arm toward the back of the room. Breathe and relax in order to twist your torso as much as possible. Keep your hips down to stretch your glutes and IT band.

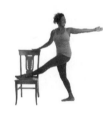

5

Windmill your arm toward the ceiling, relaxing and reaching upward.

6

Finish by straightening the knee of your standing leg. Repeat two or three times. Timing: 20 to 25 seconds per windmill. Repeat on the other side.

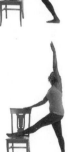

HAMSTRING AND SPINE STRETCH— CHAIR

JOINTS: spine, shoulders, hips, knees, ankles.

Ball and socket.

Hinge.

MUSCLES: latissimus dorsi, quadratus lumborum, trapezius, rhomboids, triceps, biceps, deltoids, pectorals, hamstrings, quadriceps, gluteus group, tibialis anterior and posterior, soleus, gastrocnemius.

Straight spine.

Hip hinge.

Shoulders arm rotation up.

Ankle flexion and extension.   Spine curved.   Knees bent.

1

Bend the knee of one leg and place the other leg on a chair, foot pointed.

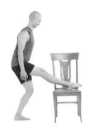

2

Raise your arms. Keep your elbows straight and hold them beside your ears while you slowly bend forward, keeping your spine straight. Timing: 5 seconds.

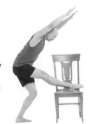

3

Hold your spine still and extend one arm behind your head. Timing: 3 seconds.

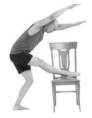

4

Hold your spine still and extend your other arm behind your head. Timing: 3 seconds.

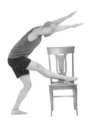

5

Flex the foot on the chair. Timing: 3 seconds.

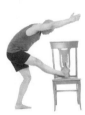

6

Relax your spine and bend the knee of the leg on the chair. Slowly roll up the spine. Timing: 5 seconds. Repeat three times maximum, then repeat the entire sequence on the other side.

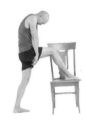

FOLDED HAMSTRING STRETCH—CHAIR

JOINTS: spine, hips, knees, toes.

Ball and socket.

Hinge.

Plane.

MUSCLES: abdominals, latissimus dorsi, erector spinae, quadratus lumborum, hamstrings, quadriceps, soleus, gastrocnemius.

Straight spine.

Knees bent.

Spine toe touch.

Heel lift with toe flexion.

1

Hold the chair slightly in front of your shoulders. Stand straight with your feet together. Relax all your muscles.

2

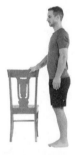

Bend your knees and lay your chest on them. Let your neck relax, dropping your head toward the floor. Hold the seat or leg of the chair with one hand and grasp your ankle with the other. Timing: 3 seconds.

3

Try to straighten your knees, keeping your chest as close to your thighs as possible. Timing: 3 seconds.

4

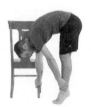

Optional: Continue to hold the chair while lifting both heels off the floor. Timing: 2 seconds.

5

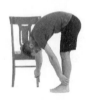

Lower your heels and try to pull your torso closer to your legs. Timing: 3 seconds.

6

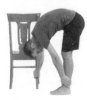

Release all the tension in your spine and hamstrings by rounding your back and bending your knees. Slowly roll up to straighten your back and repeat the stretch once more. Timing: 4 seconds. Timing for full sequence: 15 seconds.

SPINE RELEASE—CHAIR

JOINTS: spine, shoulders, elbows, hips, knees.

Ball and socket.   Hinge.

MUSCLES: abdominals, latissimus dorsi, erector spinae, quadratus lumborum, trapezius, rhomboids, triceps, biceps, deltoids, pectorals, hamstrings, quadriceps.

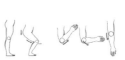

Spine curved.   Knees bent.   Bent elbows.   Spine leaning back.

1

Stand behind a chair with a relatively high back. Your feet should be comfortably apart, knees bent, spine rounded, and elbows up. Slowly wiggle your back to stretch and self-massage your spine. Timing: 5 seconds.

2

Shift your weight as far as possible in one direction and then the other. Timing: 5 seconds per direction.

3

Step far enough away from the chair to straighten your arms and spine. Keep your knees bent. Gently move in that position. Timing: 5 seconds.

4

Shift your weight as far as possible in one direction and then the other. Timing: 5 seconds per direction.

5

Return to your starting position and gently wiggle your spine. Timing: 5 seconds.

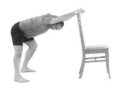

6

Step close to the chair, completely straightening your spine, and very carefully arch only the top of your back. Lift your head, making sure you're supporting your neck and not letting it crunch as it drops backward. Timing: 5 seconds. Total timing of full sequence: 40 to 60 seconds.

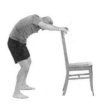

DEEP SIDE BEND AND IT BAND STRETCH—CHAIR

JOINTS: spine, shoulders, hips.

Ball and socket.

Saddle.

MUSCLES: abdominals, latissimus dorsi, obliques, intercostals, erector spinae, quadratus lumborum, pectorals, gluteus group.

Straight spine.

Arm rotation up and down.

Spine side to side.

Spine curved.

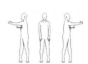

Upper body twist.

1

Stand next to a chair with your feet together. Hold the chair with one hand in front of your shoulders, your other arm straight above your head.

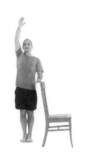

2

Move slightly away from the chair. Using the chair for balance, bend as far to the side as possible. Timing: 5 seconds.

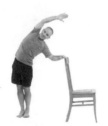

3

Step close to the chair again. Lift your arm above your head and cross your outside foot in front of your other leg. Timing: 3 seconds.

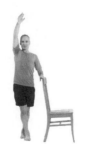

4

Bend your knees while bending forward and reaching your arm straight forward. Timing: 3 seconds.

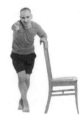

5

Imagine that you're pulling an invisible rope across your body. Timing: 3 seconds.

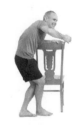

6

Finish pulling the rope across your body by rotating your torso and extending your arm directly behind. This will stretch your IT band and chest muscles. Timing: 3 seconds. Timing for the complete sequence: 17 seconds. Repeat on the other side.

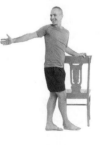

CATEGORY 11: FLOOR STRENGTHENING

STRENGTHENING QUAD RAISER—FLOOR

JOINTS: hips, ankles.

MUSCLES: hip flexors, quadriceps, hamstrings, tibialis anterior and posterior, soleus, gastrocnemius.

1

Lie flat on the floor. Place both hands beside your hips and relax your spine. Squeeze the floor with the hamstrings of one leg with your foot pointed. Timing: 3 seconds.

2

Slide that leg forward, continuing to press your hamstring into the floor. Timing: 3 seconds.

3

Lift the lengthened leg and hold, continuing to try to pull the leg away from your hip. Timing: 2 seconds.

4

Continue to pull the lifted leg away from your hip and flex your foot. Timing: 2 seconds.

5

Lower your leg to the floor and return it to the starting position. Repeat with the other leg. Timing: 12 seconds for the full sequence.

ABDUCTOR AND GLUTES STRENGTHENING—FLOOR

JOINTS: spine, hips, knees, ankles.

Ball and socket.

Hinge.

MUSCLES: abdominals, gluteus group, hip abductors, hip flexors, quadriceps, hamstrings, tibialis anterior.

Knees bent.

Hip hinge front.

Hip hinge side.

Ankle flexion.

1

Lie on your side on the floor. Place your top hand in front of you and lie on your lower arm. Do not lift your head. Bend both knees and bring your upper knee close to your chest.

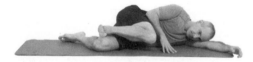

2

Kick your top leg toward your shoulder and lower it quickly. Repeat for eight to sixteen kicks. Timing: 2 seconds per kick. Total timing for the sequence: 16 to 32 seconds.

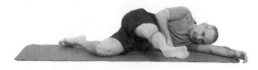

3

Raise and lower your straight leg eight times. Timing: 3 seconds per lift. Total timing for the sequence: 24 seconds.

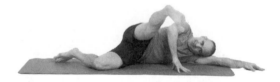

4

Twist your leg in the socket, touching your toes and then your heel to the floor. Repeat eight times. Timing: 3 seconds per complete twist. Total timing for the sequence: 24 seconds.

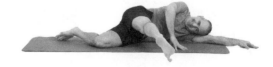

ADVANCED SPINE STRETCHING AND STRENGTHENING USING ARMS, VARIATION #1—FLOOR

JOINTS: shoulders, spine, hips, knees, ankles.

Ball and socket.

Hinge.

Plane.

MUSCLES: abdominals, triceps, biceps, deltoids, rhomboids, pectorals, trapezius, latissimus dorsi, erector spinae, quadriceps, hamstrings, tibialis anterior and posterior, soleus, gastrocnemius.

Hip hinge.   Straight spine.   Shoulder arm rotation up.

Bent elbows.   Ankle flexion and extension.

1

Sit on the floor with both arms above your head. If possible, keep your elbows, spine, and knees straight.

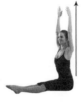

2

Modification: Bend your knees if you can't keep the them straight, or use one or more risers.

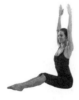

3

Reach one arm as high as possible, relaxing your shoulders to permit you to pull on your obliques. Timing: 4 seconds. Once you arrive at your maximum height, pull your arm behind your shoulders. Timing: 4 seconds. Repeat four times, alternating arms.

4

Bend your elbows at chest height, clasping your hands together. Point and flex your feet. Timing: 3 seconds.

5

Hold your hands in front of you at shoulder height and slowly bend forward from your hips, trying to keep your spine and knees straight. Point and flex your feet. Timing: 8 seconds.

6

Slowly return to an upright position with your arms bent. Timing: 5 seconds. Repeat two times, then repeat the entire sequence on the opposite side.

ADVANCED SPINE STRETCHING AND STRENGTHENING USING ARMS, VARIATION #2—FLOOR

JOINTS: shoulders, spine, hips.

Ball and socket.   Hinge.

MUSCLES: abdominals, latissimus dorsi, erector spinae, quadratus lumborum, rhomboids, trapezius, deltoids, triceps, biceps, muscles of the hand, hamstrings.

Aligned neck.   Straight spine.   Hip hinge.   Shoulder arm rotation up.

Shoulders: up, down.   Bent elbows.   Leaning forward.   Knees bent.

1

Sit on the floor, knees bent or straight depending on your flexibility. Use a riser or risers if your spine or hamstrings are tight. Lift your arms above your head.

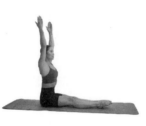

2

Slowly bend forward with your arms extended, keeping your arms beside your ears and your spine straight. Timing: 5 seconds.

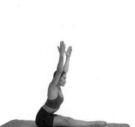

3

Return upright and pull one arm at a time behind your shoulders. Timing: 5 seconds per arm.

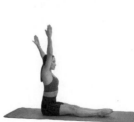

4

Make fists, bend forward slightly, and pull your bent elbows behind your shoulders. Timing: 5 seconds.

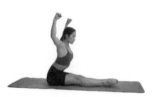

5

Rapidly release your fists and straighten your elbows, trying to open your chest more. Timing: 5 seconds.

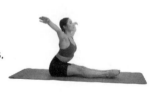

6

Release your spine into a crunch, bending your elbows and knees while relaxing all your muscles. Timing: 5 seconds. Timing for the full sequence: 25 seconds.

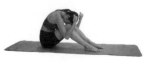

ADVANCED TRAPEZE STRENGTHENING WITH QUAD RAISERS—FLOOR

JOINTS: spine, shoulders, fingers, hips.

Ball and socket.

Hinge.

MUSCLES: abdominals, latissimus dorsi, erector spinae, quadratus lumborum, obliques, trapezius, pectorals, muscles of the hand, quadriceps, hip flexors, gluteus group, hamstrings.

Spine standing.   Hip hinge.

Shoulder arm rotation up.

Spine side to side.   Shoulders: up, down.   Fists closed.

1

Sit with your legs extended, arms above your head, knees as straight as possible, and toes pointed. Imagine that you're in the circus and are about to be lifted off the floor as you hold on to a trapeze bar.

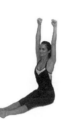

2

Keep pulling upward as you lift one leg off the floor. Hold for 3 seconds and then lower your leg carefully to the floor. Do not round your lower spine. Repeat, alternating legs, four to eight times. Timing: 5 seconds per leg.

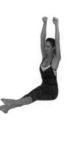

3

Bend slightly forward, keeping your spine straight.

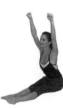

4

Pull upward as if you're being suspended off the floor and bend sideways.

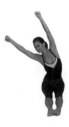

5

Return to your starting position. Repeat, alternating sides, four to eight times. Timing: 8 seconds per side bend.

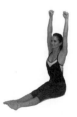

SUPERMAN SPINE STRENGTHENING— FLOOR

JOINTS: spine, shoulders, hips.

Ball and socket.

MUSCLES: abdominals, latissimus dorsi, erector spinae, quadratus lumborum, trapezius, deltoids, triceps, pectorals, biceps, gluteus group, hamstrings, hip flexors.

Spine leaning back.   Correct head posture.   Shoulder arm rotation up.

Shoulders: up, down.   Hip hinge back.

1

This sequence is excellent for

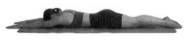

those with back pain, weak back muscles, and poor posture. Lie flat on the floor.

2

Raise one arm,

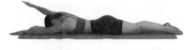

keeping both shoulders flat on the floor, then raise the other arm. Timing: 5 seconds per arm.

3

Lift your arms upward as

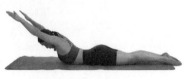

high as possible, followed by your upper back. Timing: 5 seconds. Relax back to the floor for 5 seconds, then repeat the full sequence. Timing: 20 seconds per sequence.

4

To strengthen and increase the mobility

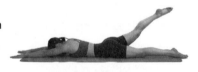

of the psoas muscles, practice this sequence daily. Raise one leg at a time. Timing: 5 seconds per leg.

5

Lift both legs together three times, holding for 5 seconds

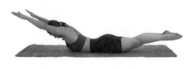

per lift. Relax back to the floor for 5 seconds between each leg lift. For more of a challenge, lift your arms and back (as in the previous sequence) along with your legs.

SLOW SIT-UPS WITH ARM VARIATIONS—FLOOR

JOINTS: spine, shoulders.

Ball and socket.

MUSCLES: abdominals, latissimus dorsi, erector spinae, obliques, pectorals, trapezius, rhomboids.

Straight spine.

Spine side to side.

Hip hinge.

Knees bent.

Shoulder arm rotation toward ceiling.

Bent elbows.

1

These are not rapid sit-ups. I want you to lift slowly and lower slowly, using your abdominal muscles and *not* momentum to do each sit-up. Lie flat with your elbows touching the floor.

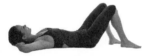

2

Variation #1: Under Head. Keep your elbows open under your head. Timing: 3 seconds per sit-up. Repeat eight times. Total time: 24 seconds.

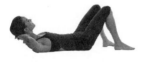

3

Variation #2: Ceiling Reach. Twist your upper back and reach toward the ceiling. Timing: 3 seconds per sit-up. Repeat eight times. Total time: 24 seconds.

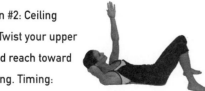

4

Variation #3: Heel Reach. Bend sideways, lifting your upper back slightly off the floor, trying to touch your heel. Timing: 3 seconds per sit-up. Repeat eight times. Total time: 24 seconds. Repeat on the other side.

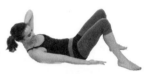

5

Variation #4: Opposite Knee Reach. Lift your body slightly off the floor and twist your upper back to touch the opposite knee. Timing: 3 seconds per sit-up. Repeat eight times. Total time: 24 seconds. Repeat on the other side.

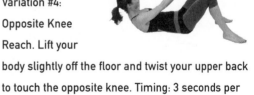

6

Incorrect. Never lift your head by pulling your elbows forward.

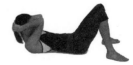

SIT-UPS WITH A WAIST TWIST—FLOOR

JOINTS: spine, shoulders, knees.

Ball and socket.

Hinge.

MUSCLES: abdominals, obliques, latissimus dorsi, erector spinae, pectorals, trapezius, rhomboids, hip flexors, quadriceps.

Straight spine.

Knees bent.

Hip hinge.

Bent elbows.

Upper torso rotation.

1

Lie flat on the floor with your elbows bent. Bend one leg, placing your foot

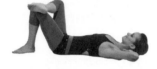

flat on the floor, and rest your other foot on the bent knee.

2

Twist your upper body, lifting your shoulder toward the opposite raised knee.

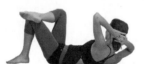

3

Repeat four times per side, lowering your body to the floor after each

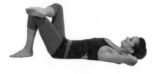

twist. Timing: 4 seconds. Total time for each side: 16 seconds.

4

Imagine you're slowly pedaling a bicycle

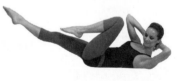

with pointed feet. With each pedal, bring your knee as close to your chest as possible while simultaneously straightening your extended leg. Twist your upper body with each pedal. Timing: 4 seconds per pedal. Repeat for sixteen to thirty-two pedals.

SIT-UPS WITH SINGLE-LEG KICKS—FLOOR

JOINTS: spine, shoulders.

Ball and socket.

MUSCLES: abdominals, obliques, latissimus dorsi, erector spinae, pectorals, trapezius, rhomboids, hip flexors, quadriceps.

Straight spine.   Knees bent.   Hip hinge.   Bent elbows.

1

Lie flat on the floor with your hands behind your head. Bend one knee and place your foot flat on the floor. Extend the other leg and point your foot.

2

Bring your other knee toward your chest, lifting your upper body slightly off the floor. Keep your elbows wide open. Timing: 3 seconds.

3

Extend your leg in front. Timing: 2 seconds. Timing for one sequence: 5 seconds. Repeat for eight sit-ups.

4

Advanced: Lie flat with your leg extended in front.

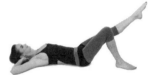

5

Advanced: Lift your upper back slightly off the floor, keeping your leg extended. Timing: 3 seconds.

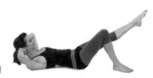

6

Advanced: Lower yourself slowly under muscle control. Timing: 2 seconds. Timing for one sequence: 5 seconds. Repeat for eight sit-ups.

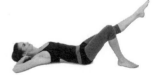

ADVANCED SIT-UPS WITH EXTENDED LEGS—FLOOR

JOINTS: spine, shoulders.

Ball and socket.

MUSCLES: abdominals, obliques, latissimus dorsi, erector spinae, trapezius, rhomboids, pectorals, hip flexors, quadriceps.

 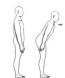

Spine standing.   Hip hinge.

Knees bent.   Shoulder arm rotation.

1

Lie flat on the floor with your arms extended over your head, both knees bent.
Use your abdominal muscles and *not* momentum as you move.

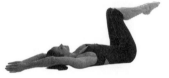

2

Lift both arms. Timing: 3 seconds.

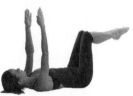

3

Straighten your legs at a 45° angle off the floor. Timing: 3 seconds.

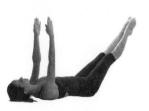

4

Lower your arms to the floor behind your head. Timing: 3 seconds.

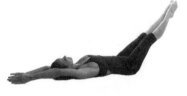

5

Bend your knees again. Timing: 3 seconds. Timing per sequence: 12 to 15 seconds. Repeat eight times.

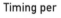

CATEGORY 12:
FLOOR STRETCHING

BUTTERFLY WITH PNF FOR HIP STRETCH—FLOOR

JOINTS: hips, knees, shoulders, spine.

MUSCLES: hip adductors, gluteus group, quadriceps, hip flexors, erector spinae, latissimus dorsi, triceps, biceps, deltoids, rhomboids, pectorals, trapezius.

These sequences use the stretching technique of PNF, known as "contract—relax—relax more—stretch."

1

Sit with your knees bent and feet together. Bend forward while resting your elbows on your knees.

2

Using your inner thigh muscles, try to bring your knees together while simultaneously forcing your knees open with your elbows. Hold for 6 to 8 seconds.

3

Completely relax your groin and hips while bending forward,

using your elbows to open your knees farther. Timing: 8 to 10 seconds. Total timing for the sequence: 15 to 20 seconds. Repeat two or three times.

4

Hip Blast: Use the full strength of your arms to squeeze your bent knees together while simultaneously trying to open them with the strength of your hips. Hold for 6 to 8 seconds.

5

Completely relax your groin and hips while bending forward, using your elbows to open your knees farther. Timing: 8 to 10 seconds. Total timing for the sequence: 15 to 20 seconds. Repeat two or three times.

BUTTERFLY WITH DEEP HIP AND SPINE STRETCH—FLOOR

JOINTS: hips, knees, shoulders, spine.

Ball and socket.

Hinge.

MUSCLES: hip adductors, gluteus group, quadriceps, hip flexors, latissimus dorsi, erector spinae, quadratus lumborum, trapezius, rhomboids, triceps, biceps, deltoids, pectorals.

Hip hinge.　　　Straight spine.　　　Spine leaning forward.

1

Sit with your spine straight and hold your shins. Sit on one or more risers if necessary.

2

Hold on to your shins and roll your spine backward. Timing: 10 seconds.

3

Reverse your position, bending as far forward as possible, still holding your shins. Place your elbows on your knees and press down to stretch your hips. Timing: 10 seconds.

4

Hold one shin with both hands. Pull away from your knee, rounding your back. Repeat on the other side. Timing: 5 seconds for each direction.

5

Place both hands on the floor in front of you and reach as far forward as possible. Timing: 5 seconds.

6

Walk your hands as far as you can to one side and then to the other to deeply stretch your glutes. Timing: 5 seconds for each direction. Time for the full sequence: 45 seconds.

SEATED HAMSTRING AND GLUTE STRETCH—FLOOR

JOINTS: hips, knees, spine, shoulders.

Ball and socket.

Hinge.

MUSCLES: hamstrings, gluteus group, soleus, gastrocnemius, quadratus lumborum, erector spinae, latissimus dorsi, obliques, rhomboids, trapezius, pectorals, deltoids, biceps, triceps.

Hip hinge.

Knees bent.

Upper body rotation.

Elbows bent.

Neck rotation left and right.

1

Sit on the floor with your legs extended. If your back or hamstrings are tight, sit on one or more risers.

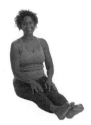

2

Bend one knee and flex your foot. Grab the flexed foot, pulling your knee closer to your chest. You can use a TheraBand or other resistance band to reach your foot if necessary. Timing: 5 seconds.

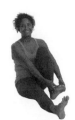

3

Hold for 5 to 7 seconds to feel the hamstring stretch.

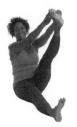

4

Bend your leg.

5

Cross the foot of your bent leg over your extended leg and place it flat on the floor. Embrace your knee with your opposite arm and pull it toward your chest. Timing: 5 to 7 seconds.

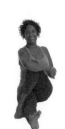

6

Rotate your spine toward the back, turning your head. Pull your spine upward and pull your knee closer to your chest. Total timing for the sequence: 20 to 25 seconds. Repeat on the other side.

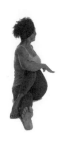

SEATED HIP STRETCH WITH SPINE ROTATION—FLOOR

JOINTS: spine, shoulders, hips, knees.

Ball and socket.

Hinge.

MUSCLES: abdominals, latissimus dorsi, erector spinae, quadratus lumborum, obliques, triceps, biceps, deltoids, rhomboids, pectorals, trapezius, gluteus group, hamstrings.

Hip hinge.

Knees bent.   Upper body rotation.

Spine side.   Spine curved.   Spine leaning back.

1

Sit on the floor with one leg extended to the front, foot pointed. Cross your other foot across your extended leg.

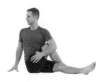

Keep your spine straight and embrace your knee with your opposite arm, pulling your knee toward your chest. Rotate your torso as much as possible toward the back of the room. Timing: 5 seconds.

2

Lift your back arm over your head and bend forward toward the front. Timing: 5 seconds.

3

Pull your bent knee toward your chest with both hands and straighten your spine. Timing: 5 seconds.

4

Hold on to your knee and round your spine, placing your forehead on your knee. Timing: 5 seconds.

5

Straighten your spine and, still holding your knee, stretch your neck, pulling your face toward the ceiling. Timing: 5 seconds.

Total timing of the sequence: 25 seconds. Repeat with the other leg.

ROW THE BOAT WITH HAMSTRING AND SPINE STRETCH—FLOOR

JOINTS: hips, spine, shoulders, ankles.

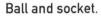

Ball and socket.   Saddle.

Plane.

MUSCLES: abdominals, hamstrings, gluteus group, latissimus dorsi, trapezius, deltoids, triceps, biceps, soleus, gastrocnemius, tibialis anterior and posterior.

Hip hinge.   Spine standing.

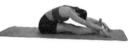

Bent elbows.   Spine leaning forward.

1

Sit on the floor with your legs extended, elbows bent and hands near your sides, preparing to row an imaginary boat. Modification: You can use one or more risers if your back is tight, or bend your knees if your hamstrings are tight.

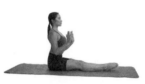

2

Slowly bend forward as if rowing a boat, pointing your feet.

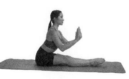

3

Timing: 5 seconds to reach maximum forward movement.

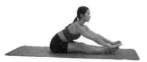

4

Relax the tension on your spine and in your arms and flex your feet. Timing: 3 seconds.

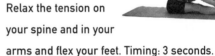

5

Bend your knees and round your back as you pull back the imaginary oars. Timing: 3 seconds.

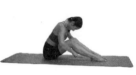

6

Return to your starting position with knees bent and feet flat on the floor. Timing: 3 seconds.

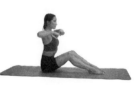

DEEP HIP FLEXOR STRETCH—FLOOR

JOINTS: hips, knees, spine, shoulders.

Saddle.

Ball and socket.

Hinge.

MUSCLES: abdominals, hip flexors, quadriceps, hamstrings, tibialis anterior and posterior, latissimus dorsi, triceps, biceps, deltoids, rhomboids, pectorals, trapezius, soleus, gastrocnemius.

Hip hinge.

Knees bent.

Ankle flexion and extension.

Bent elbows.

1

Sit with one knee bent in front and the other knee bent behind.

2

Grasp the foot of your back leg and pull your lower leg at a right angle to the floor. Try to keep your hips and torso facing forward. Gently move your leg up and down in this position. Timing: 5 to 8 seconds.

3

Very slowly pull your foot and heel toward your buttocks. This will stretch your quadriceps. Timing: 5 to 8 seconds. Repeat two times.

4

Twist your torso and hips toward the front and place the knee and toes of your flexed leg behind.

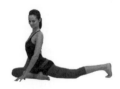

5

Straighten your back knee to lift it off the floor and stretch the psoas. Timing: 4 seconds. Straighten and lift your knee three times. Total timing: 14 to 20 seconds.

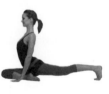

6

Point your toe while reaching

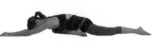

your arms forward and lying flat on the floor. Roll slowly from side to side to release all the tension in your psoas and back. Timing: 8 to 10 seconds. Total timing for the full sequence: 40 to 60 seconds. Repeat on the other side.

LONG ADDUCTOR STRETCH WITH FIGURE EIGHT—FLOOR

JOINTS: spine, shoulders, hips, knees, ankles.

Ball and socket.

Saddle.

Hinge.

Plane.

MUSCLES: abdominals, obliques, erector spinae, intercostals, latissimus dorsi, quadratus lumborum, trapezius, triceps, deltoids, rhomboids, pectorals, hip adductors, gluteus group, hamstrings, quadriceps, hip flexors, gracilis, sartorius, tibialis anterior and posterior, soleus, gastrocnemius.

Hip hinge. Knees bent. Hip hinge side.

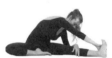

Shoulder arm rotation. Spine side bend. Spine leaning forward.

1

Sit with one leg extended to the side and the other leg bent in front. Raise the opposite arm to the extended leg. Make sure both hips are flat on the floor. Use one or more risers and a TheraBand or other resistance band if you need to.

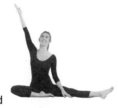

2

Look at the back of the room and reach toward it with your arm as you rotate your spine. Timing: 4 seconds.

3

Twist your arm in the socket and return your torso to the front while rounding your upper back. Timing: 4 seconds.

4

Sweep your arm toward your extended leg and try to grasp your foot. Timing: 6 seconds.

5

Let go of your foot and face sideways in a deep side bend. Timing: 4 seconds.

6

Cross your extended leg over your bent knee. Bend toward your legs, trying to place your hands as far forward as possible. Timing: 4 seconds. Total timing of the sequence: 22 seconds. Repeat on the opposite side.

CAT AND COW FOR SPINE FLEXIBILITY— FLOOR

JOINTS: spine, hips, knees, shoulders.

Ball and socket.

Hinge.

MUSCLES: abdominals, obliques, latissimus dorsi, erector spinae, quadratus lumborum, hip flexors, quadriceps, gluteus group, hamstrings, tibialis anterior, triceps, biceps, deltoids, rhomboids, pectorals, trapezius.

Hip hinge.   Spine leaning back.   Spine leaning forward.   Spine side bend.

1

Get down on your hands and knees, placing your hands directly below your shoulders. Timing: 3 seconds.

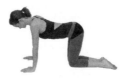

2

Arch your spine to stretch your chest and lift your tailbone. Timing: 3 to 6 seconds. Repeat two times.

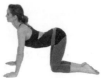

3

Round your spine as much as possible. Drop your head and tailbone and hold for 5 seconds.

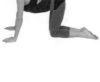

4

Try to sit on your heels, stretching your arms in front. Note: Many people have tight muscles and cannot straighten the joint between their shin and foot. That's common. Go as low as you can and hold for 5 to 8 seconds.

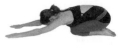

5

Walk your hands around your lower legs to embrace one side of your thighs and then the other.

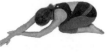

6

Walk your hands around your lower legs to embrace the right side of your knees and then the left to stretch your back, hips, and neck. Total timing for the sequence: 25 seconds.

ADVANCED SHIN STRETCH—FLOOR

JOINTS: hips, knees, spine, shoulders.

Ball and socket.

Hinge.

MUSCLES: abdominals, quadriceps, hamstrings, gluteus group, tibialis anterior, latissimus dorsi, erector spinae, quadratus lumborum, trapezius, rhomboids, pectorals.

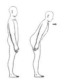

Hip hinge.   Spine leaning forward.   Spine leaning back.

1

Kneel with your torso folded forward, your head hanging toward your knees, and your hands holding your heels. Point your toes and use your hips to gently push your heels toward the floor. Timing: 5 to 10 seconds.

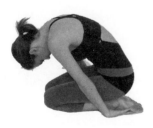

2

Slowly arch your spine to increase the pressure on your heels and create an even greater stretch of your shins. Don't force it to the point of pain. Timing: 5 to 10 seconds.

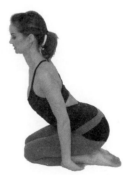

BABY STRETCH WITH DEEP HIP RELEASE—FLOOR

JOINTS: hips, knees.

Ball and socket.

Hinge.

MUSCLES: gluteus group, erector spinae, quadratus lumborum, sartorius, hip adductors.

Hip hinge.

Knees bent.

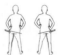

Hips: left, right.

Hip hinge side.

1

Lie on the floor and bend both knees. Raise one leg and place your foot on the opposite knee.

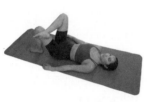

2

Hold the opposite shins with your hands or a TheraBand or other resistance band. Pull your knees as close to your chest as possible, lifting your buttocks off the floor. Twist slowly from side to side, then very slowly rock from side to side. Timing: 30 seconds.

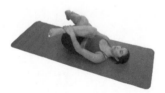

3

Replace your foot on the floor and pull your bent knee across your body, trying to place your big toe on the floor. Timing: 5 seconds.

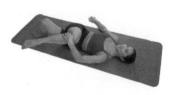

4

Keep your bent knee open to stretch your inner leg. Timing: 5 seconds. Total timing for the sequence: 40 seconds. Repeat the sequence twice, alternating legs each time. Total timing: 3 minutes.

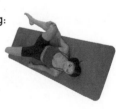

DEEP HAMSTRING, LONG ADDUCTOR, AND IT BAND STRETCH—FLOOR

JOINTS: spine, hips, ankles.

Ball and socket.

Hinge.

Plane.

MUSCLES: erector spinae, hamstrings, hip adductors, gluteus group, quadriceps, hip flexors, tibialis anterior and posterior, soleus, gastrocnemius.

Hip hinge.

Ankle flexion and extension.

Hip hinge side.

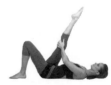

Knees bent.

1

Lie on the floor, arms resting at your sides. Bend one knee and place your foot flat on the floor while extending the other leg straight up. Rotate the extended leg within your hip joint outward and then inward. Timing: 3 to 5 seconds per rotation. Repeat four times.

2

Pull your extended leg toward the floor with your opposite hand. Use a TheraBand or other resistance band if you can't reach your leg. This will stretch your IT band. Timing: 6 to 8 seconds.

3

Change hands and open your leg sideways. Timing: 6 to 8 seconds.

4

Bend your knee and pull it toward your chest. Shake or wiggle your hips to totally relax your hip muscles. Timing: 6 to 8 seconds.

5

Point your toes and straighten your knee while carefully pulling your leg toward your chest. Timing: 6 to 8 seconds.

6

Flex your foot and pull your leg closer to your chest. Timing: 3 to 5 seconds. Repeat the sequence three times, then change legs and repeat four times. Total timing per side: 90 seconds.

ARCHING THE BACK STRETCHES—FLOOR

JOINTS: spine, shoulders, hips, knees.

Ball and socket.

Hinge.

MUSCLES: abdominals, erector spinae, latissimus dorsi, obliques, triceps, biceps, deltoids, rhomboids, pectorals, trapezius, quadriceps, hip flexors, tibialis anterior.

Straight spine.

Spine leaning back.

1

Lie facedown, bend your elbows, and place your hands close to your shoulders.

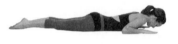

2

Without letting your shoulders lift, push away from the floor with your hands.

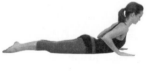

Stretch your spine, trying to roll up one vertebra at a time. Keep your neck straight. Timing: 8 seconds.

3

Try to lift your back higher, keeping your shoulders

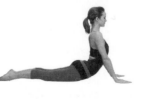

down. Continue stretching your spine, trying to roll up one vertebra at a time. Timing: 6 seconds.

4

Roll back down your spine one

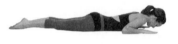

vertebra at a time, stretching it as you roll. When you're lying flat again, relax your muscles and wiggle your spine and hips. Timing: 15 seconds.

5

Incorrect. Don't sink into your shoulders.

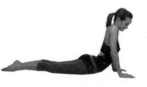

6

Incorrect. Don't sink into your shoulders or arch your neck.

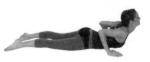

CHAPTER 9
Essentrics Routines for Every Day

Because the human body is constantly changing and adapting to everyday demands, achieving a balanced body is not a static outcome but rather a dynamic state. Just as our blood sugar levels are constantly changing throughout the day, so is the state of our muscles, joints, and tissues. To find balance in a constant state of change, we must be realistic with the demands we place on our body and do exercises that help our body adapt to our needs.

The best way to practice Essentrics routines is to start in a relaxed mode. As you get to know the exercises, and as your body becomes comfortable with them, you can put more effort and depth into the movements. Listen to your body; it will tell you when you're pushing it too hard or too far. Never push through pain! Keep moving but stay right on the edge of where pain kicks in.

This chapter offers you over sixty different routines for everyday life, sports, conditioning, and healing, as well as a warm-up routine. These routines have been carefully curated by myself and a team of master Essentrics teachers. Collectively, we have decades of experience, and we know these routines work.

We give a suggested length of time for each workout, but you should adjust it to your fitness level, physical needs, and time constraints. You may find yourself taking more time than I've suggested; take as long as you want. Never force yourself, and stop when you want. If anything, move slower rather than faster through these sequences—slower movements are safer, better at increasing strength, and better at improving flexibility.

For everyone—no matter what demands you place on your body throughout the day—integrating a rebalancing program as part of a daily routine will help you recover faster, keep you free from aches and pains, and allow you to move with strength and ease. Just as a nourishing diet and good dental care are important factors for long-term health, so is a regular program of rebalancing range-of-motion exercises.

MORNING ROUTINE

LENGTH: Twenty minutes

COMPONENTS: Standing, chair (optional)

EQUIPMENT: Mat, chair (optional)

Begin with two to four minutes of the Warm-Up Routine.

1. Zombie, page 78.

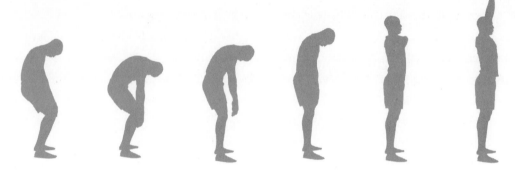

2. Embrace Yourself with Ceiling Reaches, page 82.

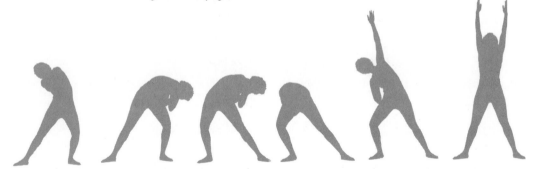

3. Triceps Stretch into Windmills, page 97.

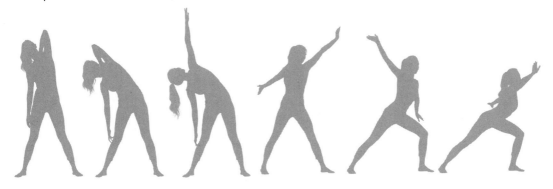

4. Double-Arm Shoulder Rotations, page 131.

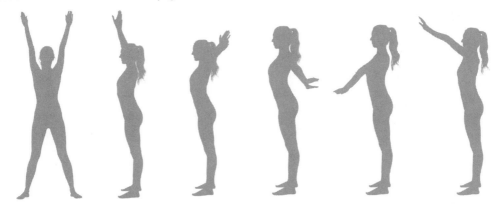

5. Pliés with Deep Side Bends, page 125.

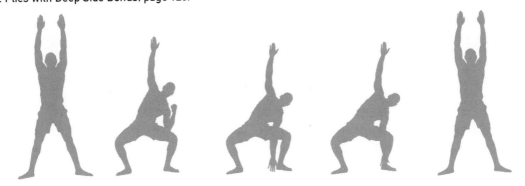

6. Musketeers Bow—IT Band and Long Adductor
Stretch, page 143.

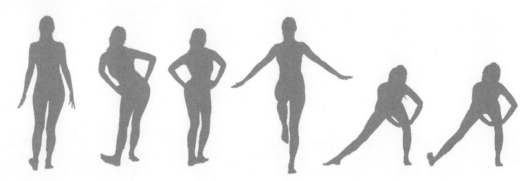

7. Standing Quad Stretch, page 142.

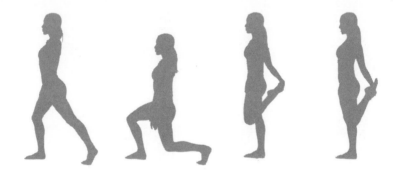

EVENING ROUTINE

LENGTH: Twenty minutes

COMPONENTS: Standing, floor

EQUIPMENT: Mat, riser, TheraBand or other resistance band, cushion

Begin with two to four minutes of the Warm-Up Routine.

1. Zombie, page 78.

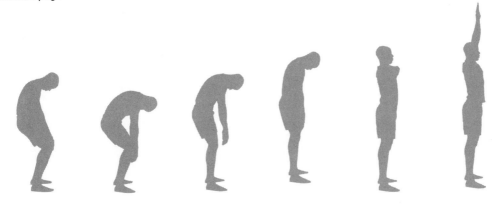

2. Diagonal Presses at Various Heights, page 93.

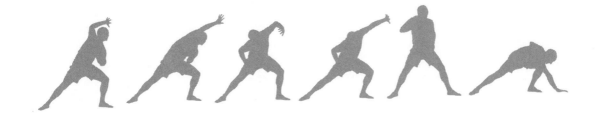

3. Washing a Small Round Table, page 89.

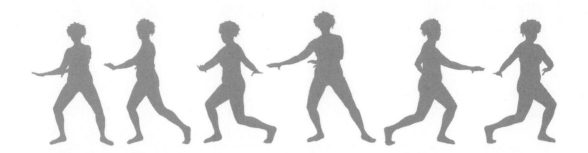

4. Lullaby and Lower a Blanket, page 80.

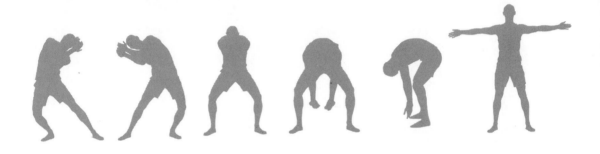

5. Hands, Fingers, and Wrists Mobility Sequence #1, page 129.

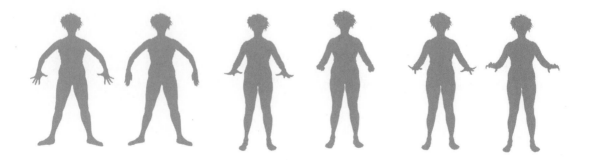

6. Butterfly with PNF for Hip Stretch—Floor,
page 173.

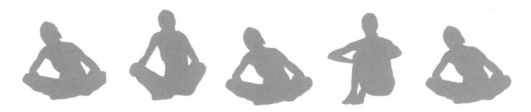

7. Long Adductor Stretch with Figure Eight—Floor,
page 179.

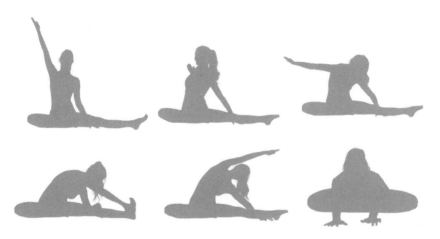

8. Row the Boat with Hamstring and Spine
Stretch—Floor, page 177.

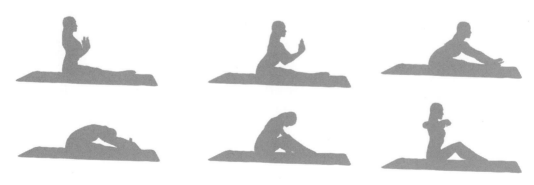

TRAVEL DAYS

LENGTH: Twenty minutes

COMPONENTS: Standing, chair

EQUIPMENT: Mat, chair

Begin with two to four minutes of the Warm-Up
Routine.

1. Double-Arm Figure Eights, page 119.

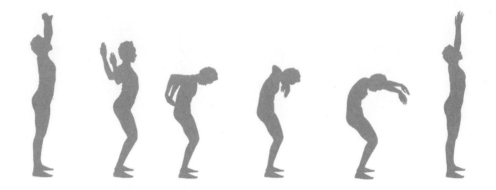

2. Ceiling Reach and Open Chest Swan, page 114.

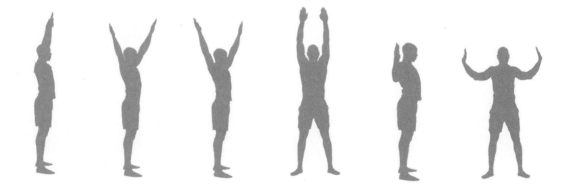

3. Windmill with Spine Flexion, page 96.

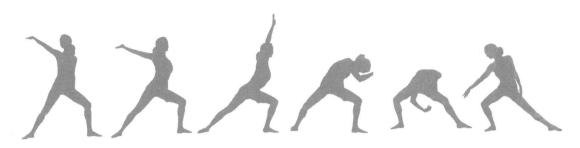

4. Fan Kicks with Lunges, page 139.

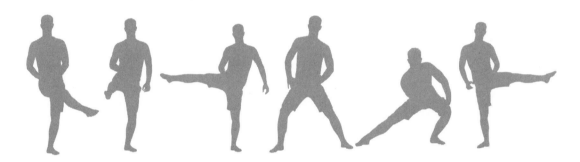

5. Hip Cleaners—Chair, page 150.

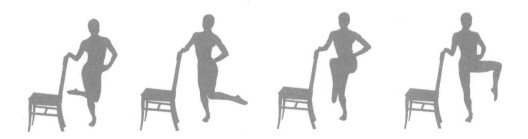

6. Four-Directional Hip Stretch—Chair, page 151.

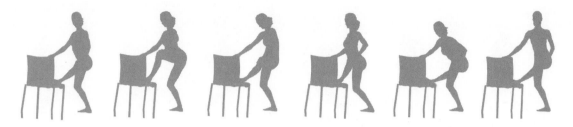

7. Preparation: Hip Flexor and Hamstring Stretch—Chair, page 152.

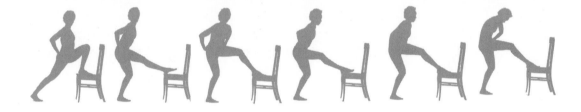

8. Hamstring and Spine Stretch—Chair, page 159.

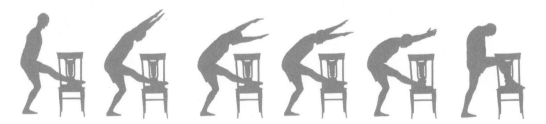

WALKING THE DOG

LENGTH: Fifteen minutes

COMPONENTS: Standing, chair

EQUIPMENT: Mat, chair

Begin with two to four minutes of the Warm-Up Routine.

1. Small Single-Arm Figure Eights, page 117.

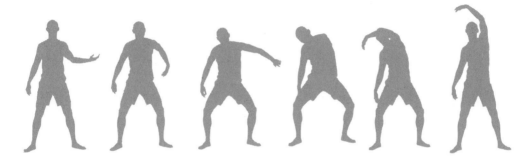

2. Sweeping behind Head into Cutting the Air, page 104.

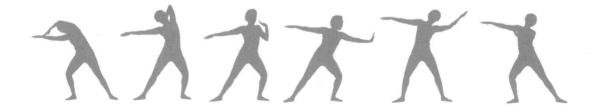

3. Hands, Fingers, and Wrists Mobility Sequence #2, page 130.

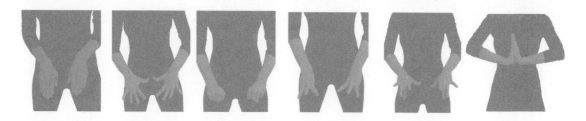

4. Squash Lunges, page 140.

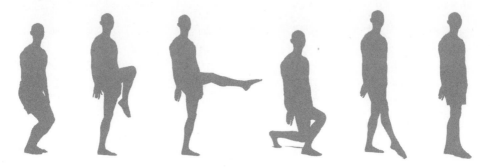

5. Calf Stretch Sequence, page 145.

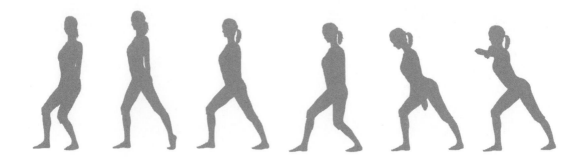

6. Hamstring Stretch—Chair, page 157.

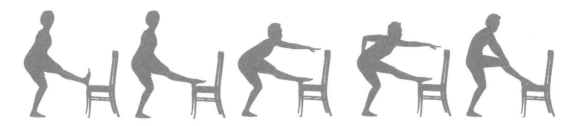

7. Hip Flexor and Hamstring Stretch—Chair,
page 156.

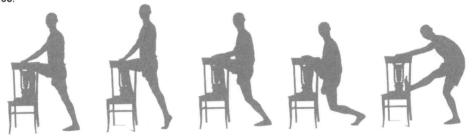

STRESS RELIEF

LENGTH: Twenty minutes

COMPONENTS: Standing, floor

EQUIPMENT: Mat, riser, TheraBand or other resistance band, cushion

Begin with two to four minutes of the Warm-Up Routine.

1. Zombie, page 78.

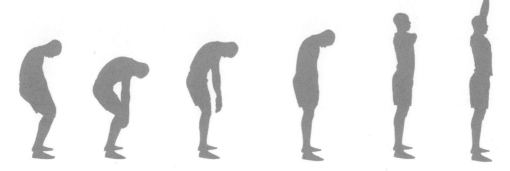

2. Small Single-Arm Figure Eights, page 117.

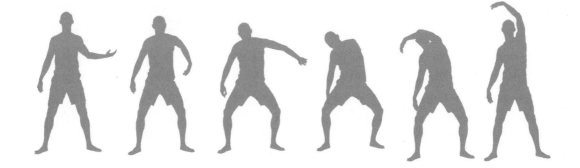

3. Shoulder Blast, page 83.

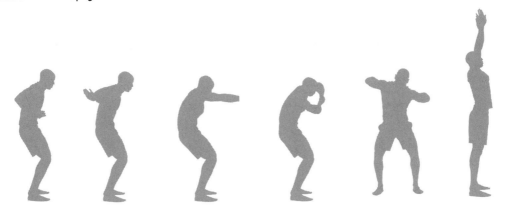

4. Washing a Small Round Table, page 89.

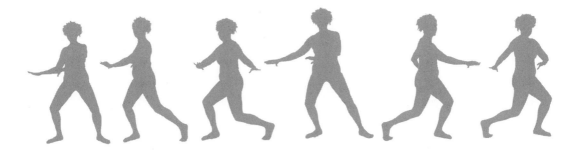

5. Butterfly with PNF for Hip Stretch—Floor, page 173.

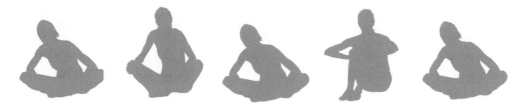

6. Cat and Cow for Spine Flexibility—Floor, page 180.

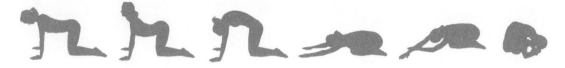

7. Deep Hamstring, Long Adductor, and IT Band
Stretch—Floor, page 183.

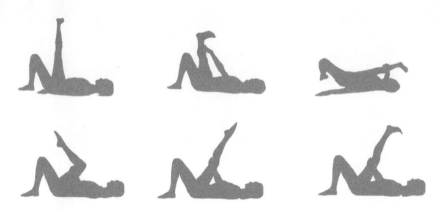

8. Baby Stretch with Deep Hip Release—Floor,
page 182.

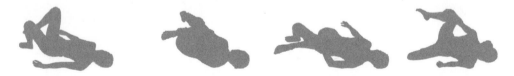

RELAXATION

LENGTH: Twenty minutes

COMPONENTS: Standing, chair

EQUIPMENT: Mat, chair

Begin with two to four minutes of the Warm-Up Routine.

1. Zombie, page 78.

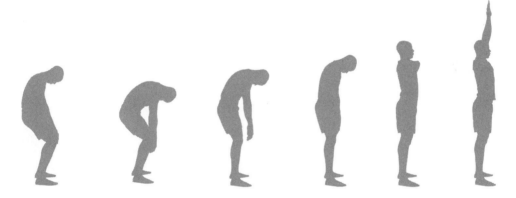

2. Ceiling Reach and Open Chest Swan, page 114.

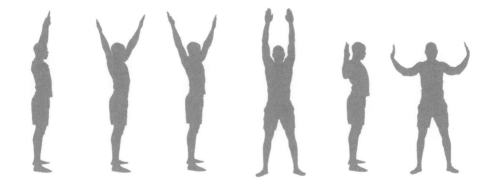

3. Remove a Sweater, page 115.

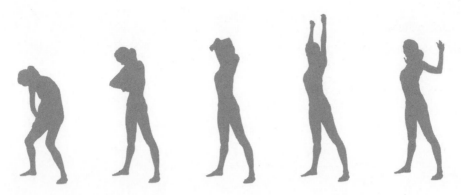

4. Sweeping behind Head into Cutting the Air, page 104.

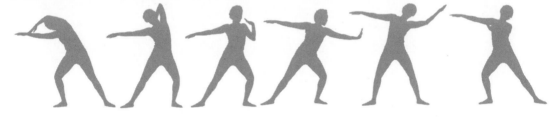

5. Diagonal Presses at Various Heights, page 93.

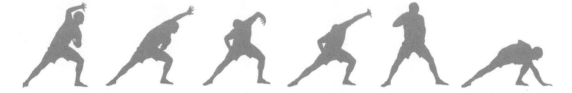

6. Hip Cleaners—Chair, page 150.

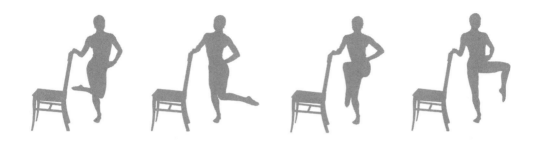

7. Spine Release—Chair, page 161.

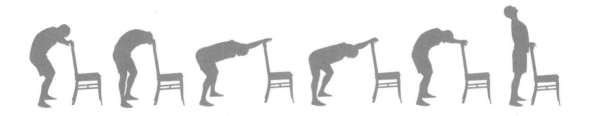

INCREASE YOUR ENERGY

LENGTH: Twenty-five minutes

COMPONENTS: Standing, chair

EQUIPMENT: Mat, chair

Begin with two to four minutes of the Warm-Up
Routine.

1. Zombie, page 78.

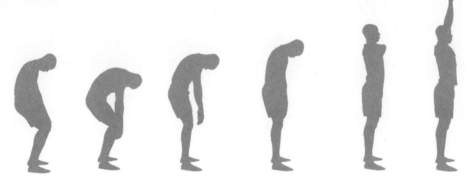

2. Arms Following the Circumference of a Beach
Ball—Ceiling to Floor, page 85.

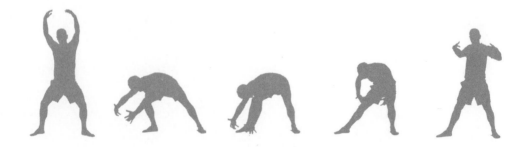

3. Deep Side Lunge Washes, page 106.

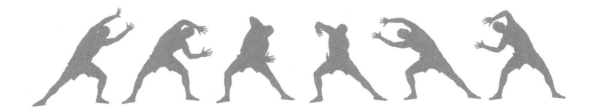

4. Pliés with Squeeze an Orange under Your Heel, page 122.

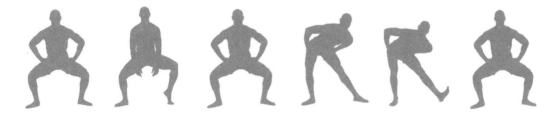

5. Squash Lunges, page 140.

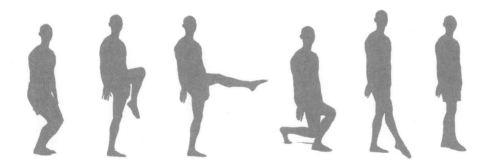

6. Karate Kicks to the Side—Chair, page 138.

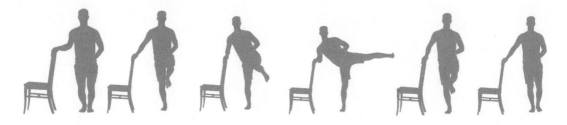

7. Shin Stretching and Strengthening—Chair, page 147.

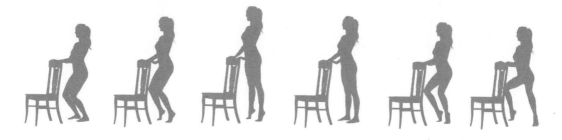

8. Calf Stretch Sequence, page 145.

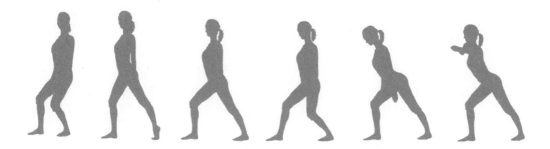

9. Musketeers Bow—IT Band and Long Adductor
Stretch, page 143.

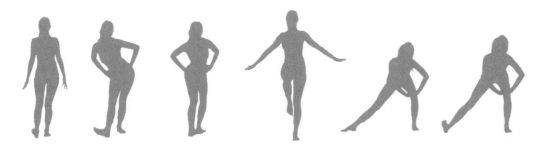

STIMULATE YOUR BRAIN

LENGTH: Twenty minutes

COMPONENTS: Standing

EQUIPMENT: Mat

Begin with two to four minutes of the Warm-Up
Routine.

1. Zombie, page 78.

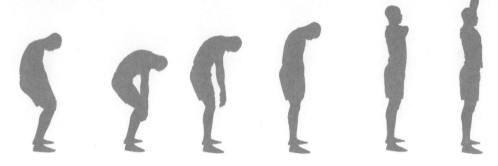

2. Waist Rotations, page 88.

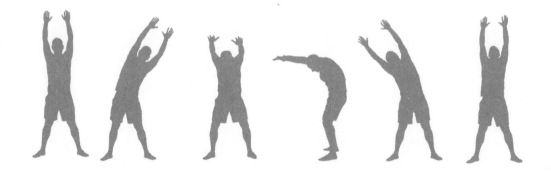

3. Push a Piano and Pull a Donkey, page 99.

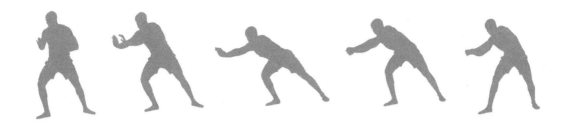

4. Washing a Small Round Table, page 89.

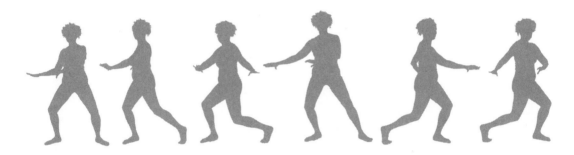

5. Ankle, Calf, and Shin Stretch, page 144.

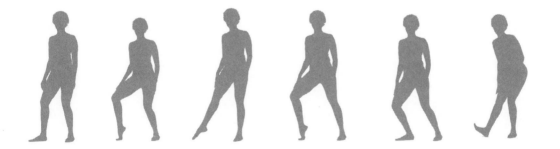

6. Hands, Fingers, and Wrists Mobility Sequence #1, page 129.

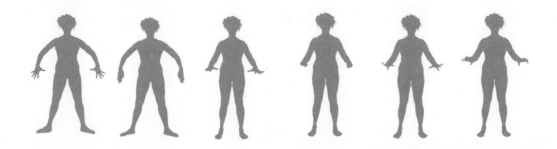

7. Fan Kicks with Lunges, page 139.

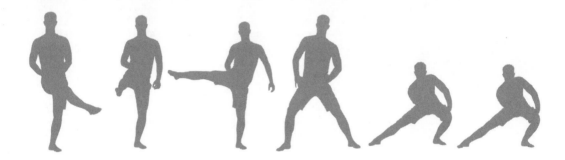

8. Calf Stretch Sequence, page 145.

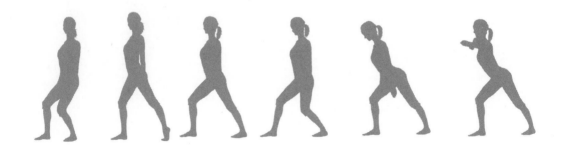

9. Musketeers Bow—IT Band and
Long Adductor Stretch, page 143.

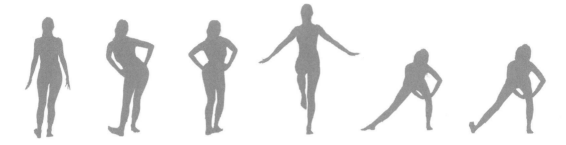

ROUTINE FOR KIDS

LENGTH: Twenty minutes

COMPONENTS: Standing, floor, chair

EQUIPMENT: Mat, chair

Begin with two to four minutes of the Warm-Up
Routine.

1. Zombie, page 78.

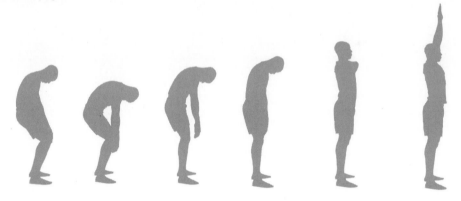

2. Embrace Yourself with Ceiling Reaches, page 82.

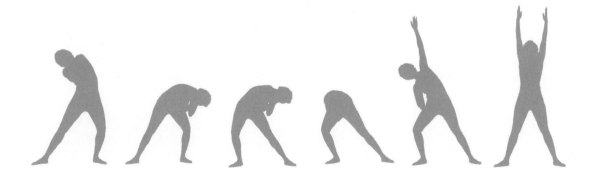

3. Single-Arm Sweeps into Celebration Arms,
page 102.

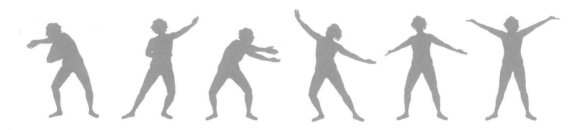

4. Single-Arm Pulling a Rope, page 92.

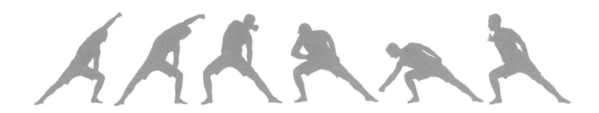

5. Pliés with Squeeze an Orange under Your Heel,
page 122.

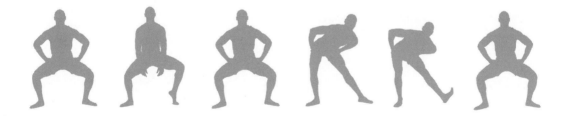

6. Karate Kicks to the Front—Chair, page 137.

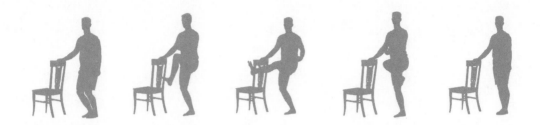

7. Karate Kicks to the Side—Chair, page 138.

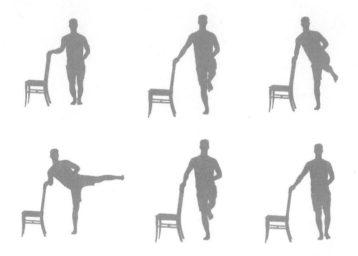

8. Superman Spine Strengthening—Floor, page 168.

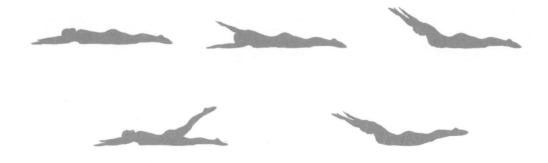

9. Cat and Cow for Spine Flexibility—Floor,
page 180.

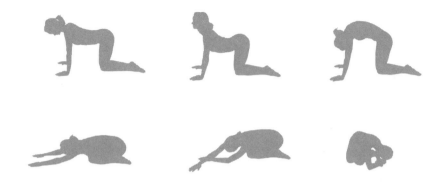

Essentrics Routines for Targeted Training

BEGINNER FLEXIBILITY (FLOOR)

LENGTH: Twenty minutes

COMPONENTS: Standing, floor

EQUIPMENT: Mat, riser, cushion

Begin with two to four minutes of the Warm-Up Routine.

1. Embrace Yourself with Single-Arm Extensions, page 81.

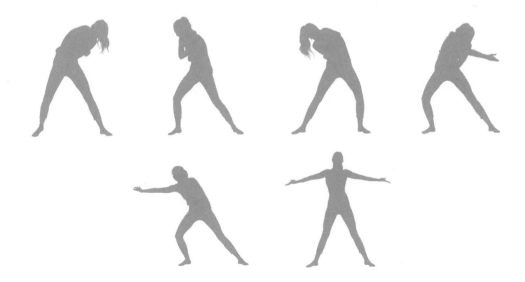

2. Waist Rotations, page 88.

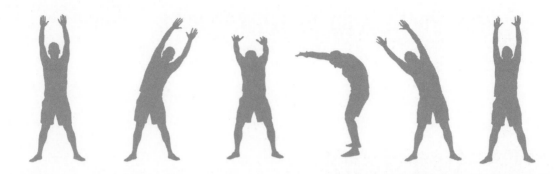

3. Double-Arm Figure Eights, page 119.

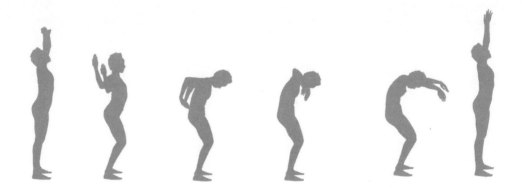

4. Pliés with Single-Arm Figure Eights, page 124.

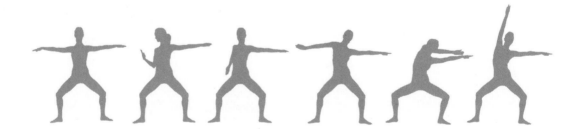

5. Hands, Fingers, and Wrists Mobility Sequence #2,
page 130.

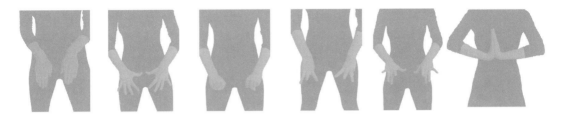

6. Ankle Mobility with Hip Rotation—Floor,
page 146.

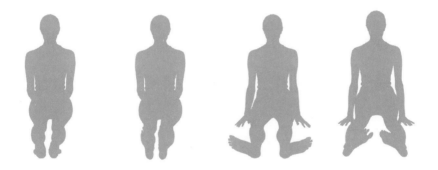

7. Butterfly with Deep Hip and Spine Stretch—Floor,
page 174.

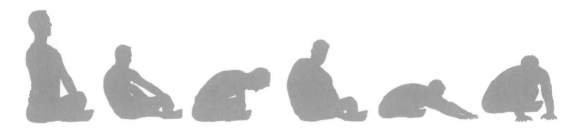

8. Row the Boat with Hamstring and Spine Stretch—
Floor, page 177.

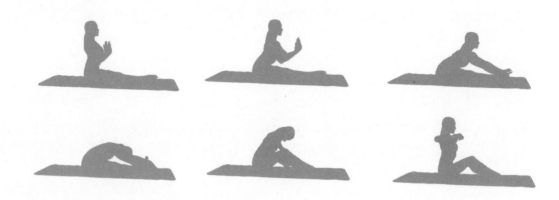

9. Seated Hip Stretch with Spine Rotation—Floor,
page 176.

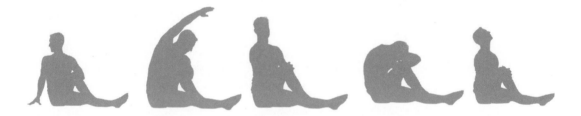

BEGINNER FLEXIBILITY (CHAIR)

LENGTH: Thirty minutes

COMPONENTS: Standing, chair

EQUIPMENT: Mat, chair

Begin with two to four minutes of the Warm-Up Routine.

1. Single-Arm Sweeps into Celebration Arms, page 102.

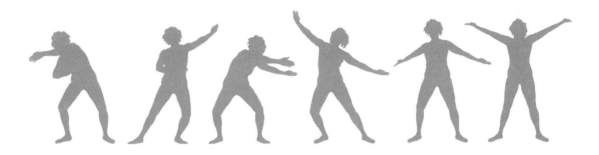

2. Ceiling Reach and Open Chest Swan, page 114.

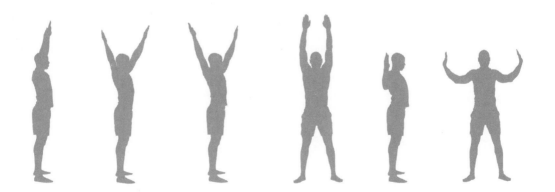

3. Sweeping behind Head into Cutting the Air,
page 104.

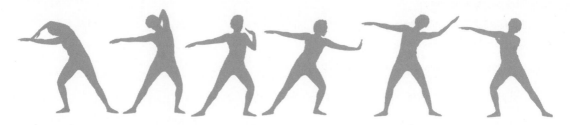

4. Deep Side Lunge Washes, page 106.

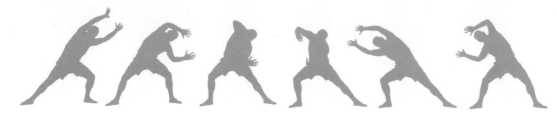

5. Preparation: Hip Flexor and Hamstring Stretch—
Chair, page 152.

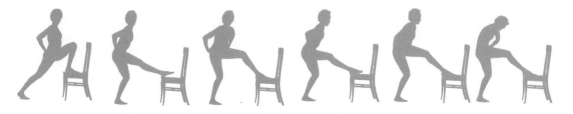

6. Hip Cleaners—Chair, page 150.

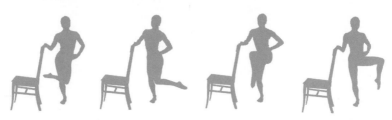

7. Four-Directional Hip Stretch—Chair, page 151.

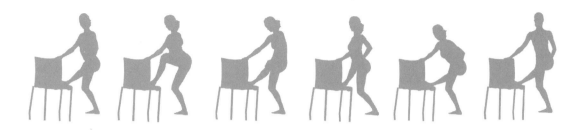

8. Inner and Outer Thigh Rotations: IT Band and
Long Adductor Stretch—Chair, page 153.

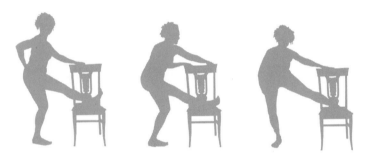

9. Deep Hamstring and Spine Stretch with
Release—Chair, page 154.

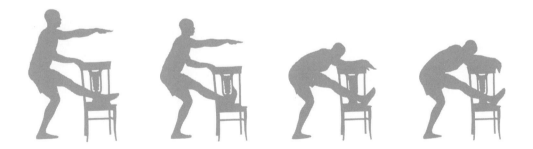

AGILITY

LENGTH: Thirty-five minutes

COMPONENTS: Standing, chair, floor

EQUIPMENT: Mat, riser, TheraBand or other resistance band, cushion, chair

Begin with two to four minutes of the Warm-Up Routine.

1. Washing Windows above the Shoulders, page 105.

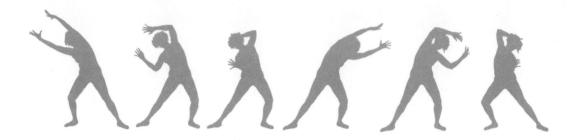

2. Large Single-Arm Figure Eights, page 118.

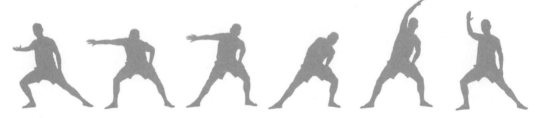

3. Embrace a Ball with Diagonal Movements, page 87.

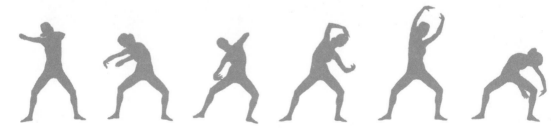

4. Shin Stretching and Strengthening—Chair,
page 147.

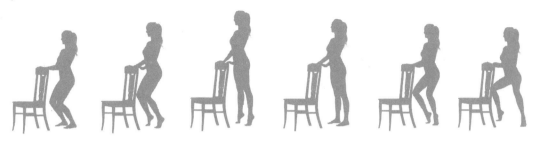

5. Calf Stretch Sequence, page 145.

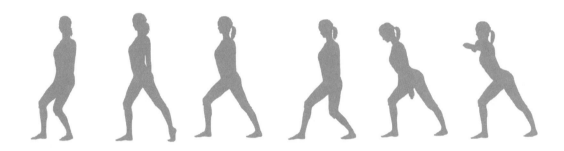

6. Butterfly with PNF for Hip Stretch—Floor,
page 173.

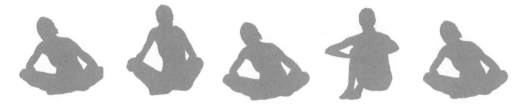

7. Deep Hip Flexor Stretch—Floor, page 178.

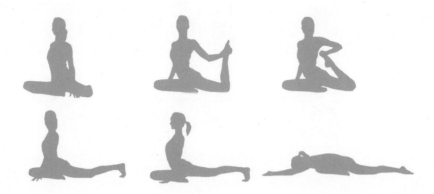

8. Long Adductor Stretch with Figure Eight—Floor, page 179.

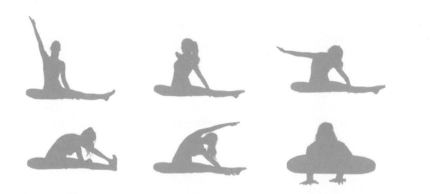

9. Deep Hamstring, Long Adductor, and IT Band Stretch—Floor, page 183.

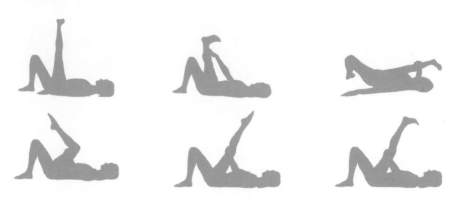

COOLDOWN OR RECOVERY

LENGTH: Twenty-five minutes

COMPONENTS: Standing, floor

EQUIPMENT: Mat, riser, cushion

Begin with two to four minutes of the Warm-Up Routine.

1. Zombie, page 78.

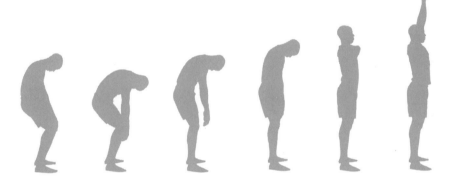

2. Ceiling Reach and Open Chest Swan, page 114.

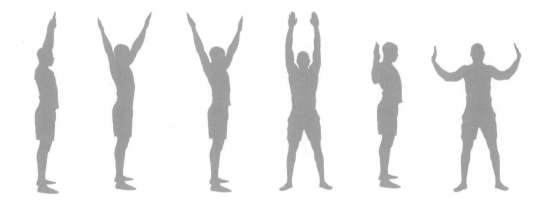

3. Windmill with Spine Flexion, page 96.

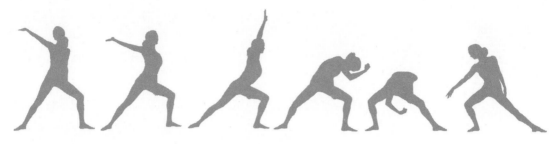

4. Calf Stretch Sequence, page 145.

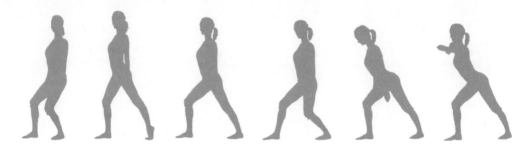

5. Musketeers Bow—IT Band and Long Adductor
Stretch, page 143.

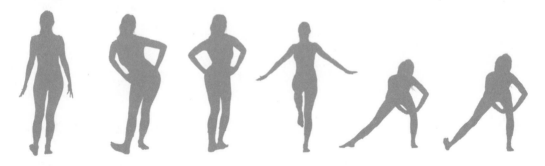

6. Butterfly with Deep Hip and Spine Stretch—
Floor, page 174.

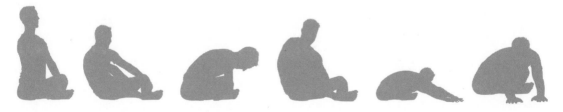

7. Deep Hip Flexor Stretch—Floor, page 178.

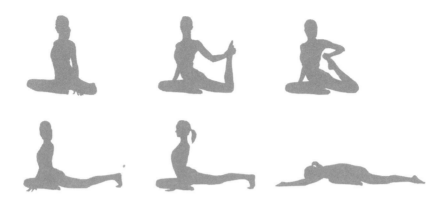

8. Long Adductor Stretch with Figure Eight—Floor,
page 179.

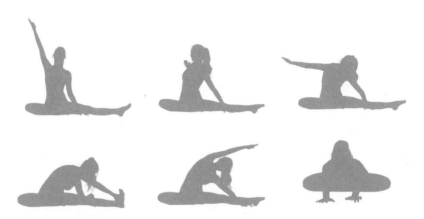

9. Baby Stretch with Deep Hip Release—Floor,
page 182.

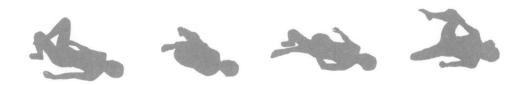

UPPER-BODY TONING

LENGTH: Thirty minutes

COMPONENTS: Standing, floor

EQUIPMENT: Mat, cushion

Begin with two to four minutes of the Warm-Up
Routine.

1. Shoulder Blast, page 83.

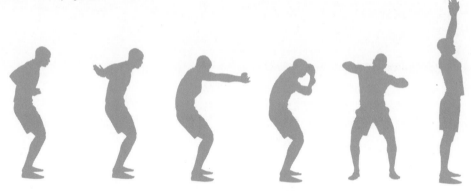

2. Single-Arm Pulling a Rope, page 92.

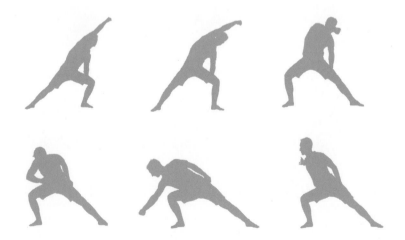

3. Double-Arm Half-Body Rotation, page 108.

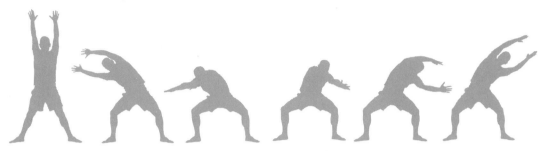

4. Advanced Clock Sequence, page 111.

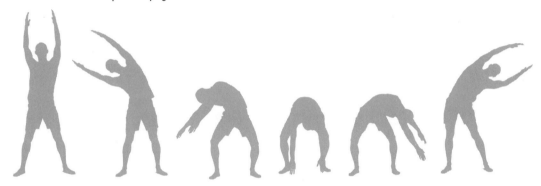

5. Lullaby and Lower a Blanket, page 80.

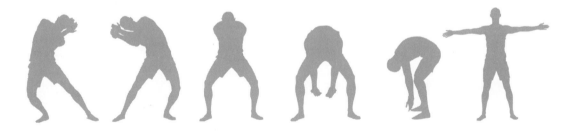

6. Arm Pumps for Posture, page 135.

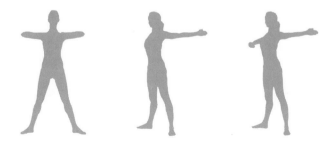

7. Slow Sit-Ups with Arm Variations—Floor,
page 169.

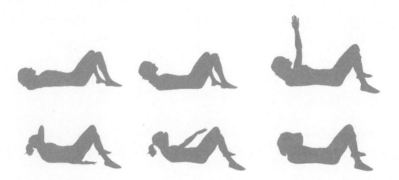

8. Advanced Sit-Ups with Extended Legs—
Floor, page 172.

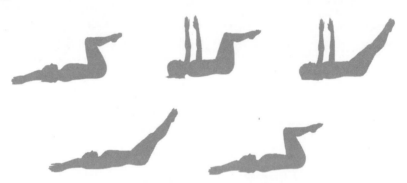

9. Superman Spine Strengthening—Floor, page 168.

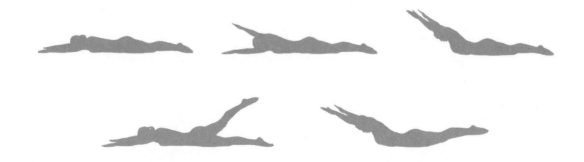

LOWER-BODY TONING

LENGTH: Thirty minutes

COMPONENTS: Standing, chair, floor

EQUIPMENT: Mat, chair, riser, cushion

Begin with two to four minutes of the Warm-Up Routine.

1. Arms Following the Circumference of a Beach Ball—Ceiling to Waist, page 84.

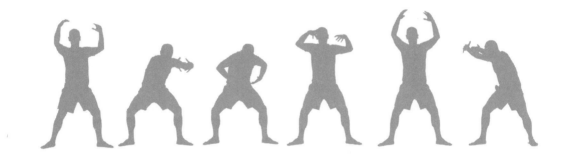

2. Deep Lunges Washing a Large Round Table, page 98.

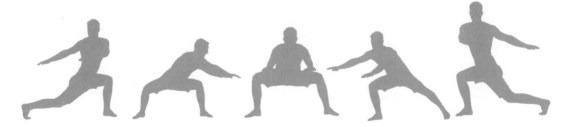

3. Pliés with Quadriceps Strengthening, page 121.

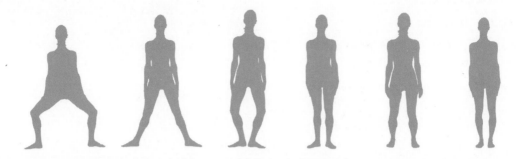

4. Low Rapid Kicks, page 136.

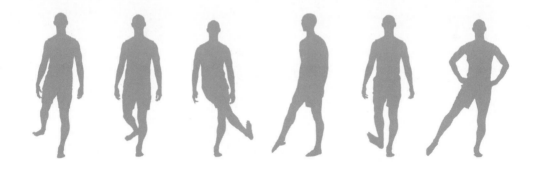

5. Advanced Ankle Strengthening—Chair, page 148.

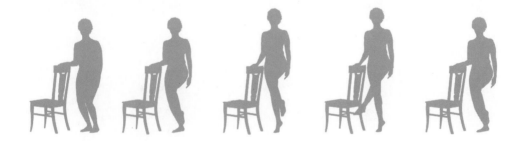

6. Karate Kicks to the Side—Chair, page 138.

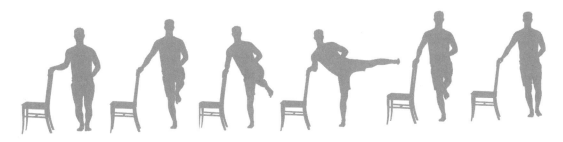

7. Butterfly with Deep Hip and Spine Stretch—
Floor, page 174.

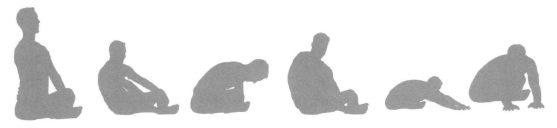

8. Abductor and Glutes Strengthening—Floor,
page 164.

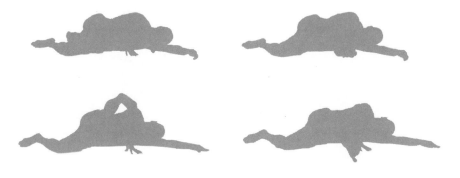

9. Strengthening Quad Raiser—Floor, page 163.

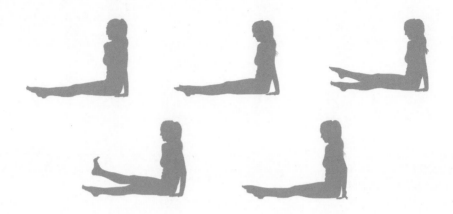

10. Baby Stretch with Deep Hip Release—Floor, page 182.

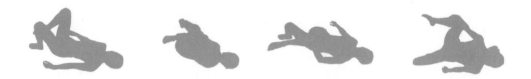

EXPLOSIVE POWER

LENGTH: Twenty-five minutes

COMPONENTS: Standing

EQUIPMENT: Mat

Begin with two to four minutes of the Warm-Up

Routine.

1. Remove a Sweater, page 115.

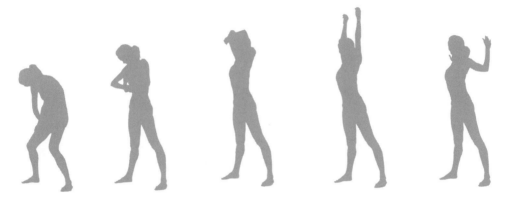

2. Washing a Small Round Table, page 89.

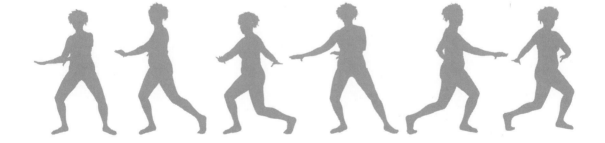

3. Ankle, Calf, and Shin Stretch, page 144.

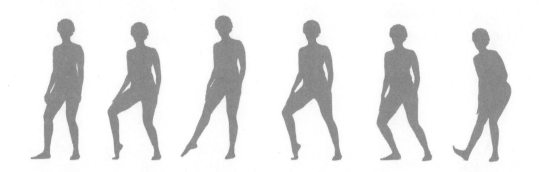

4. Pliés with Side-Bend Arm Reaches, page 128.

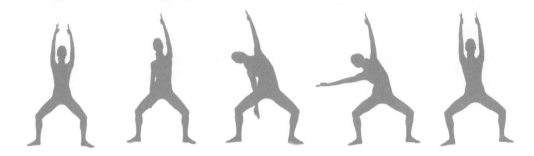

5. Low Rapid Kicks, page 136.

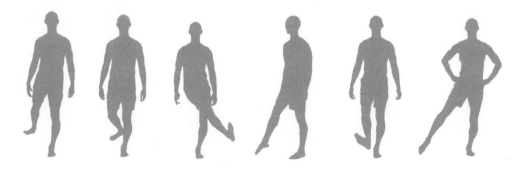

6. Triceps Stretch into Windmills, page 97.

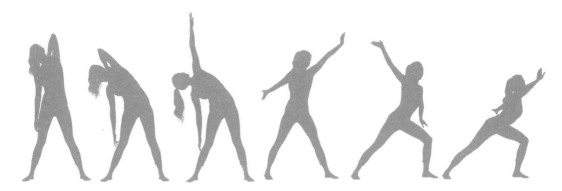

7. Fan Kicks with Lunges, page 139.

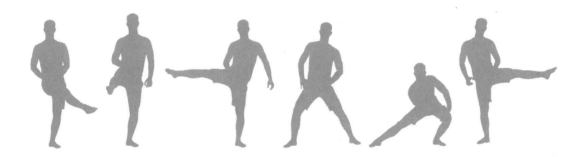

8. Deep Lunges Washing a Large Round Table, page 98.

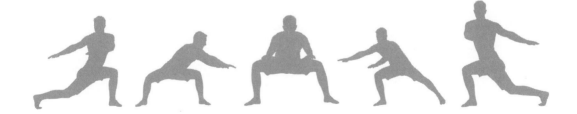

9. Double-Arm Pulling Ropes to the Floor, page 94.

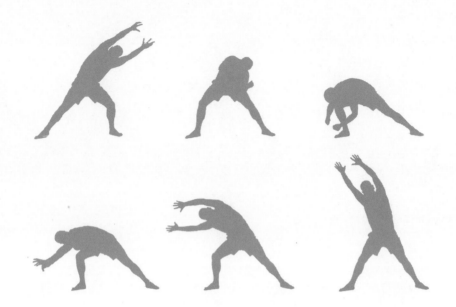

ROUTINE FOR SPEED

LENGTH: Thirty minutes

COMPONENTS: Standing, floor

EQUIPMENT: Mat, cushion, riser

Begin with two to four minutes of the Warm-Up

Routine.

1. Double-Arm Figure Eights, page 119.

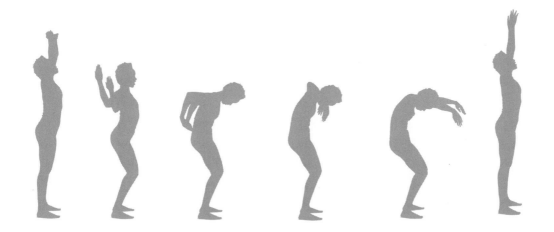

2. Large Single-Arm Figure Eights, page 118.

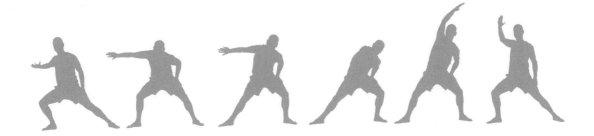

3. Pliés with Squeeze an Orange under Your Heel,
page 122.

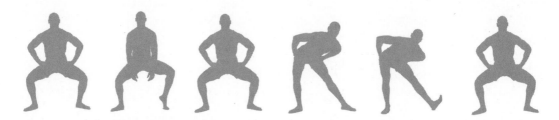

4. Arm Pumps for Shoulder Joint Liberation,
page 132.

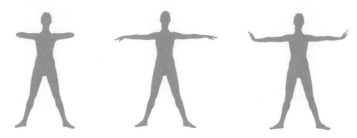

5. Squash Lunges, page 140.

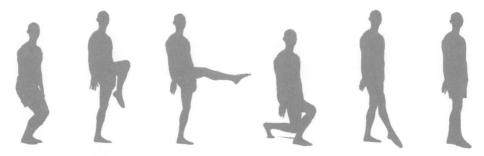

6. Calf Stretch Sequence, page 145.

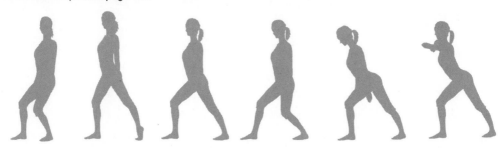

7. Abductor and Glutes Strengthening—Floor,
page 164.

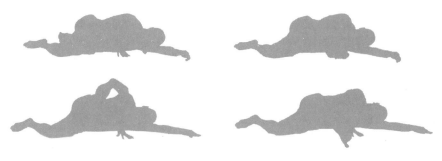

8. Sit-Ups with a Waist Twist—Floor, page 170.

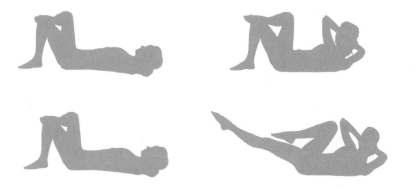

9. Advanced Trapeze Strengthening with Quad
Raisers—Floor, page 167.

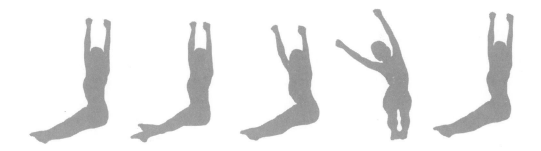

AGILITY

LENGTH: Thirty minutes

COMPONENTS: Standing, chair

EQUIPMENT: Mat, chair

Begin with two to four minutes of the Warm-Up Routine.

1. Deep Diagonal Reaches at Three Heights, page 95.

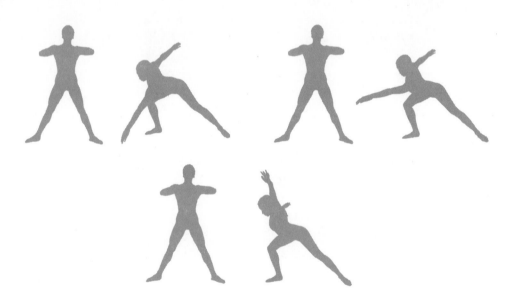

2. Lunge Hip Mobility Sequence, page 141.

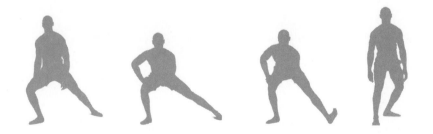

3. Pliés with Single-Arm Figure Eights, page 124.

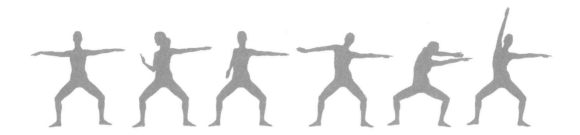

4. Fan Kicks with Lunges, page 139.

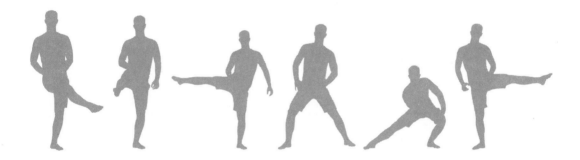

5. Squash Lunges, page 140.

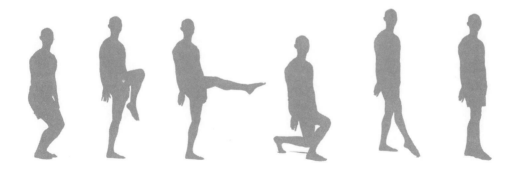

6. Bow and Arrow, page 103.

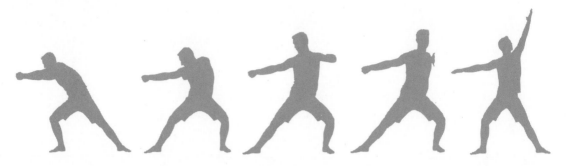

7. Shin Stretching and Strengthening—Chair, page 147.

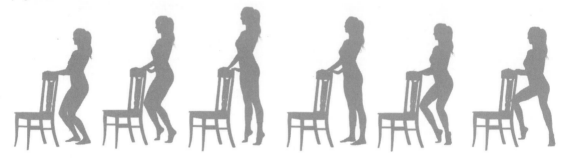

8. Karate Kicks to the Side—Chair, page 138.

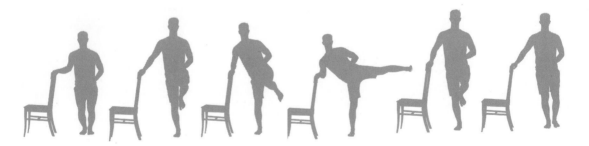

9. Hip Cleaners—Chair, page 150.

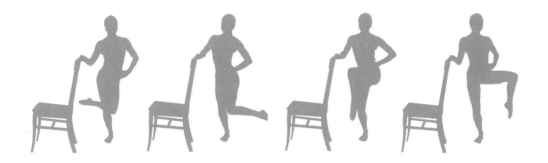

BALANCE

LENGTH: Thirty minutes

COMPONENTS: Standing

EQUIPMENT: Mat

Begin with two to four minutes of the Warm-Up
Routine.

1. Pliés with Deep Side Bends, page 125.

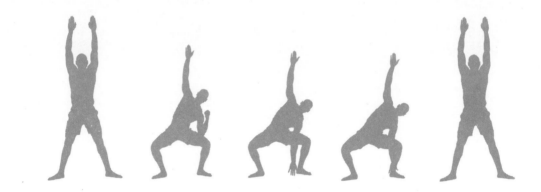

2. Calf Stretch Sequence, page 145.

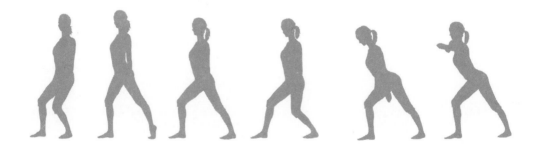

3. Low Rapid Kicks, page 136.

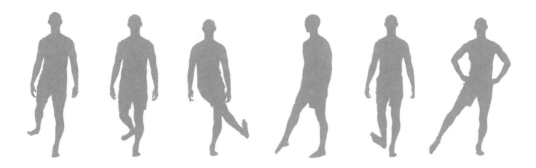

4. Fan Kicks with Lunges, page 139.

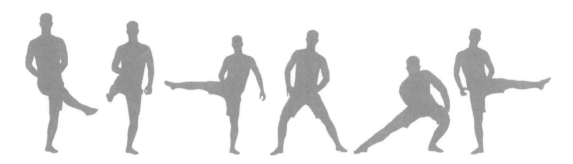

5. Large Full-Body Figure Eights with Rotation,
page 120.

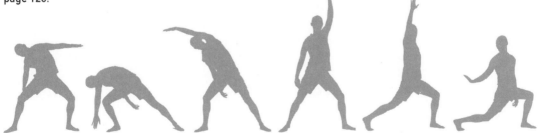

6. Triceps Stretch into Windmills, page 97.

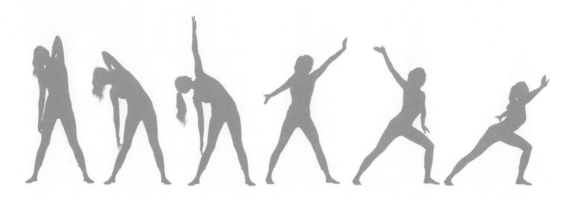

7. Deep Side Lunge Washes, page 106.

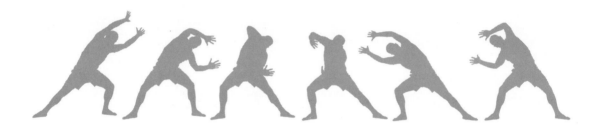

8. Ankle, Calf, and Shin Stretch, page 144.

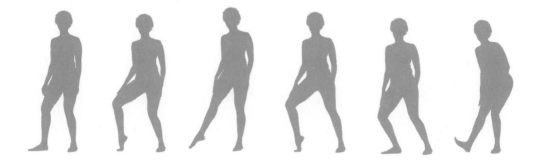

9. Calf Stretch Sequence for Balance, page 149.

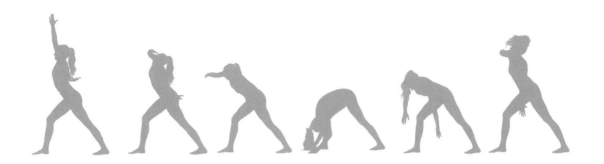

10. Musketeers Bow—IT Band and Long Adductor Stretch, page 143.

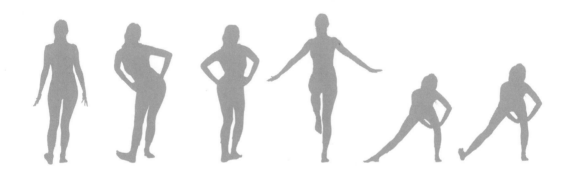

JUMPING HIGHER

LENGTH: Twenty minutes

COMPONENTS: Standing, chair

EQUIPMENT: Mat, chair

Begin with two to four minutes of the Warm-Up Routine.

1. Calf Stretch Sequence, page 145.

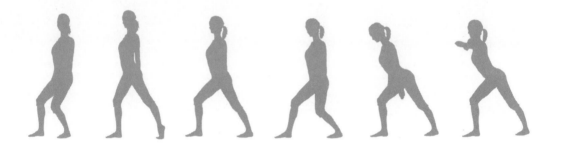

2. Pliés with Quadriceps Strengthening, page 121.

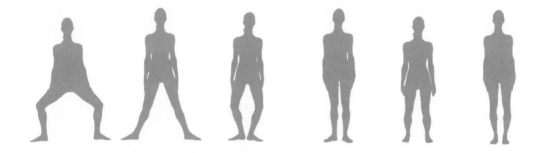

3. Lunge Hip Mobility Sequence, page 141.

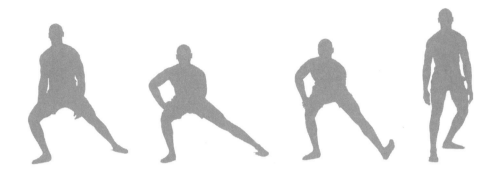

4. Pliés with Single-Arm Half-Body Rotation,
page 126.

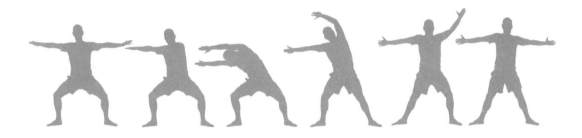

5. Shin Stretching and Strengthening—Chair,
page 147.

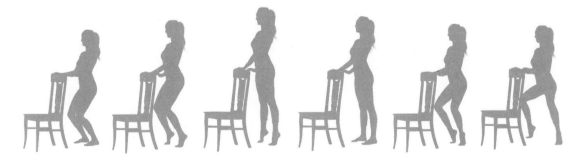

6. Four-Directional Hip Stretch—Chair, page 151.

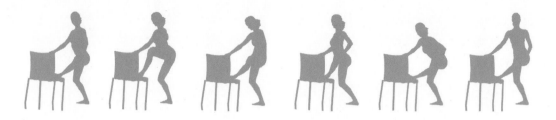

7. Hip Flexor and Hamstring Stretch—Chair, page 156.

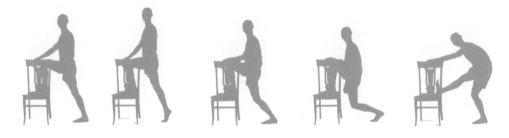

8. Hamstring and Spine Stretch—Chair, page 159.

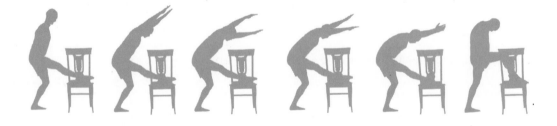

9. Inner and Outer Thigh Rotations: IT Band and Long Adductor Stretch—Chair, page 153.

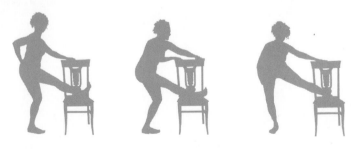

SPINE MOBILITY

LENGTH: Twenty-five minutes

COMPONENTS: Standing, floor

EQUIPMENT: Mat

Begin with two to four minutes of the Warm-Up
Routine.

1. Remove a Sweater, page 115.

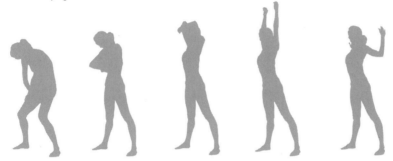

2. Fluid Spine, page 113.

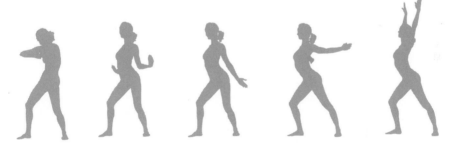

3. Washing a Small Round Table, page 89.

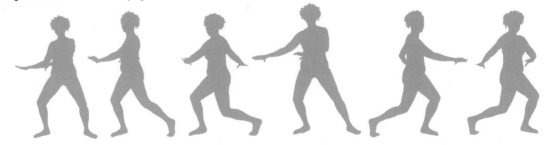

4. Sweeping behind Head into Cutting the Air,
page 104.

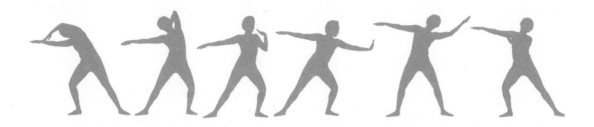

5. Pliés with Single-Arm Full-Body Rotation,
page 123.

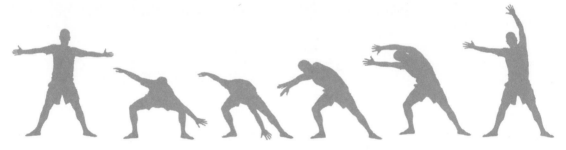

6. Embrace a Ball with Diagonal Movements,
page 87.

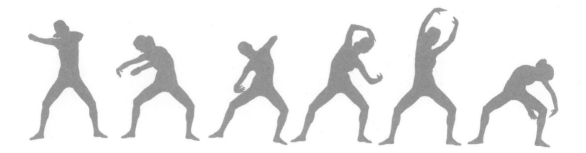

7. Superman Spine Strengthening—Floor, page 168.

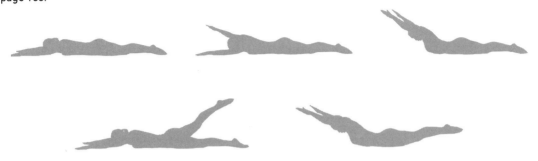

8. Arching the Back Stretches—Floor, page 184.

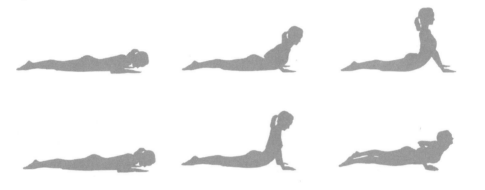

9. Cat and Cow for Spine Flexibility—Floor, page 180.

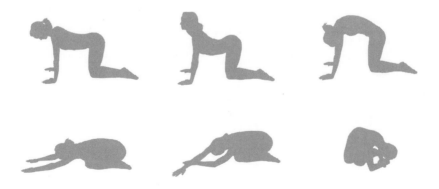

CHAPTER 11

Essentrics Routines for Sports

AMERICAN FOOTBALL

LENGTH: Twenty minutes

COMPONENTS: Standing, chair

EQUIPMENT: Mat, chair

Begin with two to four minutes of the Warm-Up
Routine.

1. Lift Imaginary Weights above Your Head,
page 116.

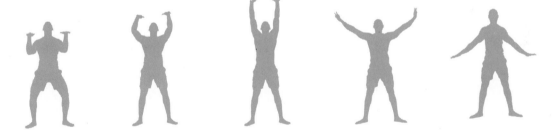

2. Simple Windmill—Feet Parallel, page 90.

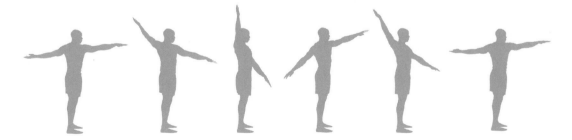

3. Pliés with Deep Side Bends, page 125.

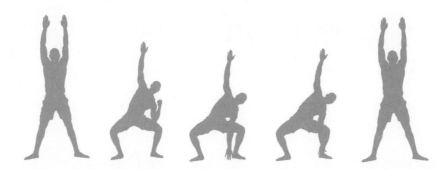

4. Deep Lunges Washing a Large Round Table,
page 98.

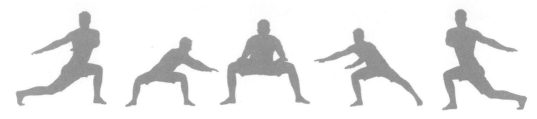

5. Squash Lunges, page 140.

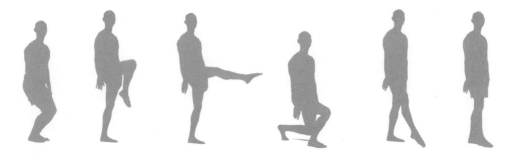

6. Calf Stretch Sequence, page 145.

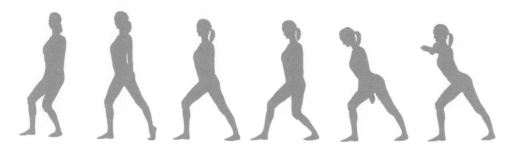

7. Hip Flexor and Hamstring Stretch—Chair, page 156.

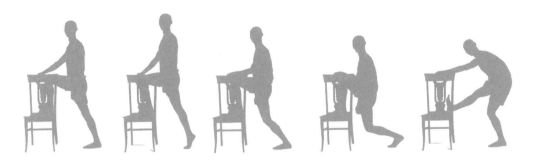

8. Deep Hamstring and Spine Stretch with Release—Chair, page 154.

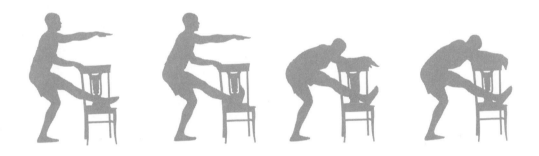

9. Inner and Outer Thigh Rotations: IT Band and Long Adductor Stretch—Chair, page 153.

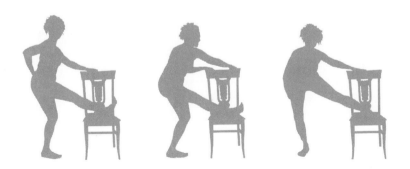

BALLET AND GYMNASTICS

LENGTH: Thirty minutes

COMPONENTS: Standing, floor, chair

EQUIPMENT: Mat, chair, TheraBand or other resistance band, cushion

Begin with two to four minutes of the Warm-Up Routine.

1 Pliés with Quadriceps Strengthening, page 121.

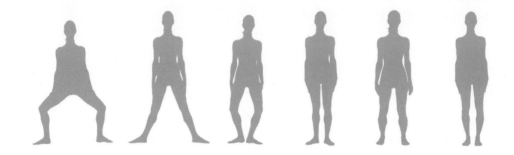

2. Shin Stretching and Strengthening—Chair, page 147.

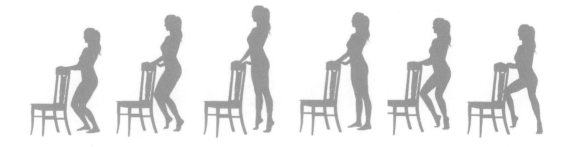

3. Calf Stretch Sequence, page 145.

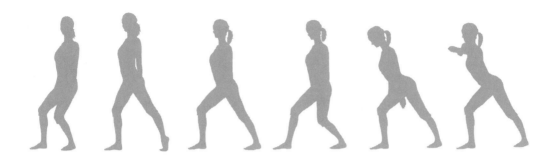

4. Large Full-Body Figure Eights with Rotation,
page 120.

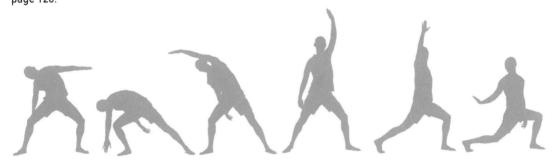

5. Arms Following the Circumference of a Beach
Ball—Ceiling to Floor, page 85.

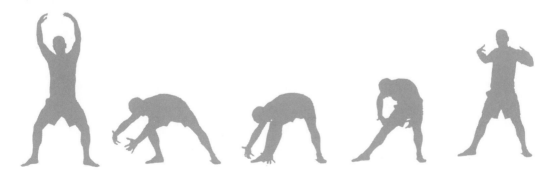

6. Advanced Clock Sequence, page 111.

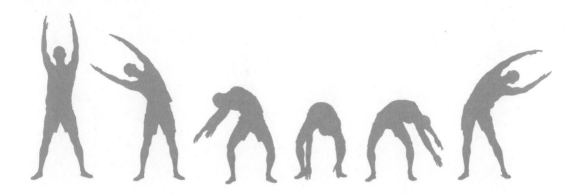

7. Butterfly with PNF for Hip Stretch—Floor,
page 173.

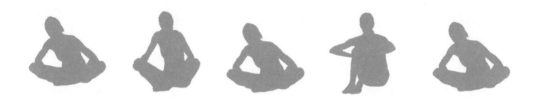

8. Deep Hip Flexor Stretch—Floor, page 178.

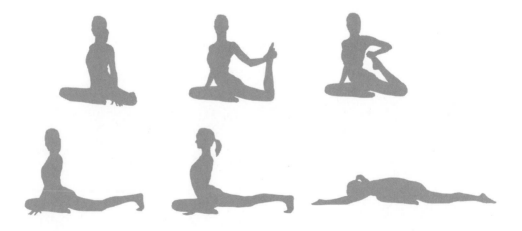

9. Deep Hamstring, Long Adductor, and IT Band
Stretch—Floor, page 183.

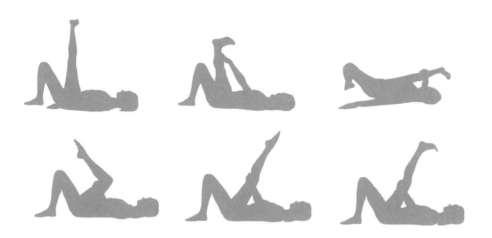

10. Superman Spine Strengthening—Floor,
page 168.

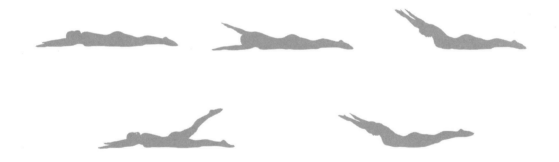

BASEBALL

LENGTH: Twenty minutes

COMPONENTS: Standing, chair

EQUIPMENT: Mat, chair

Begin with two to four minutes of the Warm-Up Routine.

1. Double-Arm Figure Eights, page 119.

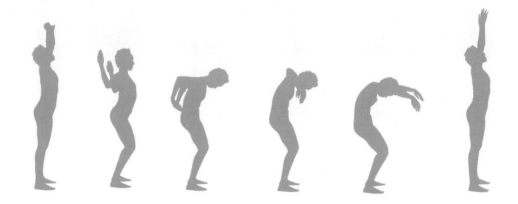

2. Large Full-Body Figure Eights with Rotation, page 120.

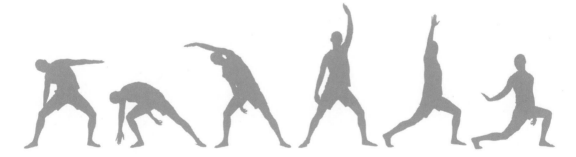

3. Shoulder Blast, page 83.

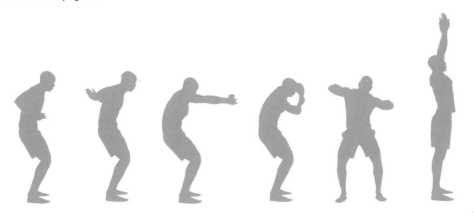

4. Fan Kicks with Lunges, page 139.

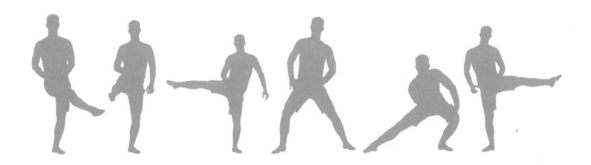

5. Arm Pumps for Pectoral Stretch, page 133.

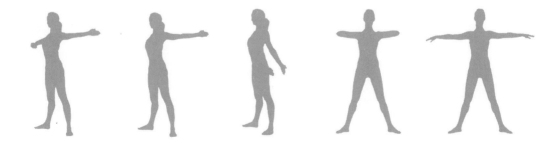

6. Calf Stretch Sequence, page 145.

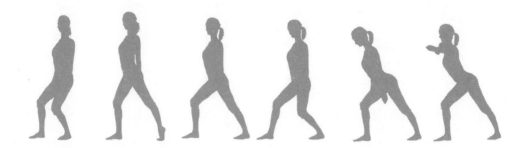

7. Four-Directional Hip Stretch—Chair, page 151.

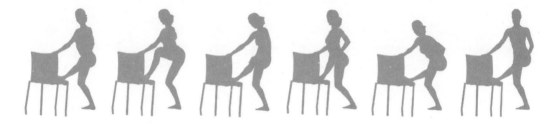

8. Preparation: Hip Flexor and Hamstring Stretch—
Chair, page 152.

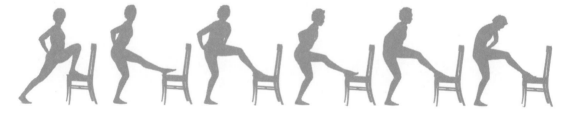

9. Inner and Outer Thigh Rotations: IT Band and
Long Adductor Stretch—Chair, page 153.

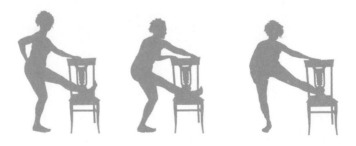

BASKETBALL

LENGTH: Twenty minutes

COMPONENTS: Standing, chair

EQUIPMENT: Mat, chair

Begin with two to four minutes of the Warm-Up Routine.

1. Shoulder Blast, page 83.

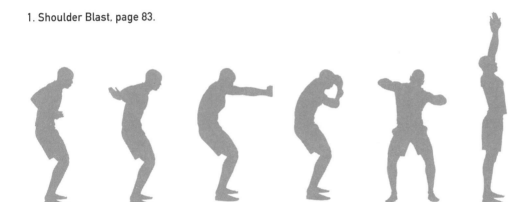

2. Hands, Fingers, and Wrists Mobility Sequence #2, page 130.

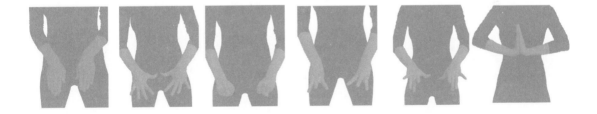

3. Diagonal Presses at Various Heights, page 93.

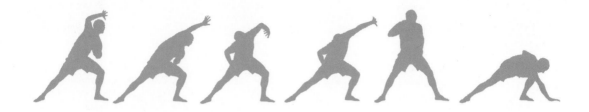

4. Pliés with Single-Arm Figure Eights, page 124.

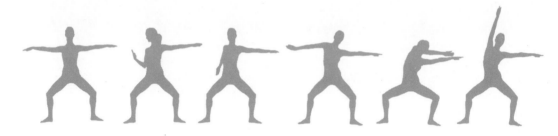

5. Ankle, Calf, and Shin Stretch, page 144.

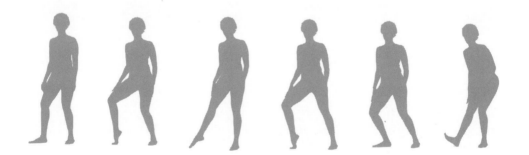

6. Calf Stretch Sequence for Balance, page 149.

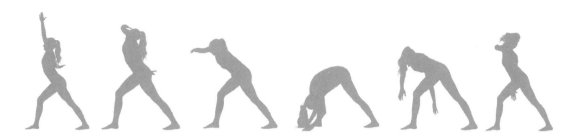

7. Hip Flexor and Hamstring Stretch—Chair, page 156.

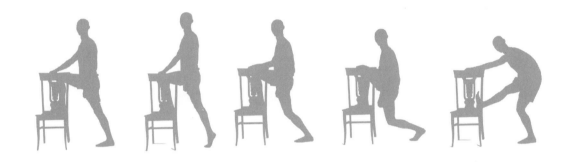

8. Deep Hamstring and Spine Stretch with Release—Chair, page 154.

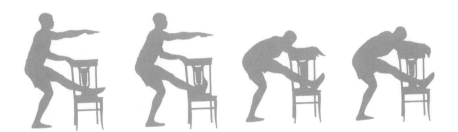

9. Pull a Rope IT Band and Hamstring Stretch—
Chair, page 155.

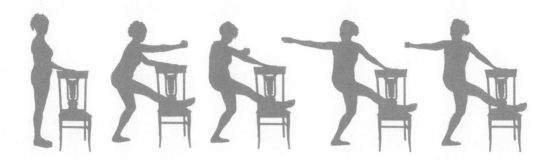

10. Advanced Pulling Sacks of Rice, page 100.

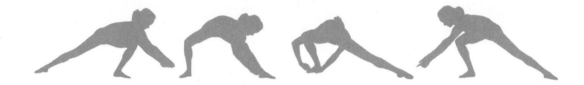

CYCLING

LENGTH: Thirty minutes

COMPONENTS: Standing, chair, floor

EQUIPMENT: Mat, chair, TheraBand or other resistance band, cushion

Begin with two to four minutes of the Warm-Up Routine.

1. Push a Piano and Pull a Donkey, page 99.

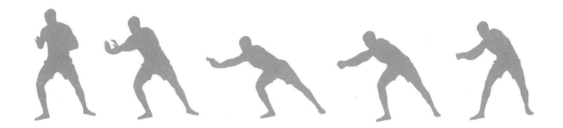

2. Washing Windows above the Shoulders, page 105.

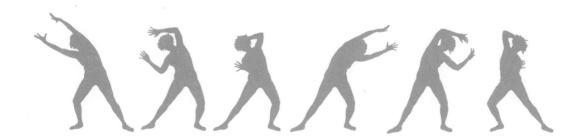

3. Hands, Fingers, and Wrists Mobility Sequence #2,
page 130.

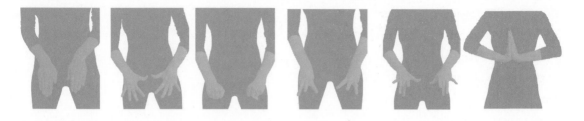

4. Pliés with Squeeze an Orange under Your Heel,
page 122.

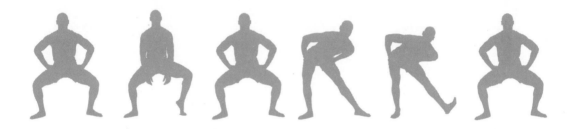

5. Shin Stretching and Strengthening—Chair,
page 147.

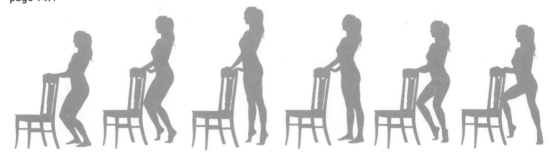

6. Hip Flexor and Hamstring Stretch—Chair,
page 156.

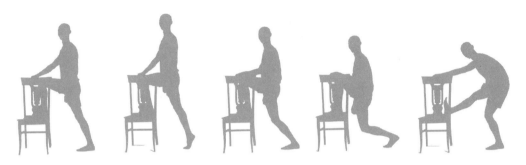

7. Deep Hamstring, Long Adductor, and IT Band
Stretch—Floor, page 183.

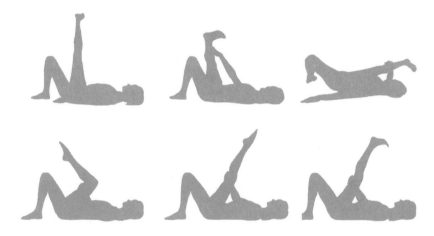

8. Baby Stretch with Deep Hip Release—Floor,
page 182.

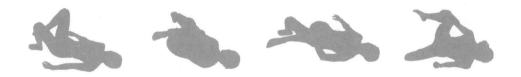

9. Cat and Cow for Spine Flexibility—Floor,
page 180.

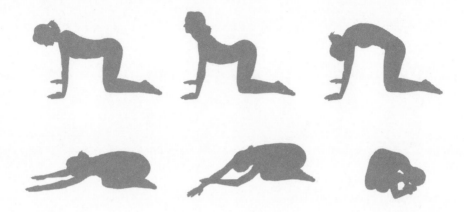

THE MIRACLE OF FLEXIBILITY

LENGTH: Thirty minutes

COMPONENTS: Standing

EQUIPMENT: Mat

Begin with two to four minutes of the Warm-Up
Routine.

1. Shoulder Blast, page 83.

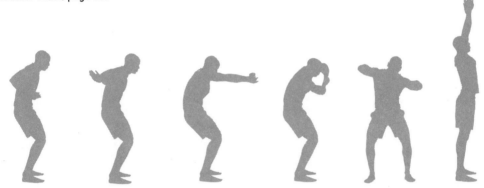

2. Open Chest Swan, page 112.

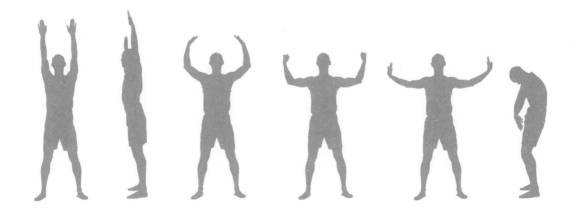

3. Waist Rotations, page 88.

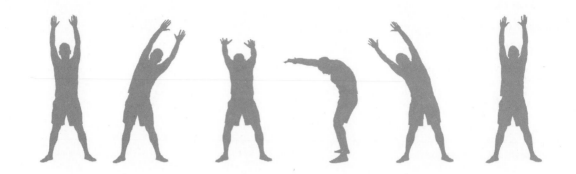

4. Small Single-Arm Figure Eights, page 117.

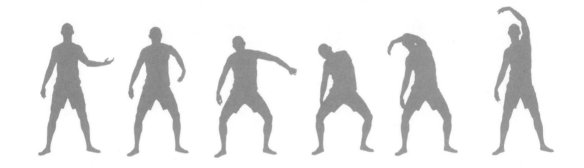

5. Fluid Spine, page 113.

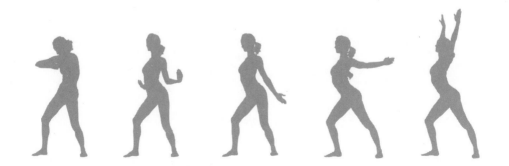

6. Pliés with Side-Bend Arm Reaches, page 128.

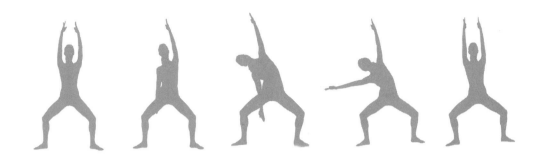

7. Calf Stretch Sequence, page 145.

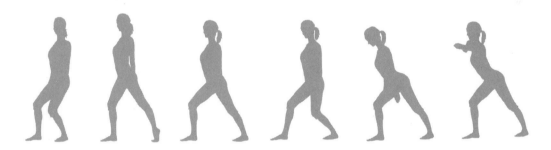

8. Advanced Clock Sequence, page 111.

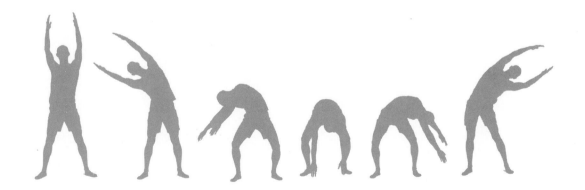

9. Fan Kicks with Lunges, page 139.

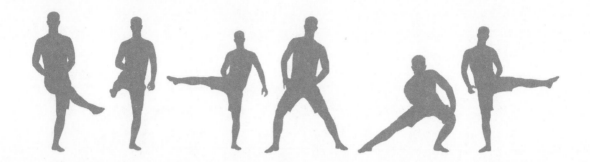

THE MIRACLE OF FLEXIBILITY

DIVING

LENGTH: Twenty minutes

COMPONENTS: Standing, chair

EQUIPMENT: Mat, chair

Begin with two to four minutes of the Warm-Up
Routine.

1. Zombie, page 78.

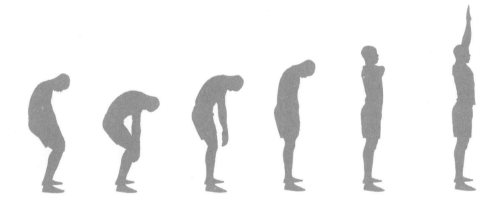

2. Shoulder Blast, page 83.

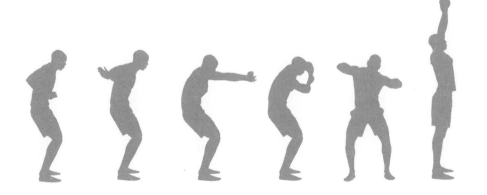

3. Large Full-Body Figure Eights with Rotation, page 120.

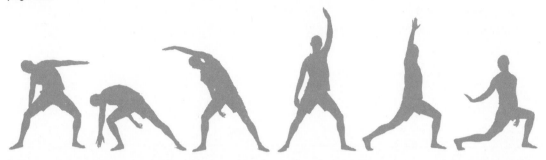

4. Double-Arm Pulling Ropes to the Floor, page 94.

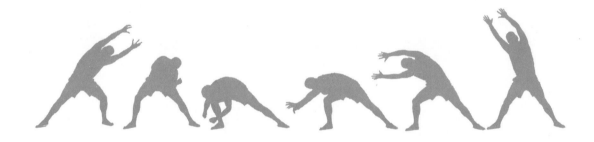

5. Shin Stretching and Strengthening—Chair, page 147.

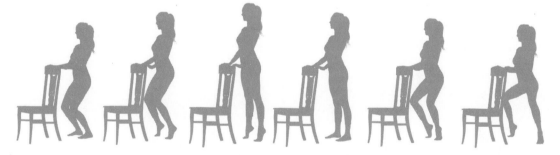

6. Hip Flexor and Hamstring Stretch—Chair.
page 156.

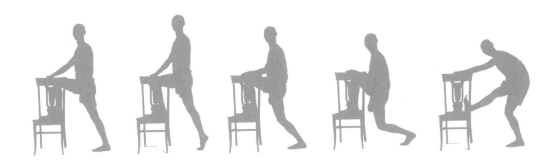

7. Inner and Outer Thigh Rotations: IT Band and
Long Adductor Stretch—Chair, page 153.

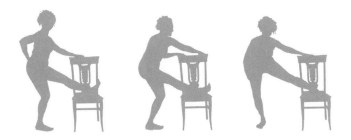

8. Hamstring and Spine Stretch—Chair, page 159.

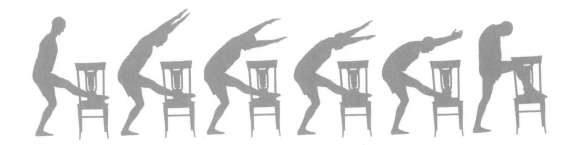

9. Folded Hamstring Stretch—Chair, page 160.

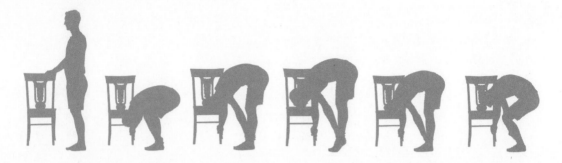

THE MIRACLE OF FLEXIBILITY

FIGURE SKATING

LENGTH: Thirty minutes

COMPONENTS: Standing, floor, chair

EQUIPMENT: Mat, chair, TheraBand or other resistance band, cushion

Begin with two to four minutes of the Warm-Up Routine.

1. Shin Stretching and Strengthening—Chair, page 147.

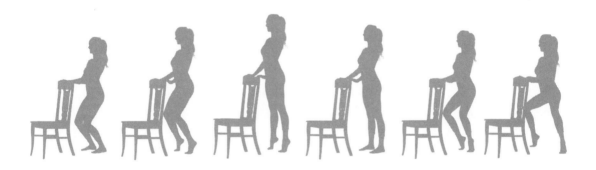

2. Pliés with Quadriceps Strengthening, page 121.

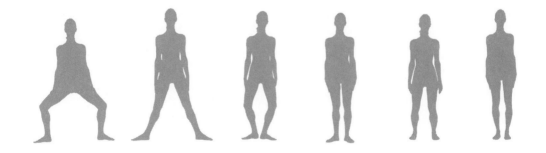

3. Calf Stretch Sequence, page 145.

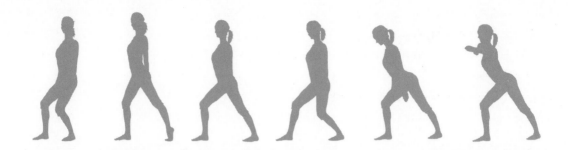

4. Large Full-Body Figure Eights with Rotation, page 120.

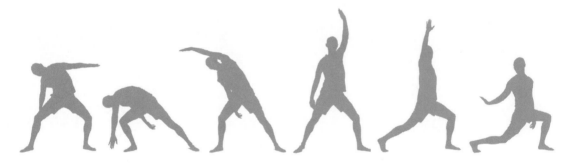

5. Superman Spine Strengthening—Floor, page 168.

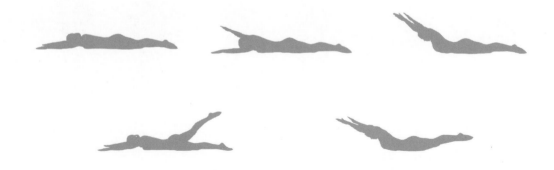

6. Baby Stretch with Deep Hip Release—Floor,
page 182.

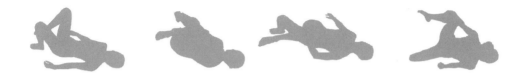

7. Deep Hamstring, Long Adductor, and IT Band
Stretch—Floor, page 183.

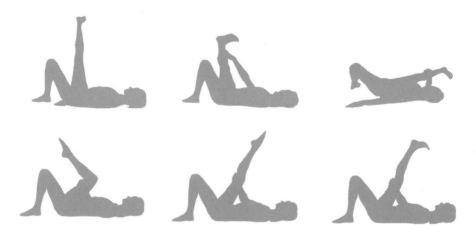

8. Deep Hip Flexor Stretch—Floor, page 178.

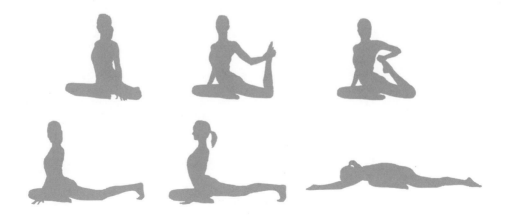

GOLF

LENGTH: Twenty-five minutes

COMPONENTS: Standing, chair

EQUIPMENT: Mat, chair

Begin with two to four minutes of the Warm-Up
Routine.

1. Zombie, page 78.

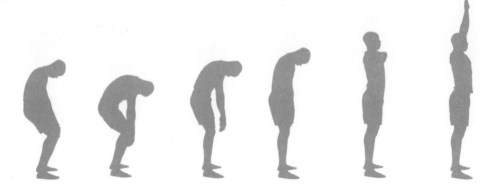

2. Shoulder Blast, page 83.

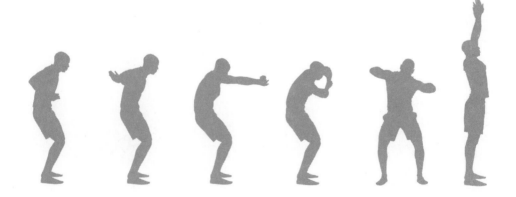

3. Diagonal Presses at Various Heights, page 93.

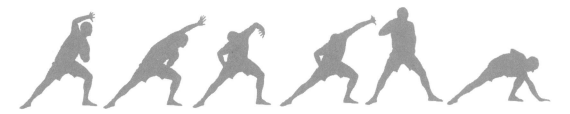

4. Washing a Small Round Table, page 89.

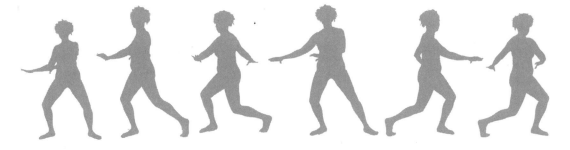

5. Wraparound Arms, page 91.

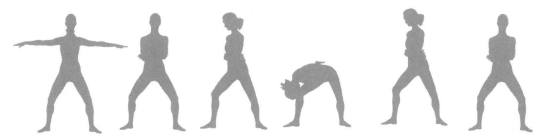

6. Calf Stretch Sequence, page 145.

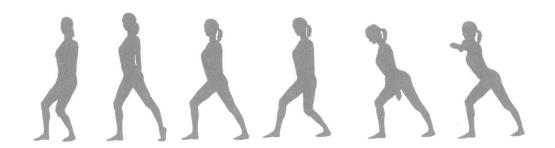

7. Pliés with Hip and Groin Stretch, page 127.

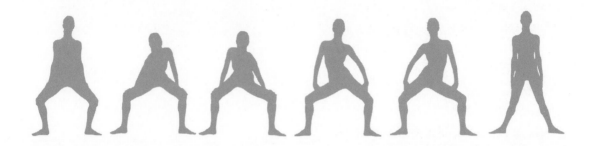

8. Inner and Outer Thigh Rotations: IT Band and
Long Adductor Stretch—Chair, page 153.

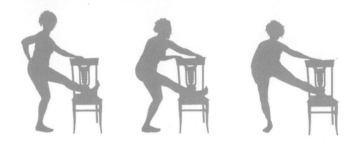

9. Spine Release—Chair, page 161.

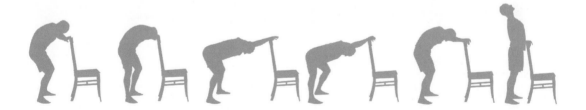

HIKING

LENGTH: Twenty minutes

COMPONENTS: Standing, floor, chair

EQUIPMENT: Mat, TheraBand or other resistance
band, riser, cushion, chair

Begin with two to four minutes of the Warm-Up
Routine.

1. Shoulder Blast, page 83.

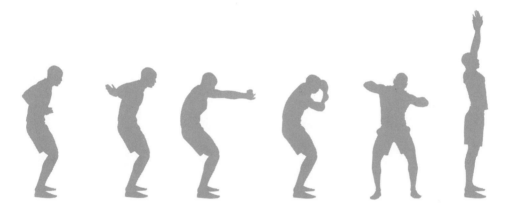

2. Diagonal Presses at Various Heights, page 93.

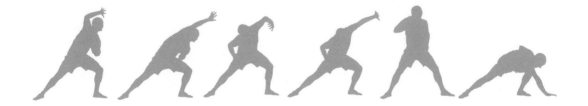

3. Pliés with Hip and Groin Stretch, page 127.

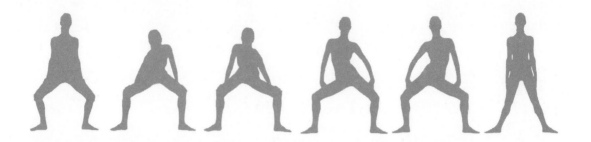

4. Low Rapid Kicks, page 136.

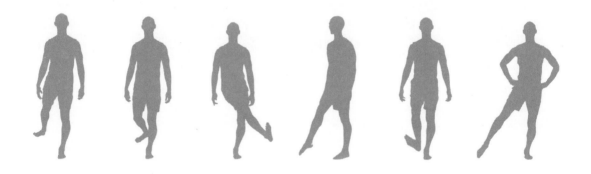

5. Butterfly with PNF for Hip Stretch—Floor, page 173.

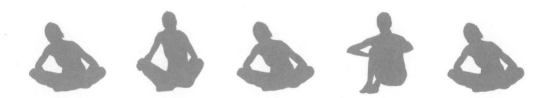

6. Baby Stretch with Deep Hip Release—Floor, page 182.

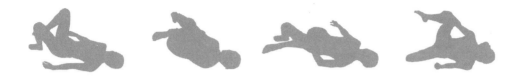

7. Deep Hamstring, Long Adductor, and IT Band Stretch—Floor, page 183.

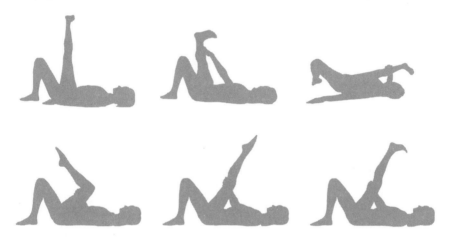

8. Spine Release—Chair, page 161.

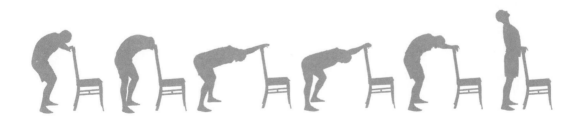

HOCKEY

LENGTH: Twenty minutes

COMPONENTS: Standing, floor, chair

EQUIPMENT: Mat, cushion, chair

Begin with two to four minutes of the Warm-Up Routine.

1. Small Single-Arm Figure Eights, page 117.

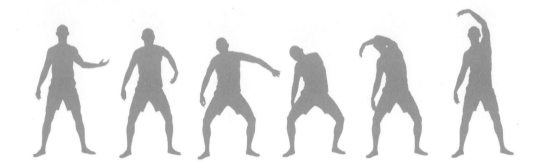

2. Pliés with Squeeze an Orange under Your Heel, page 122.

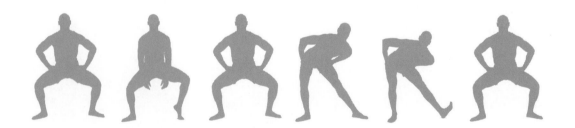

3. Simple Windmill—Feet Parallel, page 90.

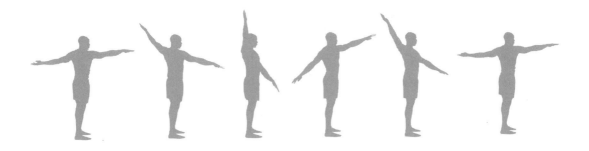

4. Calf Stretch Sequence, page 145.

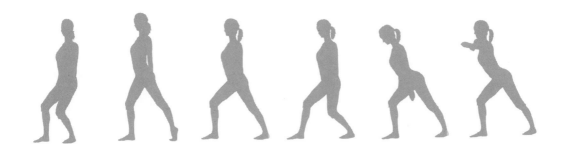

5. Baby Stretch with Deep Hip Release—Floor, page 182.

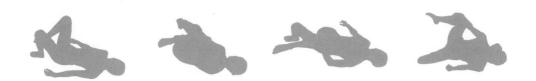

6. Hip Flexor and Hamstring Stretch—Chair, page 156.

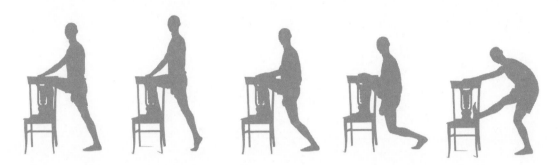

7. Four-Directional Hip Stretch—Chair, page 151.

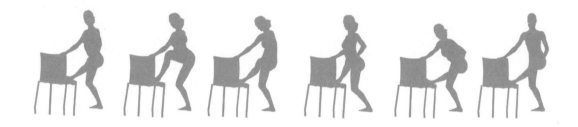

8. Inner and Outer Thigh Rotations: IT Band and Long Adductor Stretch—Chair, page 153.

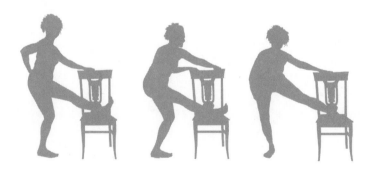

9. Pull a Rope IT Band and Hamstring Stretch—
Chair, page 155.

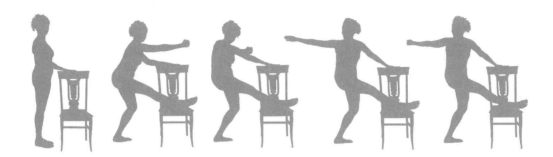

HORSEBACK RIDING

LENGTH: Thirty minutes

COMPONENTS: Standing, floor, chair

EQUIPMENT: Mat, chair, cushion, riser

Begin with two to four minutes of the Warm-Up Routine.

1. Zombie, page 78.

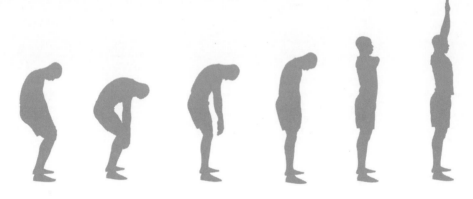

2. Waist Rotations, page 88.

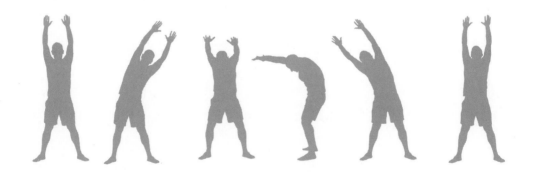

3. Double-Arm Shoulder Rotations, page 131.

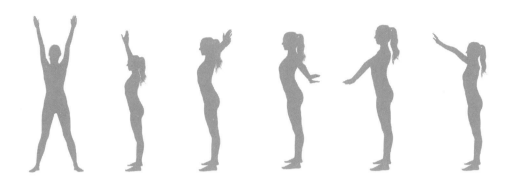

4. Sweeping behind Head into Cutting the Air, page 104.

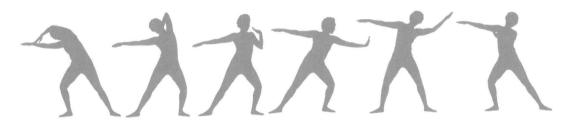

5. Simple Windmill—Feet Parallel, page 90.

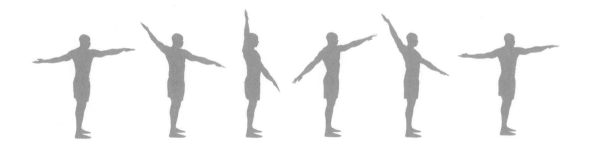

6. Hands, Fingers, and Wrists Mobility Sequence #1,
page 129.

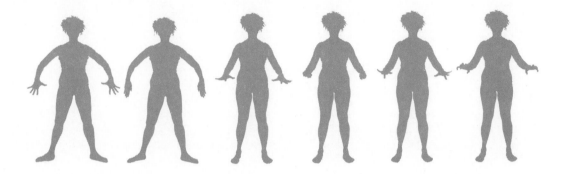

7. Wraparound Arms, page 91.

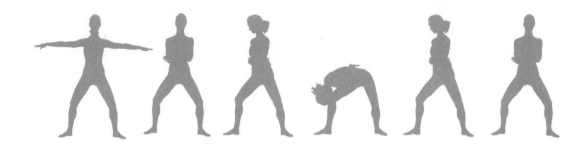

8. Pliés with Hip and Groin Stretch, page 127.

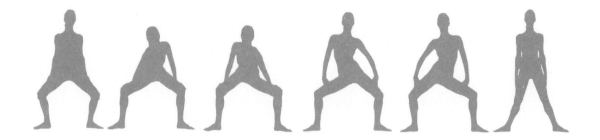

9. Butterfly with PNF for Hip Stretch—Floor,
page 173.

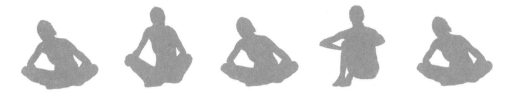

10. Inner and Outer Thigh Rotations: IT Band and
Long Adductor Stretch—Chair, page 153.

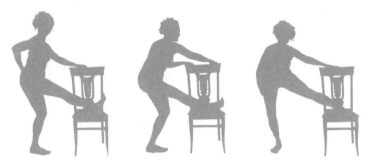

11. Hip Flexor and Hamstring Stretch—Chair,
page 156.

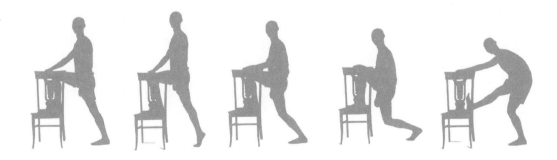

MARTIAL ARTS

LENGTH: Twenty minutes

COMPONENTS: Standing, floor, chair

EQUIPMENT: Mat, chair

Begin with two to four minutes of the Warm-Up Routine.

1. Pliés with Single-Arm Half-Body Rotation, page 126.

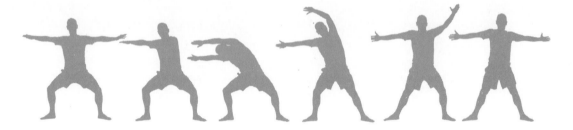

2. Arm Pumps for Pectoral Stretch, page 133.

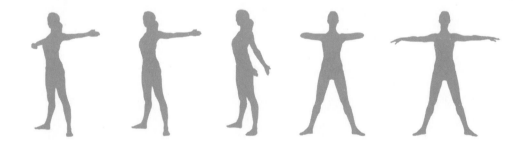

3. Double-Arm Pulling Ropes to the Floor, page 94.

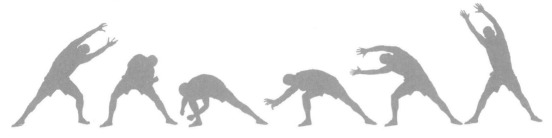

4. Butterfly with PNF for Hip Stretch—Floor,
page 173.

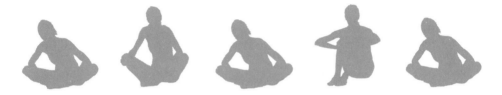

5. Shin Stretching and Strengthening—Chair,
page 147.

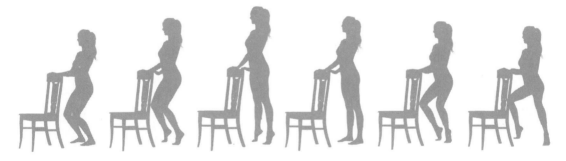

6. Karate Kicks to the Side—Chair, page 138.

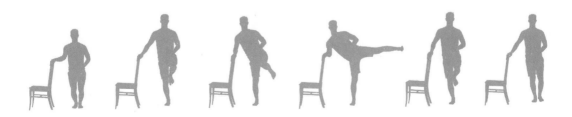

**7. Hip Flexor and Hamstring Stretch—Chair,
page 156.**

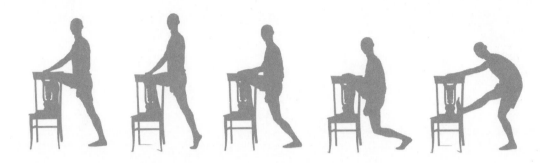

**8. Inner and Outer Thigh Rotations: IT Band and
Long Adductor Stretch—Chair, page 153.**

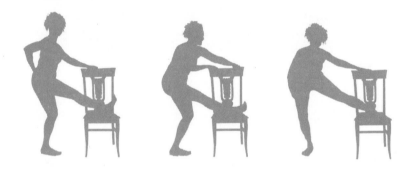

**9. Deep Hamstring and Spine Stretch with
Release—Chair, page 154.**

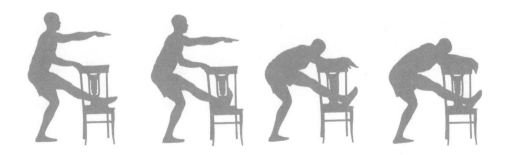

RACKET SPORTS (TENNIS, SQUASH, BADMINTON, RACQUETBALL, PICKLEBALL)

LENGTH: Twenty minutes

COMPONENTS: Standing, floor, chair

EQUIPMENT: Mat, chair

Begin with two to four minutes of the Warm-Up Routine.

1. Small Single-Arm Figure Eights, page 117.

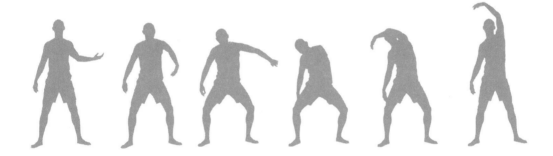

2. Shoulder Blast, page 83.

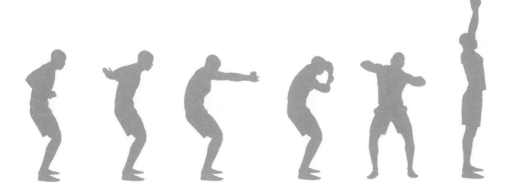

3. Diagonal Presses at Various Heights, page 93.

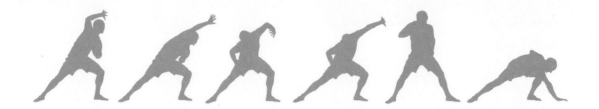

4. Pliés with Quadriceps Strengthening, page 121.

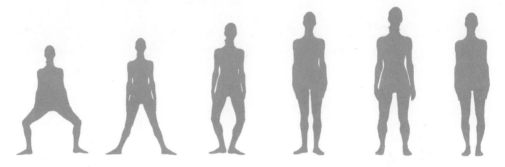

5. Calf Stretch Sequence, page 145.

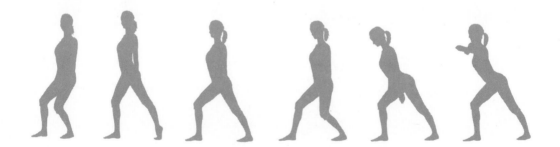

6. Ankle, Calf, and Shin Stretch, page 144.

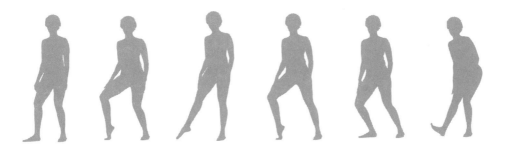

7. Hip Flexor and Hamstring Stretch—Chair, page 156.

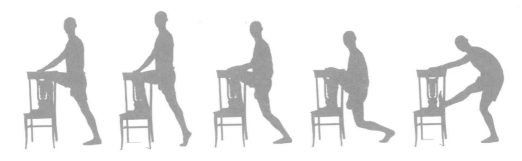

8. Inner and Outer Thigh Rotations: IT Band and Long Adductor Stretch—Chair, page 153.

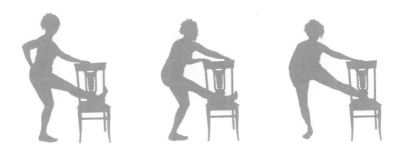

9. Hamstring and Spine Stretch—Chair, page 159.

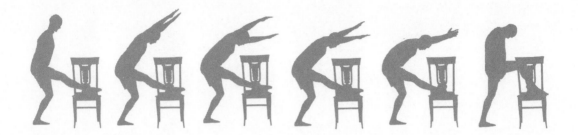

ROWING, KAYAKING, CANOEING

LENGTH: Twenty minutes

COMPONENTS: Standing, floor, chair

EQUIPMENT: Mat, chair

Begin with two to four minutes of the Warm-Up
Routine.

1. Shoulder Blast, page 83.

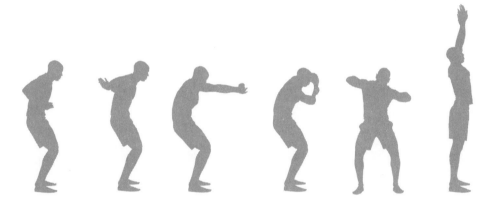

2. Simple Windmill—Feet Parallel, page 90.

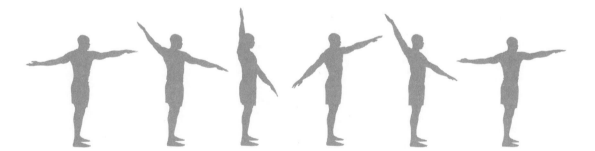

3. Lift Imaginary Weights above Your Head, page 116.

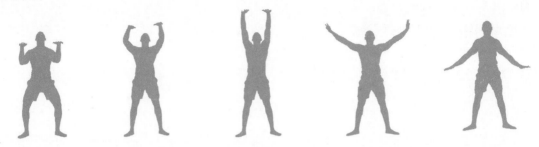

4. Pliés with Hip and Groin Stretch, page 127.

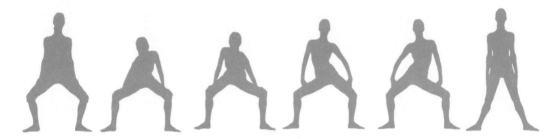

5. Karate Kicks to the Front—Chair, page 137.

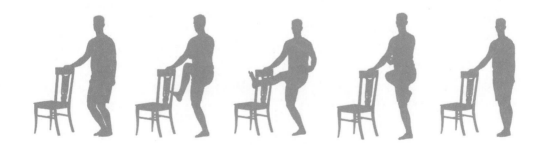

6. Four-Directional Hip Stretch—Chair, page 151.

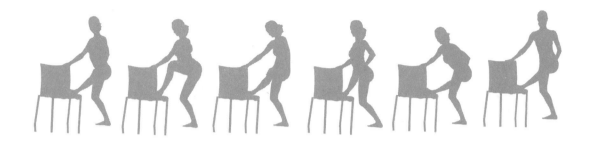

7. Hip Flexor and Hamstring Stretch—Chair, page 156.

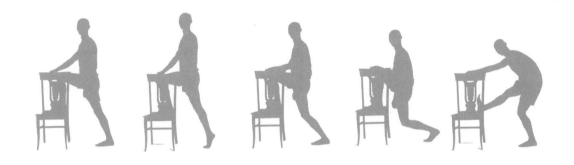

8. Inner and Outer Thigh Rotations: IT Band and Long Adductor Stretch—Chair, page 153.

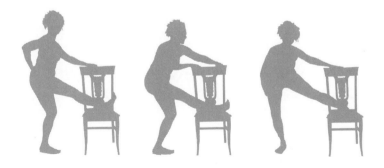

9. Hamstring and Spine Stretch—Chair, page 159.

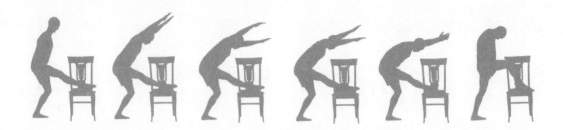

10. Spine Release—Chair, page 161.

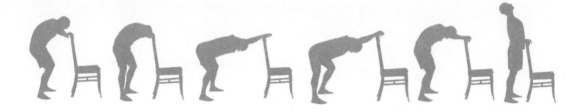

RUNNING

LENGTH: Twenty-five minutes

COMPONENTS: Standing, chair

EQUIPMENT: Mat, chair

Begin with two to four minutes of the Warm-Up
Routine.

1. Ankle, Calf, and Shin Stretch, page 144.

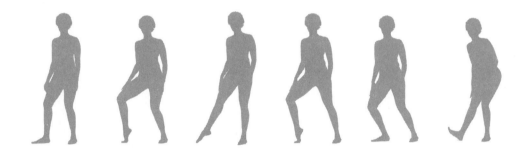

2. Pliés with Side-Bend Arm Reaches, page 128.

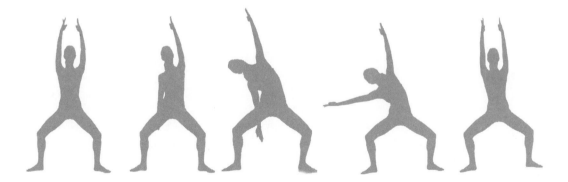

3. Calf Stretch Sequence, page 145.

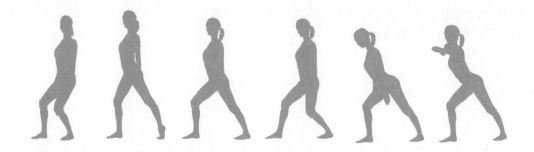

4. Squash Lunges, page 140.

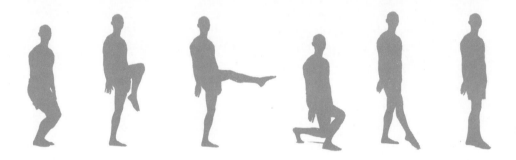

5. Preparation: Hip Flexor and Hamstring Stretch—
Chair, page 152.

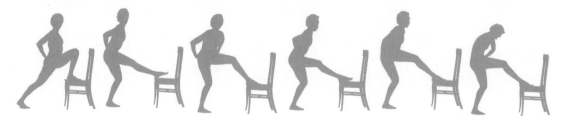

6. Inner and Outer Thigh Rotations: IT Band and
Long Adductor Stretch—Chair, page 153.

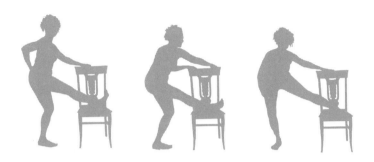

7. Hamstring and Spine Stretch—Chair, page 159.

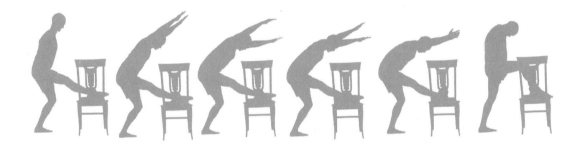

8. Large Full-Body Figure Eights with Rotation,
page 120.

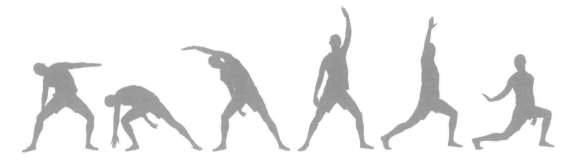

SKIING

LENGTH: Twenty minutes

COMPONENTS: Standing, chair

EQUIPMENT: Mat, chair

Begin with two to four minutes of the Warm-Up Routine.

1. Remove a Sweater, page 115.

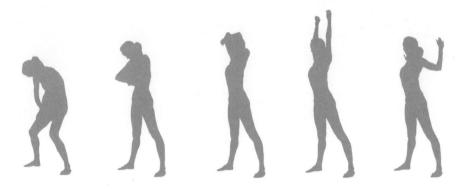

2. Deep Side Lunge Washes, page 106.

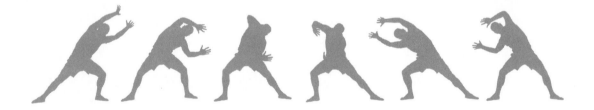

3. Pliés with Single-Arm Full-Body Rotation, page 123.

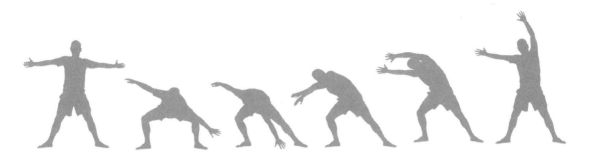

4. Shin Stretching and Strengthening—Chair, page 147.

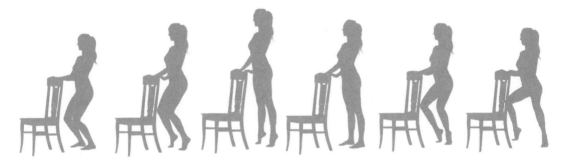

5. Calf Stretch Sequence, page 145.

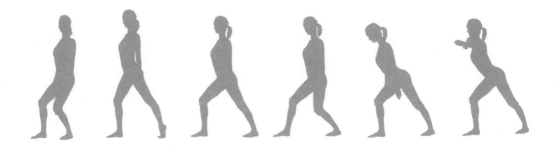

6. Hip Cleaners—Chair, page 150.

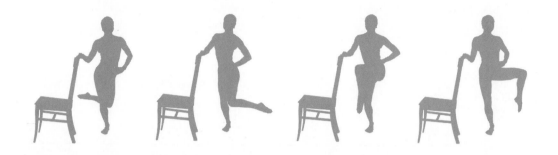

7. Hamstring and Spine Stretch—Chair, page 159.

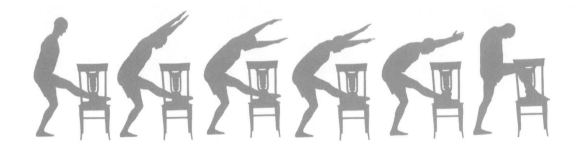

8. Inner and Outer Thigh Rotations: IT Band and
Long Adductor Stretch—Chair, page 153.

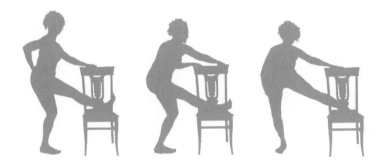

SNOWBOARDING

LENGTH: Twenty-five minutes

COMPONENTS: Standing, chair, floor

EQUIPMENT: Mat, chair, TheraBand or other resistance band, cushion

Begin with two to four minutes of the Warm-Up Routine.

1. Shoulder Blast, page 83.

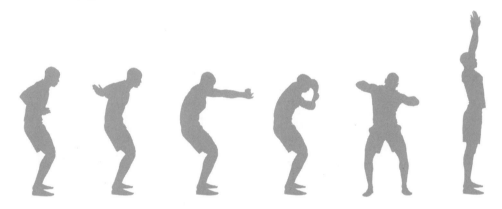

2. Diagonal Presses at Various Heights, page 93.

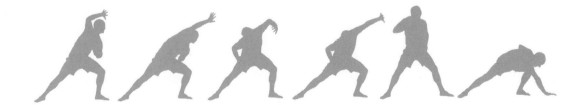

3. Pliés with Hip and Groin Stretch, page 127.

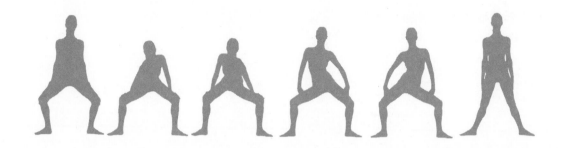

4. Simple Windmill—Feet Parallel, page 90.

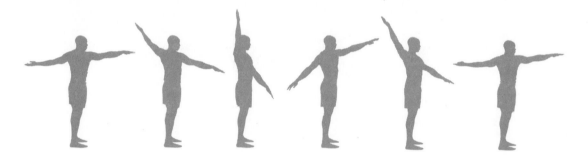

5. Calf Stretch Sequence, page 145.

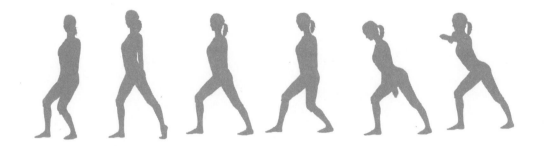

6. Four-Directional Hip Stretch—Chair, page 151.

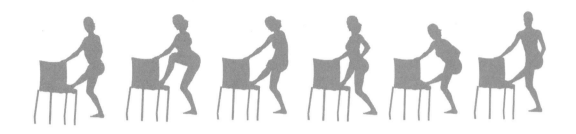

7. Hip Flexor and Hamstring Stretch—Chair,
page 156.

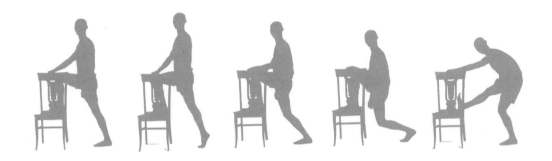

8. Baby Stretch with Deep Hip Release—Floor,
page 182.

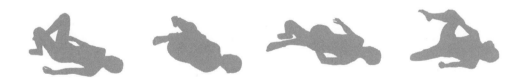

9. Deep Hamstring, Long Adductor, and IT Band
Stretch—Floor, page 183.

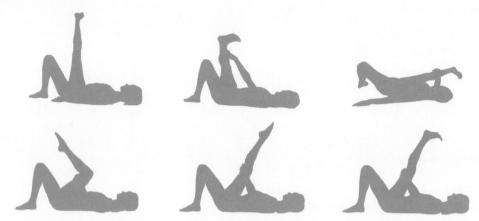

SOCCER

LENGTH: Twenty minutes

COMPONENTS: Standing, chair

EQUIPMENT: Mat, chair

Begin with two to four minutes of the Warm-Up
Routine.

1. Hip Cleaners—Chair, page 150.

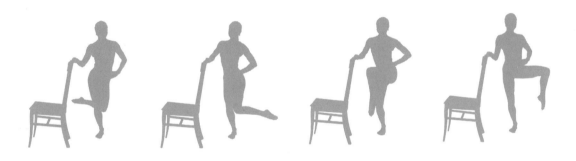

2. Large Full-Body Figure Eights with Rotation,
page 120.

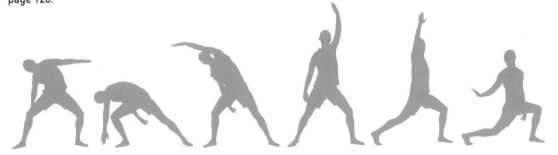

3. Pliés with Quadriceps Strengthening, page 121.

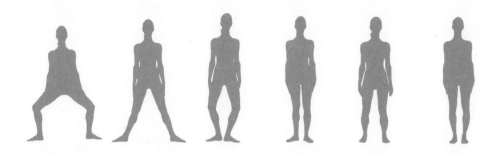

4. Squash Lunges, page 140.

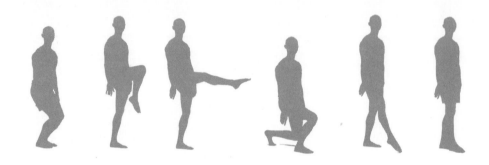

5. Ankle, Calf, and Shin Stretch, page 144.

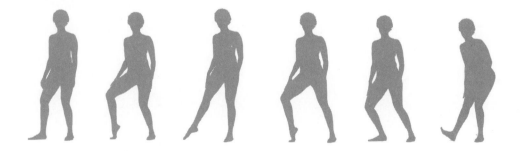

6. Calf Stretch Sequence, page 145.

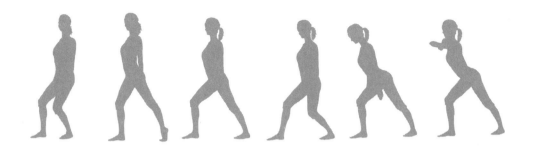

7. Hip Flexor and Hamstring Stretch—Chair, page 156.

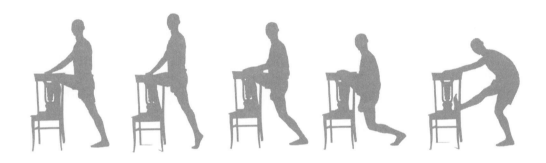

8. Inner and Outer Thigh Rotations: IT Band and Long Adductor Stretch—Chair, page 153.

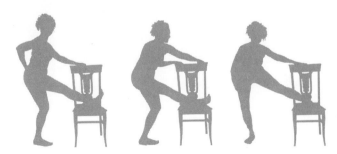

SURFING

LENGTH: Twenty minutes

COMPONENTS: Standing, floor, chair

EQUIPMENT: Mat, chair

Begin with two to four minutes of the Warm-Up Routine.

1. Zombie, page 78.

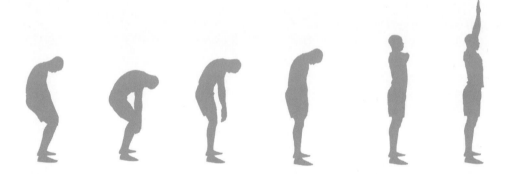

2. Shoulder Blast, page 83.

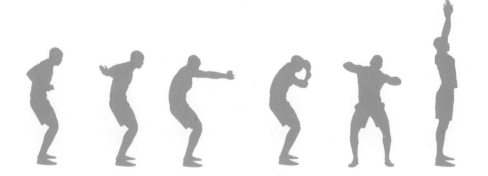

3. Windmill with Spine Flexion, page 96.

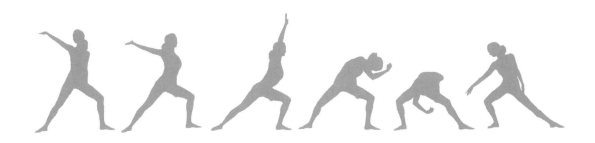

4. Pliés with Quadriceps Strengthening, page 121.

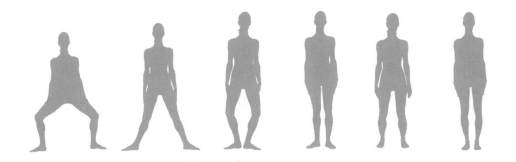

5. Fan Kicks with Lunges, page 139.

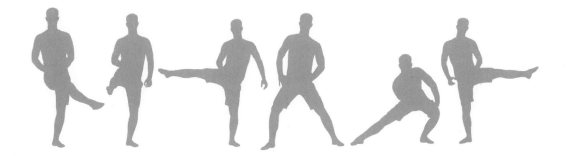

6. Shin Stretching and Strengthening—Chair,
page 147.

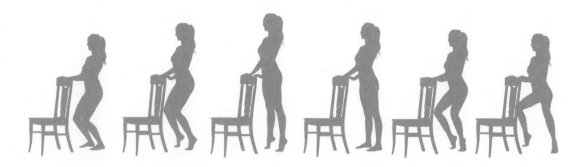

7. Calf Stretch Sequence, page 145.

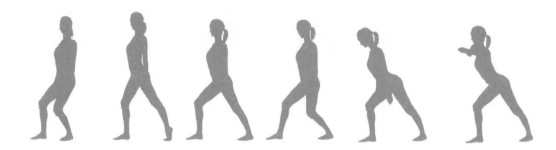

8. Hip Flexor and Hamstring Stretch—Chair,
page 156.

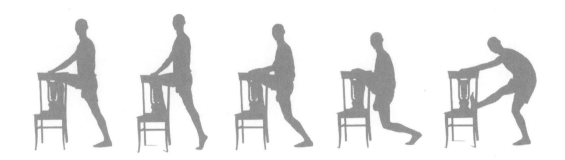

9. Inner and Outer Thigh Rotations: IT Band and
Long Adductor Stretch—Chair, page 153.

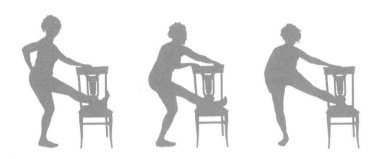

10. Folded Hamstring Stretch—Chair, page 160.

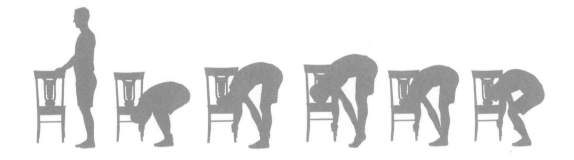

SWIMMING

LENGTH: Twenty minutes

COMPONENTS: Standing, floor, chair

EQUIPMENT: Mat, TheraBand or other resistance
band, chair

Begin with two to four minutes of the Warm-Up
Routine.

1. Double-Arm Figure Eights, page 119.

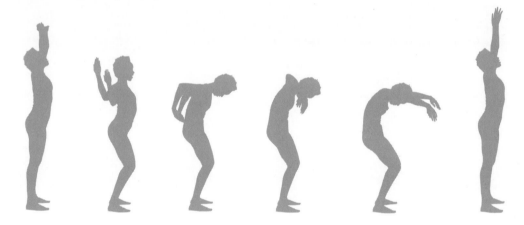

2. Deep Side Lunge Washes, page 106.

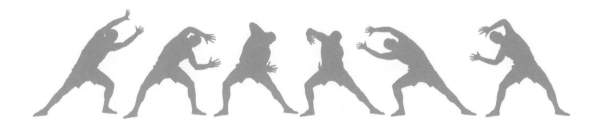

3. Windmill with Spine Flexion, page 96.

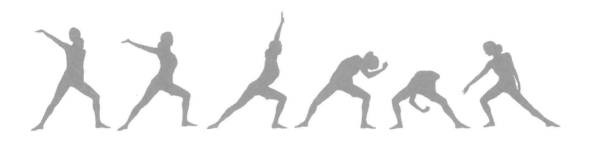

4. Shin Stretching and Strengthening—Chair, page 147.

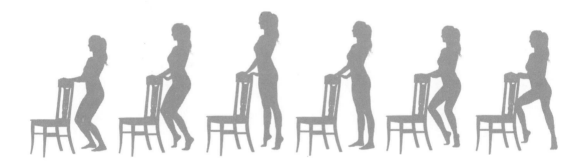

5. Standing Quad Stretch, page 142.

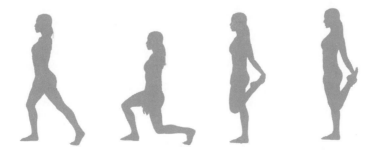

6. Arching the Back Stretches—Floor, page 184.

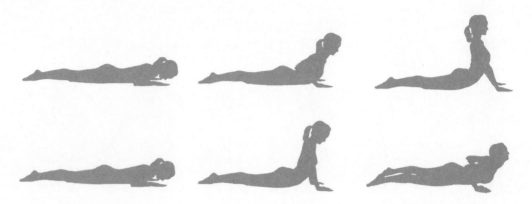

7. Deep Hip Flexor Stretch—Floor, page 178.

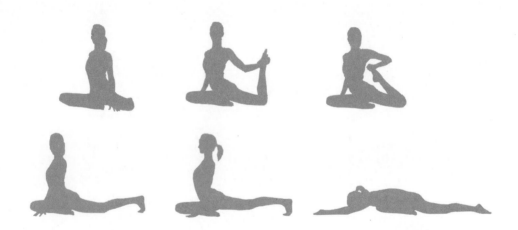

8. Long Adductor Stretch with Figure Eight—Floor,
page 179.

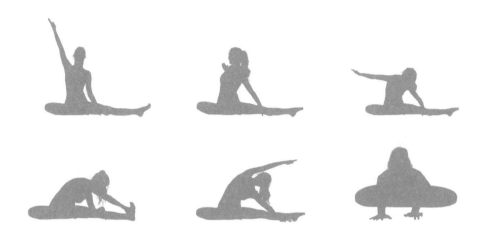

9. Row the Boat with Hamstring and Spine Stretch—
Floor, page 177.

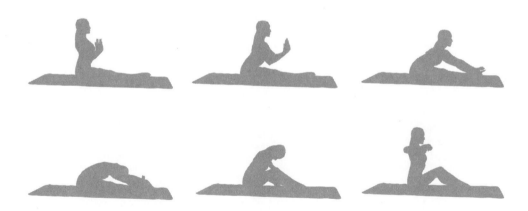

VOLLEYBALL

LENGTH: Twenty minutes

COMPONENTS: Standing, chair

EQUIPMENT: Mat, chair

Begin with two to four minutes of the Warm-Up
Routine.

1. Small Single-Arm Figure Eights, page 117.

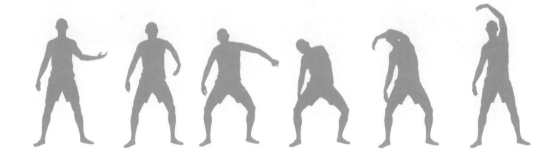

2. Arm Pumps for Pectoral Stretch,
page 133.

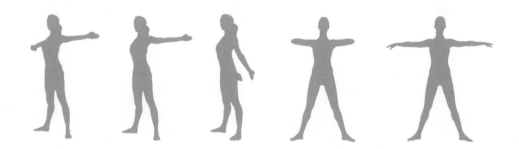

3. Pliés with Quadriceps Strengthening. page 121.

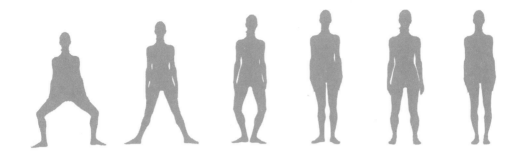

4. Windmill with Spine Flexion. page 96.

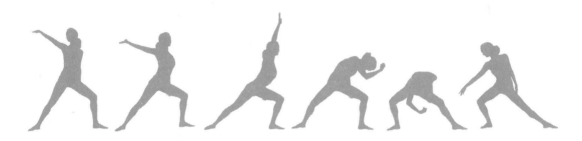

5. Advanced Clock Sequence. page 111.

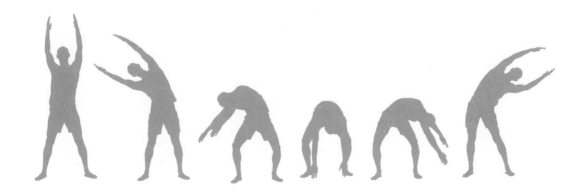

6. Fan Kicks with Lunges, page 139.

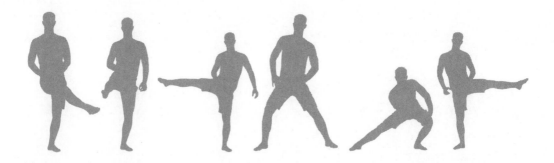

7. Advanced Pulling Sacks of Rice, page 100.

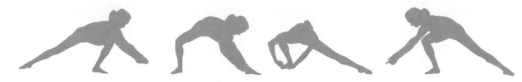

8. Shin Stretching and Strengthening—Chair, page 147.

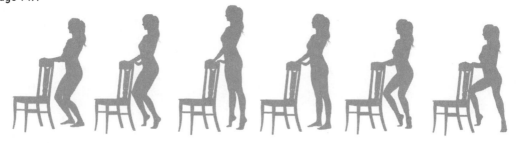

9. Preparation: Hip Flexor and Hamstring Stretch— Chair, page 152.

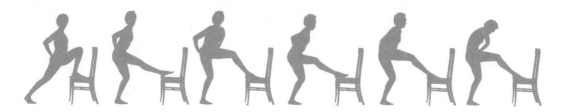

YOGA AND PILATES

LENGTH: Twenty to twenty-five minutes

COMPONENTS: Standing, floor

EQUIPMENT: Mat

Begin with two to four minutes of the Warm-Up Routine.

1. Arm Pumps for Shoulder Joint Liberation, page 132.

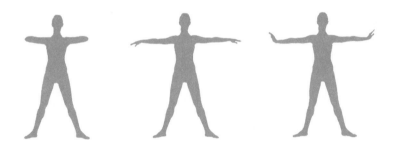

2. Hands, Fingers, and Wrists Mobility Sequence #1, page 129.

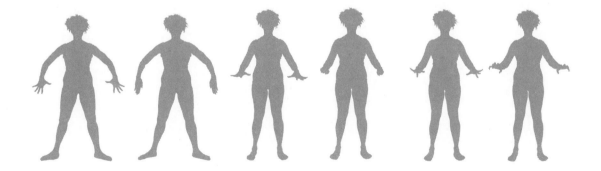

3. Pliés with Single-Arm Half-Body Rotation,
page 126.

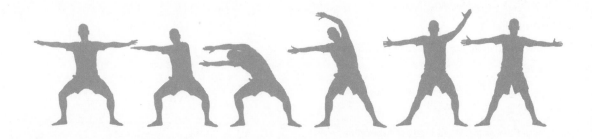

4. Large Full-Body Figure Eights with Rotation,
page 120.

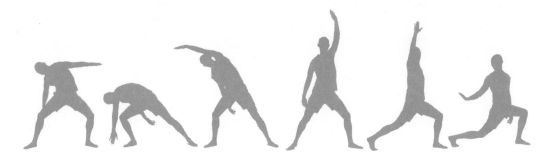

5. Butterfly with PNF for Hip Stretch—Floor,
page 173.

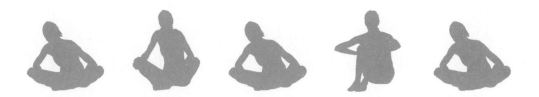

6. Deep Hip Flexor Stretch—Floor, page 178.

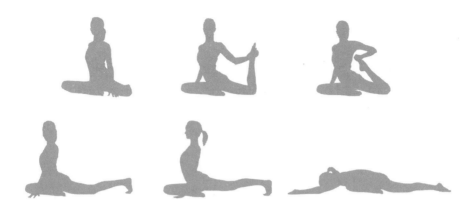

7. Baby Stretch with Deep Hip Release—Floor, page 182.

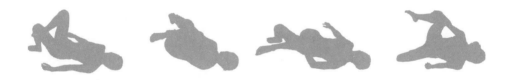

8. Deep Hamstring, Long Adductor, and IT Band Stretch—Floor, page 183.

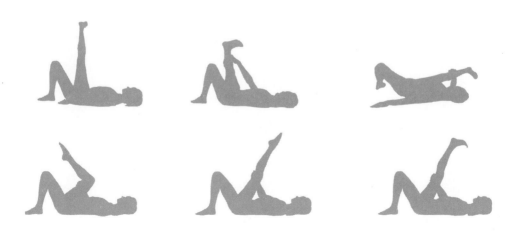

9. Advanced Trapeze Strengthening with Quad
Raisers—Floor, page 167.

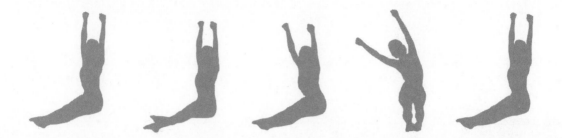

CHAPTER 12
Essentrics Routines for the Workplace

LENGTH: Twenty minutes

COMPONENTS: Standing, chair, floor

EQUIPMENT: Mat

Begin with two to four minutes of the Warm-Up

Routine.

1. Ankle, Calf, and Shin Stretch, page 144.

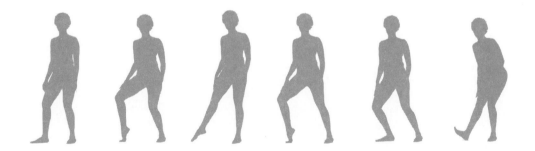

2. Squash Lunges, page 140.

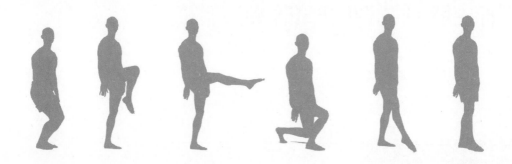

3. Calf Stretch Sequence, page 145.

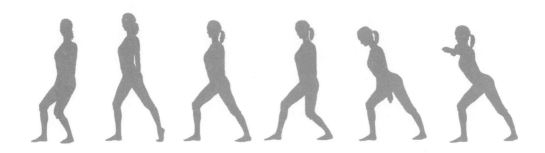

4. Shin Stretching and Strengthening—Chair, page 147.

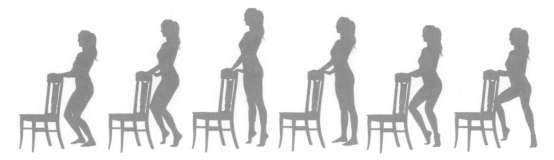

5. Advanced Ankle Strengthening—Chair, page 148.

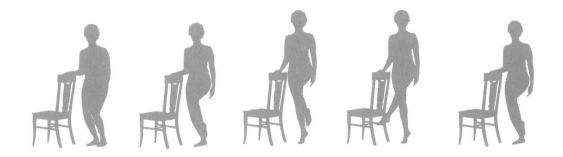

6. Ankle Mobility with Hip Rotation—Floor,
page 146.

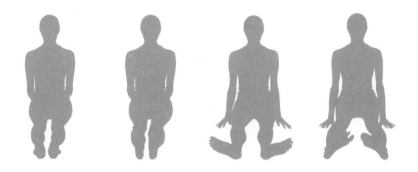

7. Advanced Shin Stretch—Floor, page 181.

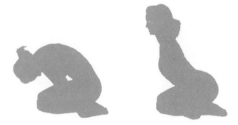

AT A DESK ALL DAY

LENGTH: Fifteen minutes

COMPONENTS: Standing, chair

EQUIPMENT: Mat, chair

Begin with two to four minutes of the Warm-Up
Routine.

1. Ceiling Reach and Open Chest Swan, page 114.

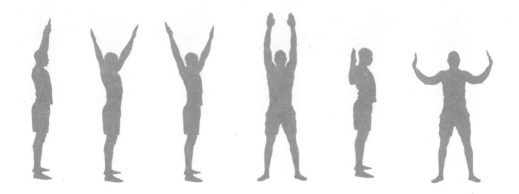

2. Shoulder Blast, page 83.

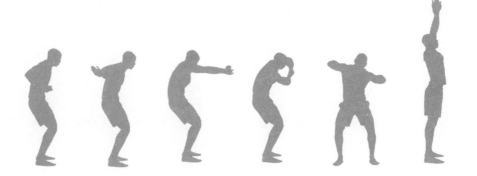

3. Diagonal Presses at Various Heights, page 93.

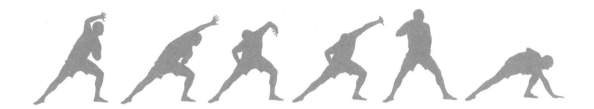

4. Triceps Stretch into Windmills, page 97.

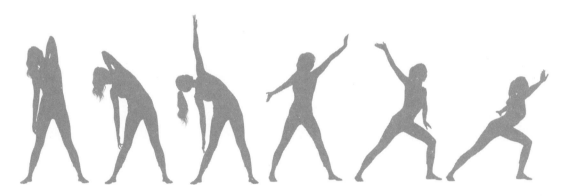

5. Wraparound Arms, page 91.

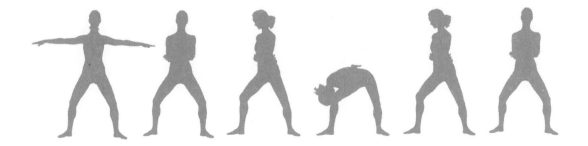

6. Karate Kicks to the Front—Chair, page 137.

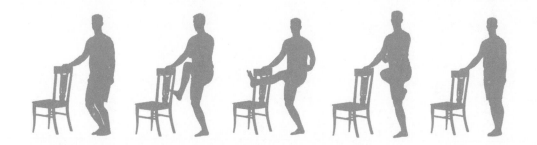

7. Karate Kicks to the Side—Chair, page 138.

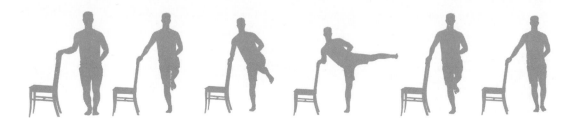

8. Calf Stretch Sequence, page 145.

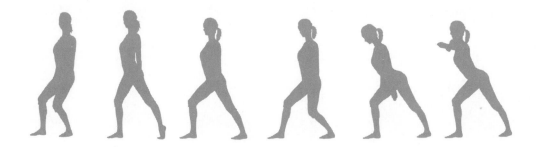

MANUAL LABOR/CONSTRUCTION/ LANDSCAPING

LENGTH: Fifteen minutes

COMPONENTS: Standing, chair

EQUIPMENT: Mat, chair

Begin with two to four minutes of the Warm-Up Routine.

1. Hands, Fingers, and Wrists Mobility Sequence #1, page 129.

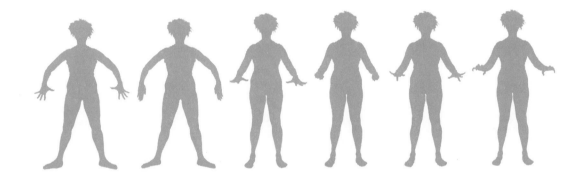

2. Hands, Fingers, and Wrists Mobility Sequence #2, page 130.

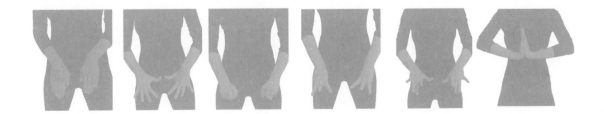

3. Ceiling Reach and Open Chest Swan, page 114.

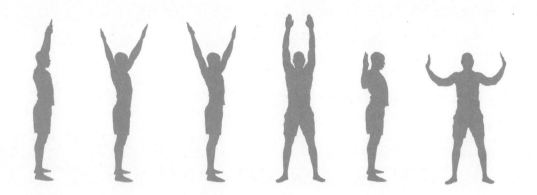

4. Washing a Small Round Table, page 89.

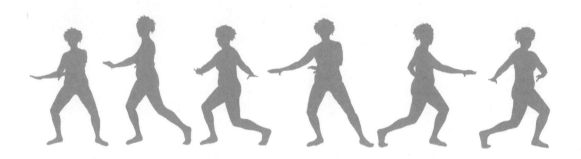

5. Simple Windmill—Feet Parallel, page 90.

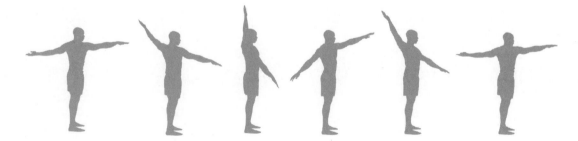

6. Arm Pumps for Shoulder Joint Liberation, page 132.

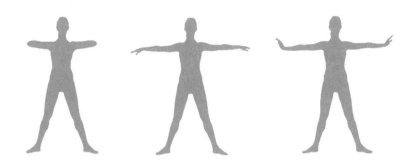

7. Four-Directional Hip Stretch—Chair, page 151.

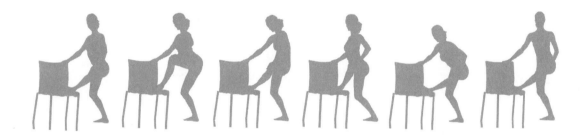

8. Spine Release—Chair, page 161.

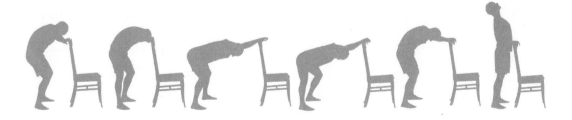

FLIGHT ATTENDANTS

LENGTH: Twenty minutes

COMPONENTS: Standing, chair

EQUIPMENT: Mat, chair

Begin with two to four minutes of the Warm-Up
Routine.

1. Ceiling Reach and Open Chest Swan, page 114.

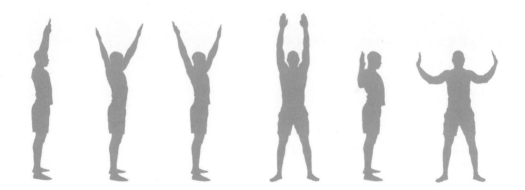

2. Small Single-Arm Figure Eights, page 117.

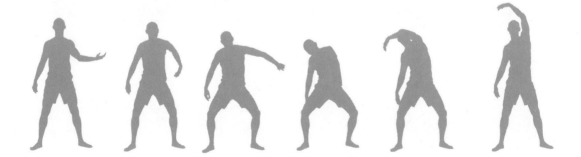

3. Lift Imaginary Weights above Your Head,
page 116.

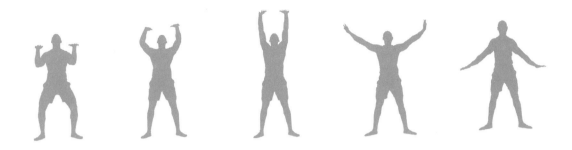

4. Diagonal Presses at Various Heights, page 93.

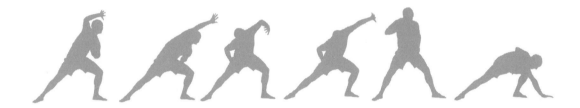

5. Ankle, Calf, and Shin Stretch, page 144.

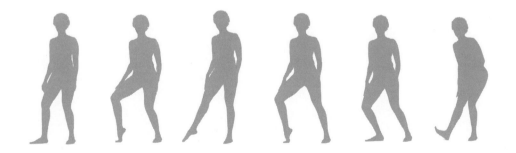

6. Calf Stretch Sequence, page 145.

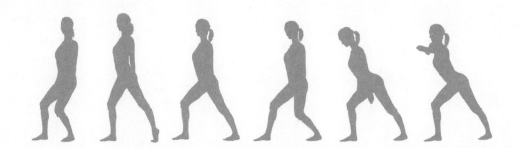

7. Standing Quad Stretch, page 142.

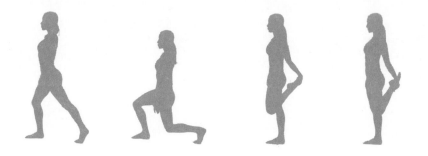

8. Four-Directional Hip Stretch—Chair, page 151.

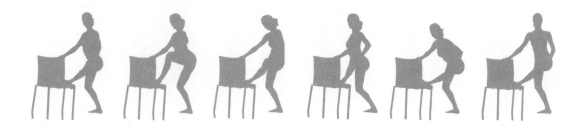

9. Windmill Hamstring and Spine Stretch—Chair,
page 158.

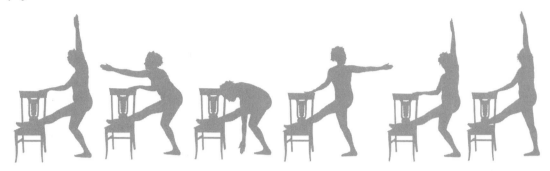

10. Hip Flexor and Hamstring Stretch—Chair,
page 156.

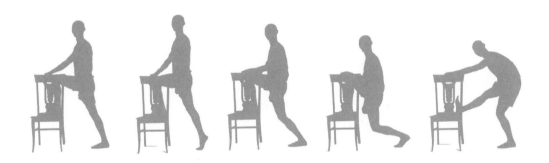

HOUSEKEEPING

LENGTH: Twenty-five minutes

COMPONENTS: Standing, chair

EQUIPMENT: Mat, chair

Begin with two to four minutes of the Warm-Up
Routine.

1. Zombie, page 78.

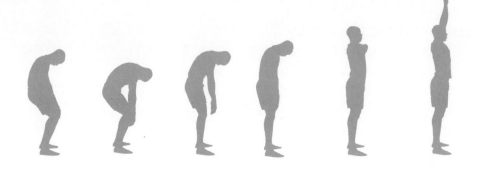

2. Waist Rotations, page 88.

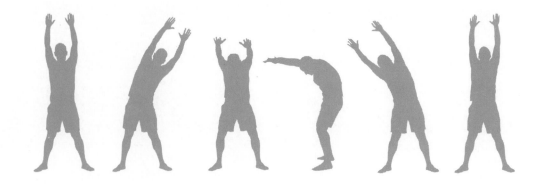

3. Washing a Small Round Table, page 89.

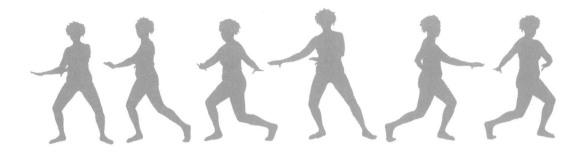

4. Diagonal Presses at Various Heights, page 93.

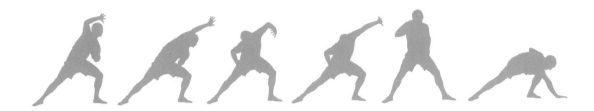

5. Simple Windmill—Feet Parallel, page 90.

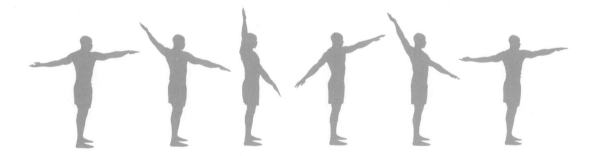

6. Advanced Ankle Strengthening—Chair, page 148.

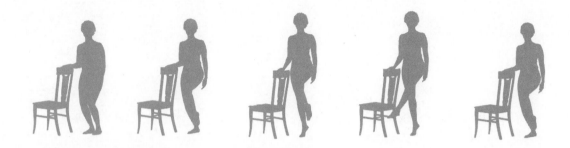

7. Hamstring and Spine Stretch—Chair, page 159.

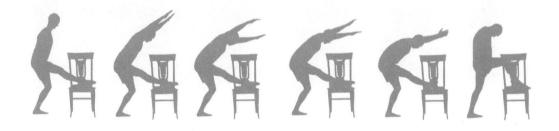

8. Inner and Outer Thigh Rotations: IT Band and
Long Adductor Stretch—Chair, page 153.

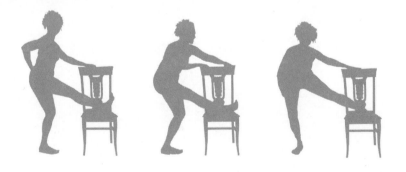

9. Spine Release—Chair, page 161.

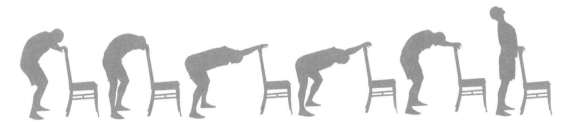

HAIRDRESSING

LENGTH: Twenty minutes

COMPONENTS: Standing, chair

EQUIPMENT: Mat, chair

Begin with two to four minutes of the Warm-Up
Routine.

1. Ceiling Reach and Open Chest Swan, page 114.

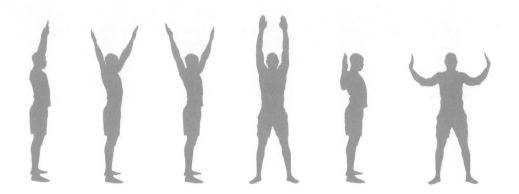

2. Shoulder Blast, page 83.

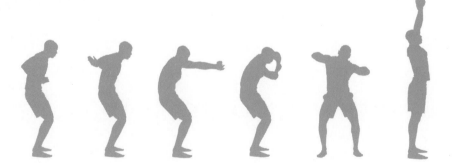

3. Fingers Walking Down the Arm, page 107.

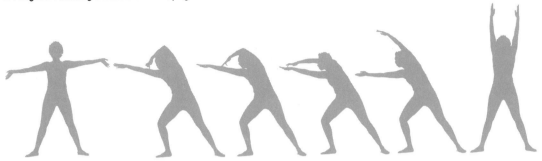

4. Hands, Fingers, and Wrists Mobility Sequence #1, page 129.

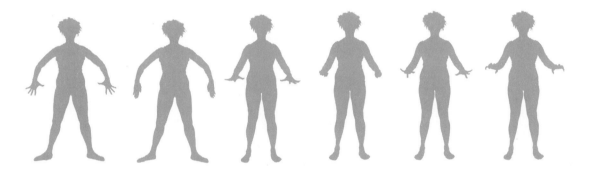

5. Hands, Fingers, and Wrists Mobility Sequence #2, page 130.

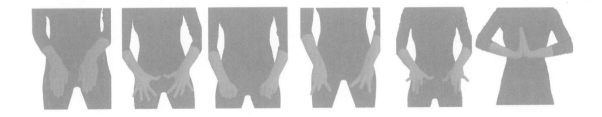

6. Arm Pumps for Pectoral Stretch, page 133.

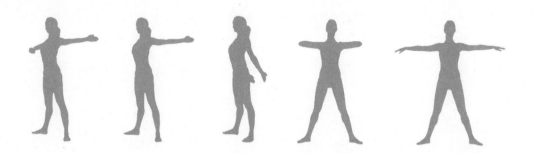

7. Rock the Baby, page 79.

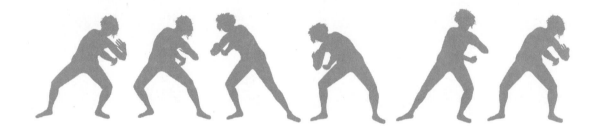

8. Single-Arm Sweeps into Celebration Arms, page 102.

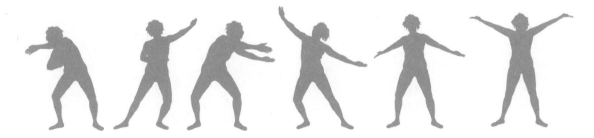

9. Spine Release—Chair, page 161.

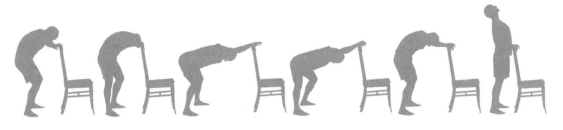

CHAPTER 13

Essentrics Routines for Chronic Pain

BACK PAIN

LENGTH: Twenty minutes

COMPONENTS: Standing, floor, chair

EQUIPMENT: Mat, chair, cushion, TheraBand or other

resistance band

Begin with two to four minutes of the

Warm-Up Routine.

1. Spine Release—Chair, page 161.

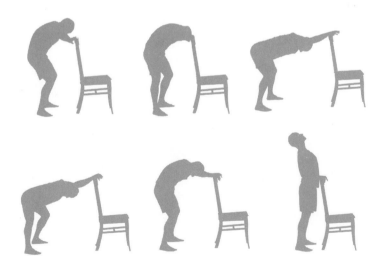

2. Wraparound Arms, page 91.

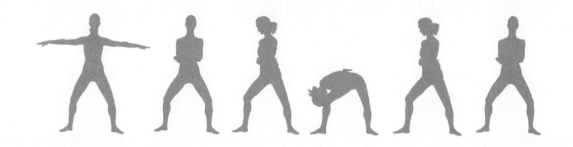

3. Remove a Sweater, page 115.

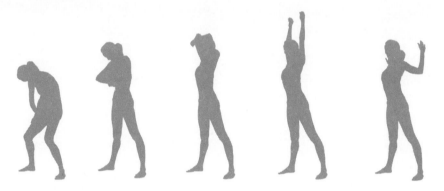

4. Open Chest Swan, page 112.

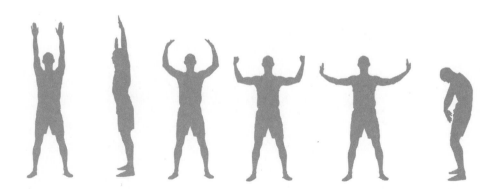

5. Arms Following the Circumference of a Beach
Ball—Ceiling to Waist, page 84.

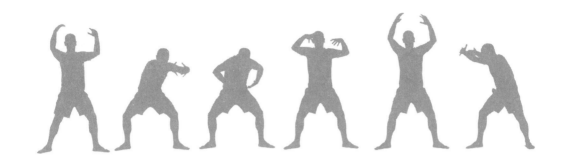

6. Four-Directional Hip Stretch—Chair, page 151.

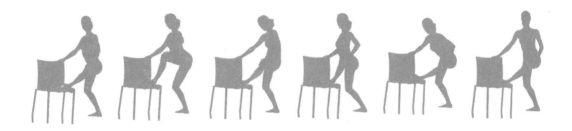

7. Preparation: Hip Flexor and Hamstring Stretch—
Chair, page 152.

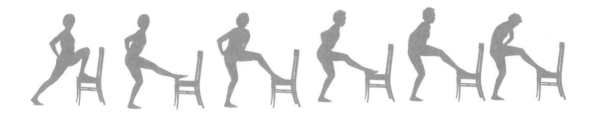

8. Baby Stretch with Deep Hip Release—Floor,
page 182.

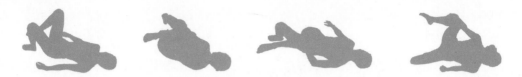

9. Deep Hamstring, Long Adductor, and IT Band
Stretch—Floor, page 183.

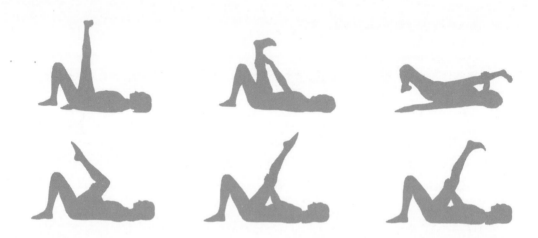

KNEE PAIN

LENGTH: Twenty-five minutes

COMPONENTS: Standing, chair

EQUIPMENT: Mat, chair

Begin with two to four minutes of the Warm-Up Routine.

1. Ankle, Calf, and Shin Stretch, page 144.

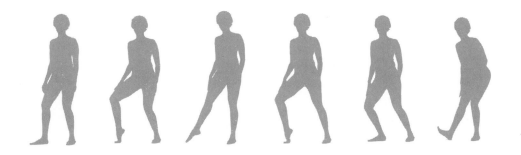

2. Calf Stretch Sequence, page 145.

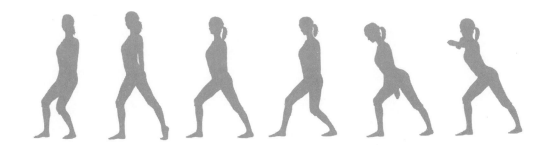

3. Musketeers Bow—IT Band and Long Adductor Stretch, page 143.

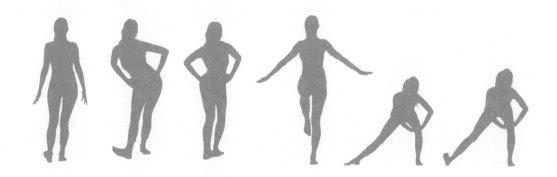

4. Pliés with Hip and Groin Stretch, page 127.

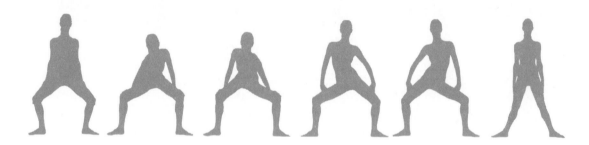

5. Hip Flexor and Hamstring Stretch—Chair, page 156.

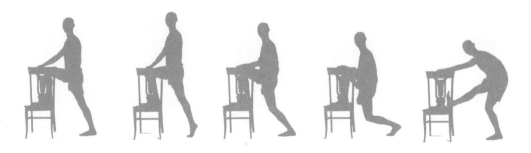

6. Inner and Outer Thigh Rotations: IT Band and
Long Adductor Stretch—Chair, page 153.

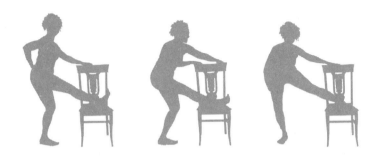

7. Shin Stretching and Strengthening—Chair,
page 147.

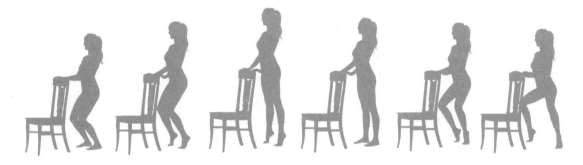

FOOT AND CALF PAIN (PLANTAR FASCIITIS AND ACHILLES TENDONITIS)

LENGTH: Twenty minutes

COMPONENTS: Standing, chair

EQUIPMENT: Mat, chair

Begin with two to four minutes of the Warm-Up Routine.

1. Zombie, page 78.

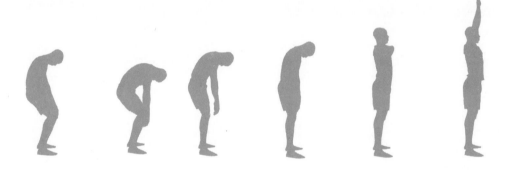

2. Open Chest Swan, page 112.

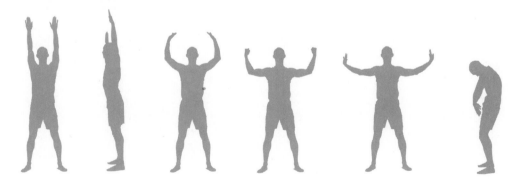

3. Push a Piano and Pull a Donkey, page 99.

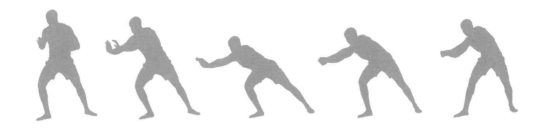

4. Deep Side Lunge Washes, page 106.

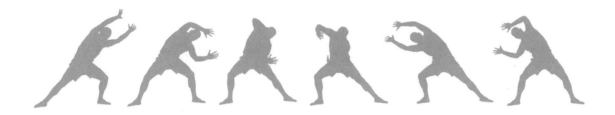

5. Calf Stretch Sequence, page 145.

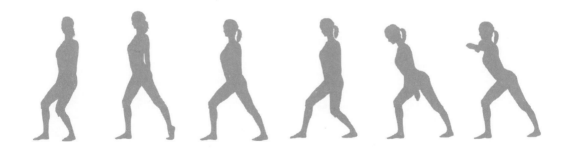

6. Fan Kicks with Lunges, page 139.

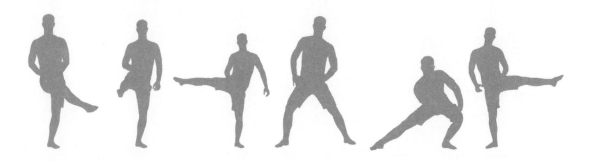

7. Ankle, Calf, and Shin Stretch, page 144.

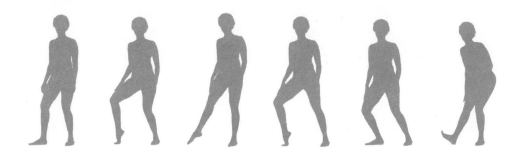

8. Hip Cleaners—Chair, page 150.

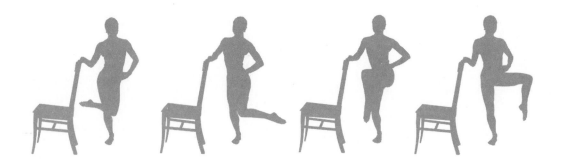

9. Shin Stretching and Strengthening—Chair,
page 147.

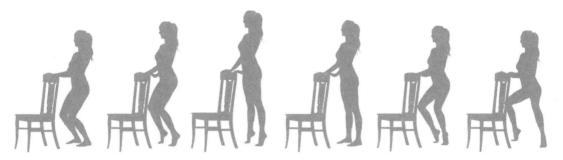

HIP PAIN

LENGTH: Twenty minutes

COMPONENTS: Standing, chair, floor

EQUIPMENT: Mat, chair, riser, cushion, TheraBand
or other resistance band

Begin with two to four minutes of the Warm-Up
Routine.

1. Wraparound Arms, page 91.

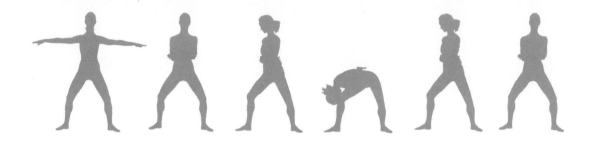

2. Fluid Spine, page 113.

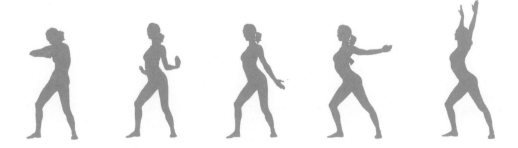

3. Pliés with Hip and Groin Stretch, page 127.

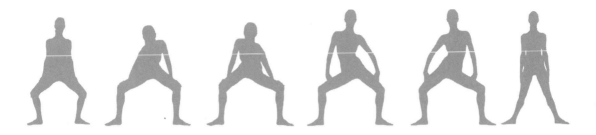

4. Lunge Hip Mobility Sequence, page 141.

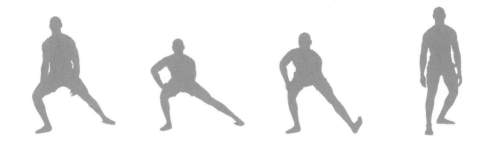

5. Preparation: Hip Flexor and Hamstring Stretch—
Chair, page 152.

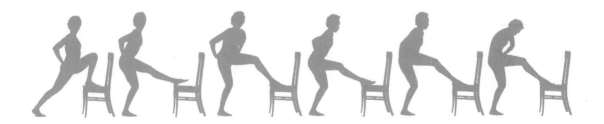

6. Butterfly with Deep Hip and Spine Stretch—Floor,
page 174.

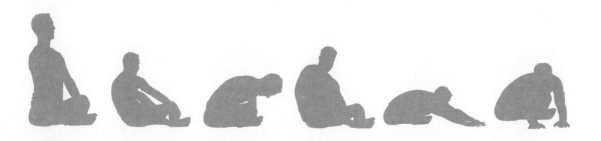

7. Abductor and Glutes Strengthening—Floor,
page 164.

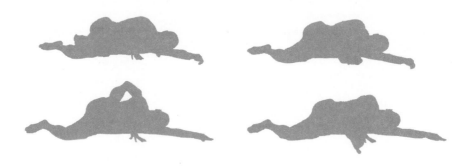

8. Baby Stretch with Deep Hip Release—Floor,
page 182.

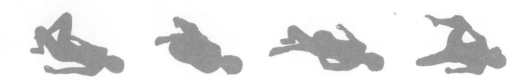

9. Deep Hamstring, Long Adductor, and IT Band
Stretch—Floor, page 183.

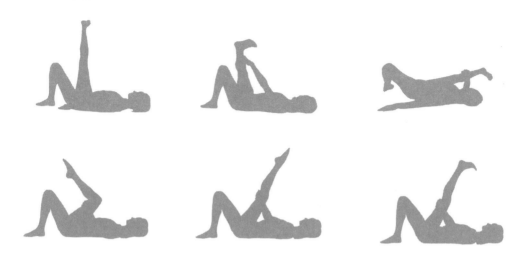

SHOULDER PAIN

LENGTH: Twenty minutes

COMPONENTS: Standing, chair

EQUIPMENT: Mat, chair

Begin with two to four minutes of the Warm-Up
Routine.

1. Double-Arm Figure Eights, page 119.

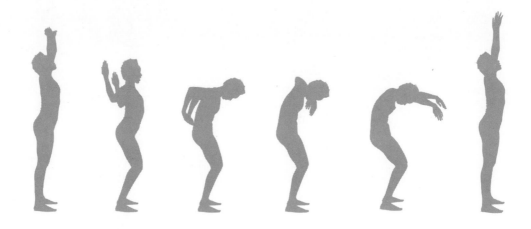

2. Shoulder Blast, page 83.

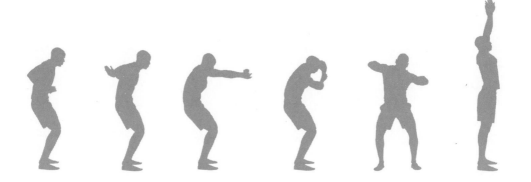

3. Waist Rotations, page 88.

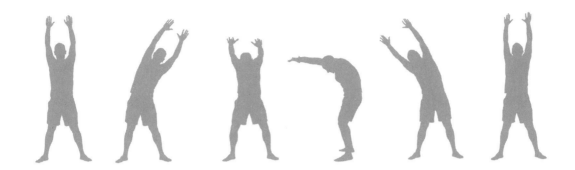

4. Simple Windmill—Feet Parallel, page 90.

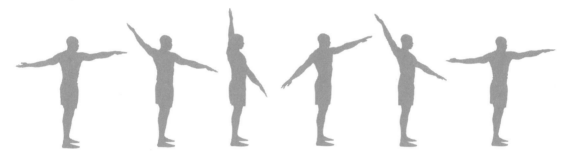

5. Lullaby and Lower a Blanket, page 80.

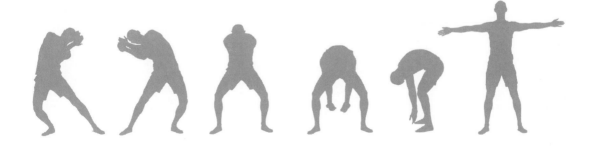

6. Small Single-Arm Figure Eights, page 117.

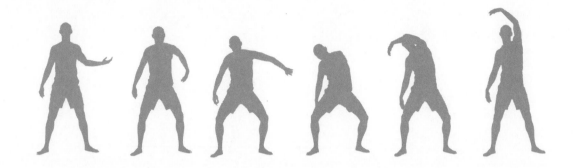

7. Double-Arm Shoulder Rotations, page 131.

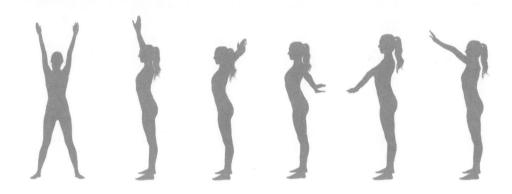

8. Spine Release—Chair, page 161.

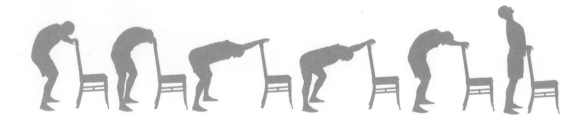

FIBROMYALGIA AND IBS

It's common for people with IBS or fibromyalgia to experience symptoms of the other condition. Both benefit from a gentle full-body routine as presented here.

LENGTH: Twenty to thirty minutes

COMPONENTS: Standing

EQUIPMENT: Mat

Begin with two to four minutes of the Warm-Up Routine.

1. Pliés with Single-Arm Half-Body Rotation, page 126.

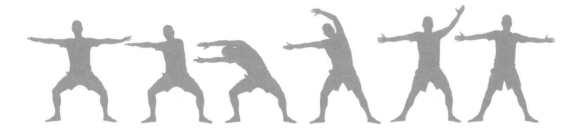

2. Ankle, Calf, and Shin Stretch, page 144.

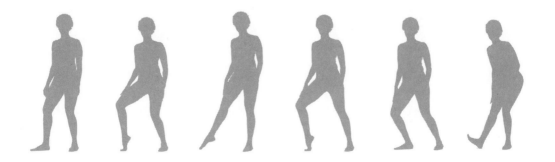

3. Hands, Fingers, and Wrists Mobility Sequence #2, page 130.

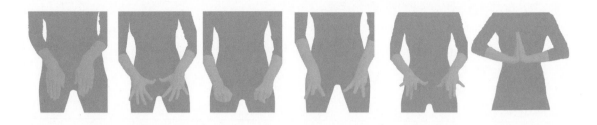

4. Arm Pumps for Pectoral Stretch, page 133.

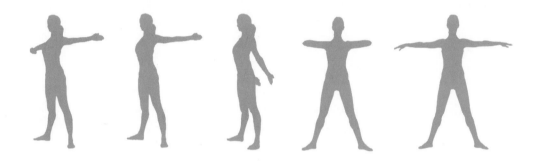

5. Fan Kicks with Lunges, page 139.

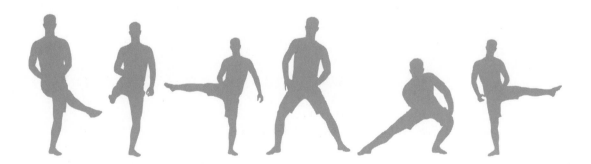

6. Double-Arm Pulling Ropes to the Floor, page 94.

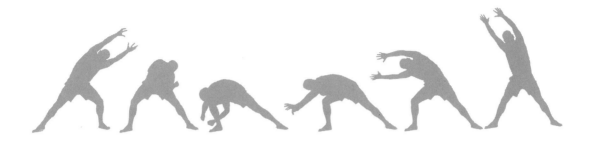

7. Washing a Small Round Table, page 89.

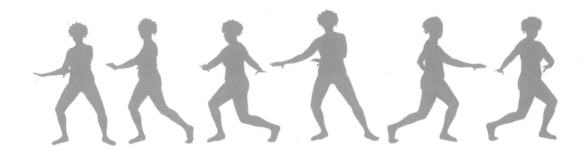

8. Low Rapid Kicks, page 136.

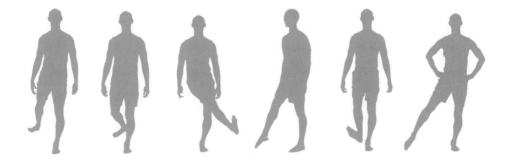

9. Calf Stretch Sequence, page 145.

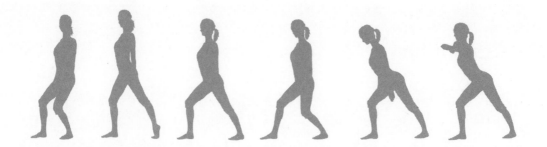

NECK PAIN

LENGTH: Ten to fifteen minutes

COMPONENTS: Standing

EQUIPMENT: Mat

Begin with two to four minutes of the Warm-Up
Routine.

1. Shoulder Blast, page 83.

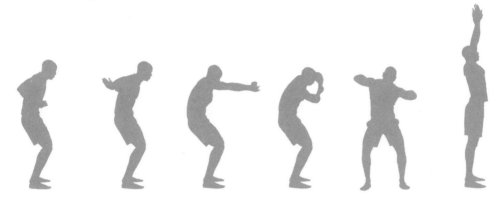

2. Embrace Yourself with Single-Arm Extensions,
page 81.

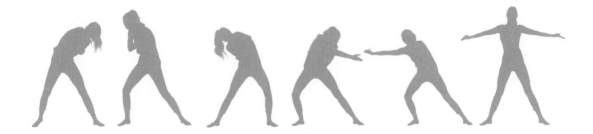

3. Small Single-Arm Figure Eights, page 117.

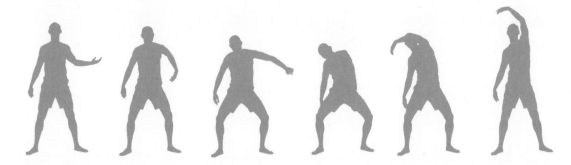

4. Wraparound Arms, page 91.

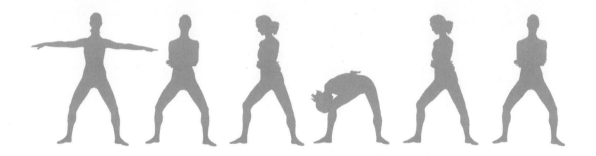

5. Swinging Both Arms Forward and Back
(Warm-Up section), page 59.

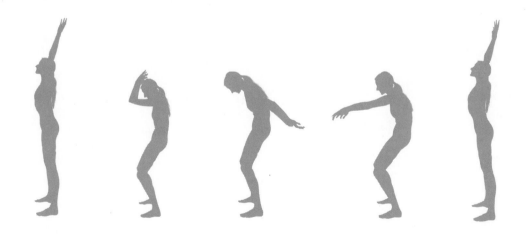

6. Tai Chi Spine Rotations (Warm-Up section), page 66.

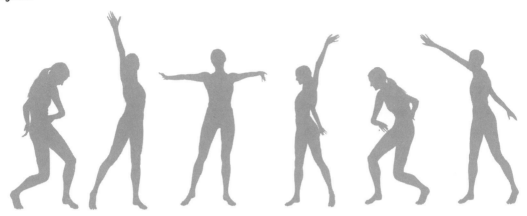

7. Double-Arm Swings, Side to Side (Warm-Up section), page 61.

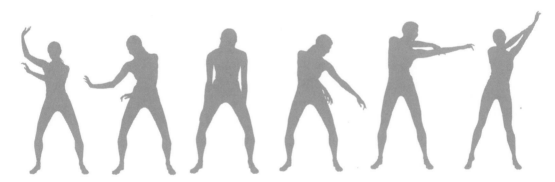

FINGER, WRIST, AND ELBOW PAIN

LENGTH: Ten to fifteen minutes

COMPONENTS: Standing

EQUIPMENT: Mat

Begin with two to four minutes of the Warm-Up
Routine.

1. Swinging Both Arms Forward and Back
(Warm-Up section), page 59.

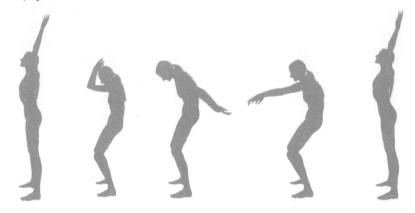

2. Double-Arm Swings, Side to Side (Warm-Up
section), page 61.

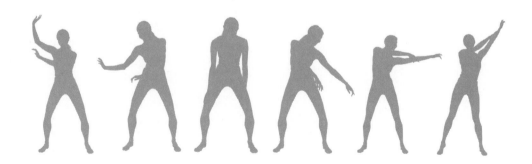

3. Double-Arm Shoulder Rotations, page 131.

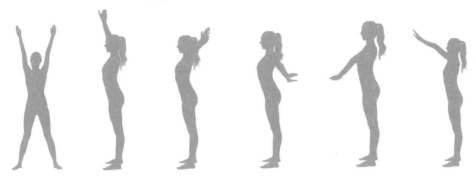

4. Hands, Fingers, and Wrists Mobility Sequence #1,
page 129.

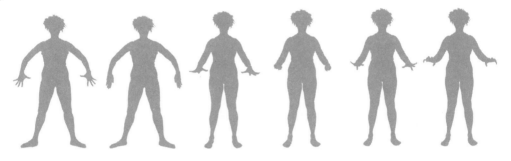

5. Hands, Fingers, and Wrists Mobility Sequence #2,
page 130.

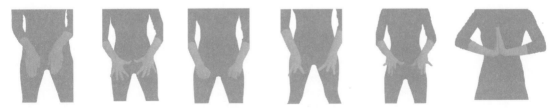

6. Arm Pumps for Shoulder Joint Liberation,
page 132.

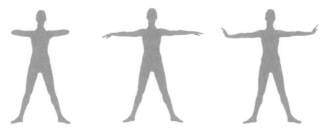

CHAPTER 14
Essentrics Routine for Better Posture

This Posture Routine is designed to stretch, strengthen, and liberate every muscle and joint in your body. It will leave you stronger, straighter, more mobile, and healthier! In order to reverse poor posture, do this routine three times a week. If you find this workout challenging, start slowly and do as many of the sequences as you can. Never force your muscles, as that is counterintuitive and often leads to inflammation and injury. Take your time, be patient—and before you know it, your posture will have improved.

Poor posture is defined by an inability to support the spine in its natural and upright position. People with poor posture tend to sink in their hips and lower back and round their shoulders and upper back. There is a spectrum to poor posture that ranges from minor issues that are easily reversible to more major concerns involving atrophied muscles that are harder to reverse.

If you can straighten your spine with ease but feel more comfortable in a slouched position, that is likely classified as minor. This level of poor posture can quickly be reversed with a few weeks to a month of doing this sixty-minute routine daily. I've seen hundreds of people rapidly reverse this minor degree of poor posture within weeks.

If you cannot straighten your spine on your own and need someone (like a therapist) to pull it straight for you, then you can assume that your muscles and fascia are in various stages of atrophy. Don't despair! In most cases, atrophy can be reversed—if not fully, then to a great deal. The only way to reverse atrophy is with daily gentle stretching and strengthening; do only thirty to sixty minutes a day, not more. Listen to your body; it will tell you when it has had enough. I've seen people push too hard and injure themselves, which only slows the process down. Don't be afraid to stop and start again tomorrow. Before you know it, you'll be well on the way toward a strong, mobile body and good posture.

THE POSTURE ROUTINE

You'll note that the Posture Routine consists of thirty-six sequences, including five warm-up sequences, fourteen standing sequences, five chair sequences, and twelve floor work sequences. Once you become familiar with these thirty-six sequences, the routine should take between fifty and sixty minutes to complete.

WARM-UP

Shoulder Rotations

1. Stand straight, arms relaxed at your sides.

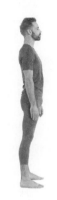

4. Roll your shoulders upward toward your ears, letting your arms move to the front of your body and keeping your spine straight. Timing: 3 seconds.

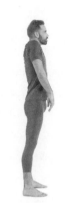

2. Roll your shoulders back and downward. Imagine that you're slipping your shoulder blades into a back pocket. Timing: 3 seconds.

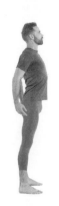

5. Relax your shoulders so that you can lift them as high as possible. Timing: 3 seconds.

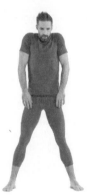

3. Roll your shoulders upward as high as possible, keeping your arms behind your body.

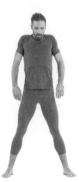

6. Roll your shoulders downward and backward to start another rotation. Timing: 3 seconds. Repeat two times in each direction. Timing for each full shoulder rotation: 12 seconds.

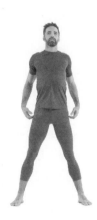

Single-Arm Swings

1. Bend slightly sideways and swing your arm down toward the floor and up to the other side. Bend one knee and extend the other leg, getting ready to shift your weight onto it.

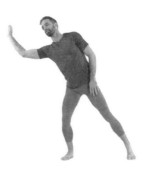

4. Let your arm swing right up to the diagonal corner. Timing: 2 seconds for half of one swing.

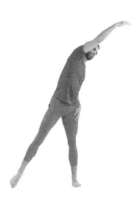

2. Shift your weight onto your extended leg, swing your arm downward, and bend forward.

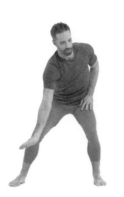

5. Return to the starting side and repeat.

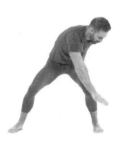

3. Shift your weight onto your other leg while swinging your arm up to the other side.

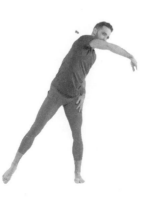

6. Timing for one cycle: 4 seconds. Repeat on the other side.

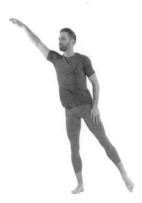

Relaxed Washes

1. For this exercise, imagine that you're sweeping away a cloud or moving your arms through warm water. Sweep from side to side at shoulder height. Repeat for four to eight sweeps. Timing: 1 second per sweep.

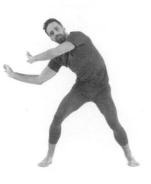

2. Sweep down toward the floor and then up the other side.

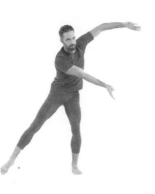

3. Sweep your arms toward the floor. Repeat four to eight times. Timing: 1 second per sweep.

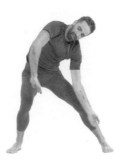

4. Imagine you're sweeping your fingers across the ceiling.

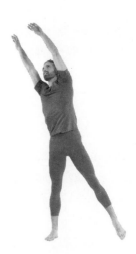

5. Move your arms from side to side above your head.

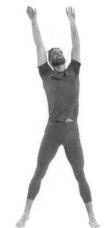

6. Repeat four to eight times. Timing: 1 second per sweep.

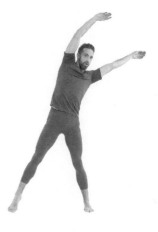

Full-Body Diagonal Reaches

1. Stand with your knees bent, feet apart, and arms bent at shoulder height.

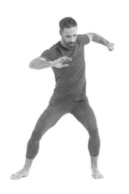

2. Rapidly twist your torso, reaching one arm on a diagonal toward the upper corner of the room and shifting your weight onto your front leg while pointing your back foot. Timing: 2 seconds.

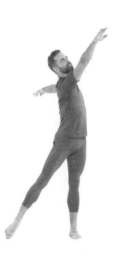

3. Return to your starting position. Timing: 2 seconds. Repeat the high diagonal reach four times in one direction and four times in the other direction. Timing for the full sequence: 16 seconds.

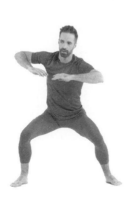

4. Repeat the diagonal reach at shoulder height four times on each side. Timing for the full sequence: 16 seconds.

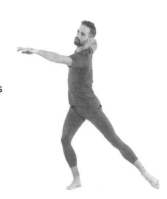

5. Preparation for diagonal reaches toward the corner of the floor.

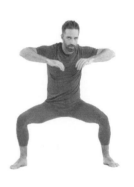

6. Repeat the diagonal reach toward the floor four times on each side. Timing for the full sequence: 16 seconds. Timing for all three heights: 48 seconds.

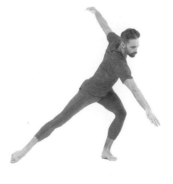

Knee Kicks while Twisting

1. Rapidly lift one knee across your body, bending your standing leg, and gently slap your knee and hip with your hands. Timing: 1 second.

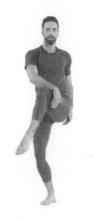

4. Kick one leg straight in a diagonal across your body while twisting your spine and hitting your hips. Timing: 1 second.

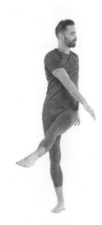

2. Return to this neutral position—feet apart and arms to your sides—between each lift. Timing: ½ second.

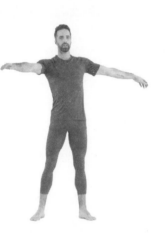

5. Return to this position between each kick: arms relaxed above your head and knees bent. Timing: ½ second.

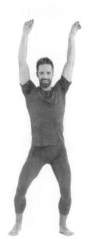

3. Repeat for four kicks on each side.

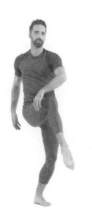

6. Repeat for four kicks on each side.

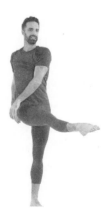

STANDING

Zombie and Open Chest Swan

1. Tuck your tailbone under, round your upper back, and drop your head so your neck is hanging. Slowly roll down your spine with your hands touching your thighs until they pass over your knees. Sway from side to side to relax your spine. Timing: 8 seconds.

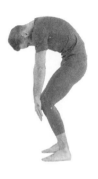

4. Keep your spine straight, and don't arch your back. Bend your elbows and pull them behind your shoulders. Timing: 3 seconds.

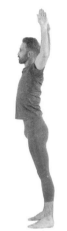

2. Slowly roll up, one vertebra at a time, with your hands touching the front of your body. Timing: 4 seconds.

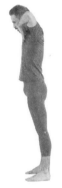

5. Straighten your elbows. Timing: 3 seconds.

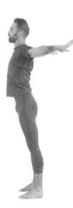

3. Raise your arms above your head, keeping them beside your ears. Relax your shoulders and lift your arms higher. Timing: 4 seconds.

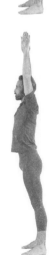

6. Lower your arms and get ready to repeat the sequence. Timing: 1 second. Total timing for the sequence: 23 seconds.

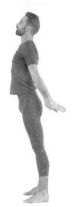

Ceiling Reaches with Overextensions

1. Stand straight with your feet apart and your arms straight and beside your ears.

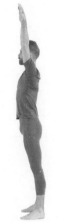

4. Don't let your upper back arch while you try to stretch the shoulder joint as you pull your arm. Timing: 6 seconds.

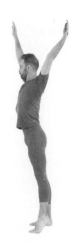

2. Reach toward the ceiling with one arm by relaxing your shoulders and back muscles. Let your shoulders lift as much as possible. Timing: 8 seconds.

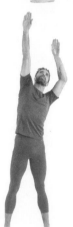

5. Repeat the stretch with your other arm. Timing: 6 seconds. Timing for the full sequence: 30 seconds.

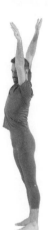

3. Repeat with the other arm. Timing: 8 seconds.

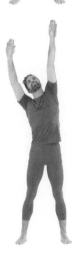

Waist Rotations

1. Stand with your feet comfortably apart and your arms held straight above your head.

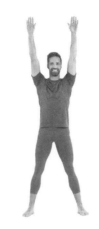

4. Keep rotating to the other side. Timing: 6 seconds.

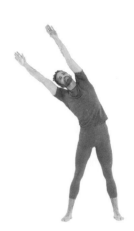

2. Reach toward the ceiling, relaxing your shoulders and letting them lift as much as they can. Pull your torso away from your hips as you bend sideways. Timing: 6 seconds.

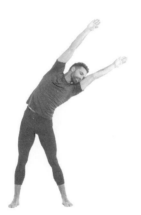

5. Keep rotating toward the front, bending your knees. Timing: 6 seconds. Timing for the full rotation: 24 seconds. Repeat in the other direction.

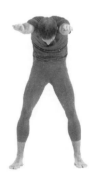

3. Arch from the waist upward and rotate your body toward the back of the room. Timing: 6 seconds.

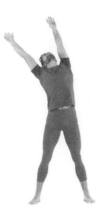

6. When arching backward, keep your lower spine lifted. Don't sink into your vertebrae.

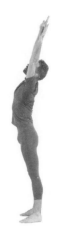

Full-Body Lift: Heavy Weights

1. Imagine that you're lifting heavy weights from the floor up over your head. Stand with your legs apart in a deep plié. Round your back and contract your muscles, preparing to lift the weights.

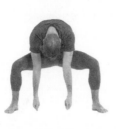

4. Bend your knees and flip your hands as if readying them to lift the weights. Timing: 2 seconds.

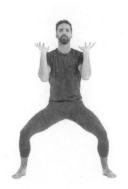

2. Lift the weights close to your body, straightening your legs as you do so. Timing: 4 seconds.

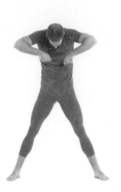

5. Contract all your back muscles and slowly lift the weights. Timing: 4 seconds.

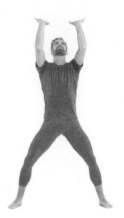

3. Perform a shoulder joint rotation to straighten your spine and prepare to engage your shoulder muscles in the lift. Timing: 3 seconds.

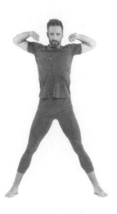

6. Release the imaginary weights, relax your back and arm muscles, straighten your knees, and stretch your arms as high as possible toward the ceiling. Timing: 4 seconds. Timing of the full sequence: 17 seconds. Repeat two times.

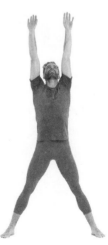

Full-Body Figure Eights

1. In this sequence, you'll be drawing a large figure eight with your arm. Stand in a front lunge with your back arm raised, and rotate the arm within the shoulder socket.

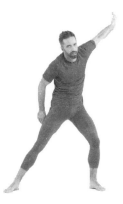

2. Sweep your arm in a large circle toward the floor. Timing: 3 seconds.

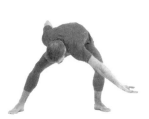

3. Continue sweeping the floor as you shift your lunge onto your other leg. Timing: 3 seconds.

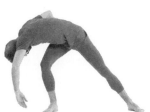

4. Follow the circumference of the circle upward. Timing: 3 seconds.

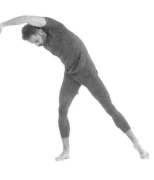

5. When you reach the top, shift your weight onto your other leg and rotate toward the back. Timing: 3 seconds.

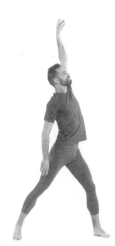

6. Draw the other half of the figure eight behind your body. Twist completely to face the back of the room and bend your back knee, raising your heel to facilitate the rotation. Timing of the full sequence: 12 seconds. Repeat on the other side.

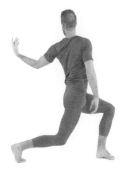

Shin and Ankle Flexibility

1. Stand with your feet apart and put one foot in front of the other. Bend your knees and sit on your back heel, putting pressure on the heel. Timing: 6 seconds.

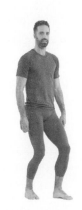

4. Flex your toes. Timing: 2 to 4 seconds.

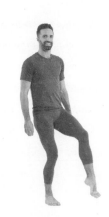

2. Lift the heel of your front leg, leaving your toes on the floor. This will stretch the shin, arch, and toe muscles. Timing: 4 seconds.

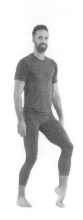

5. Flex the entire foot and ankle, feeling the stretch in your calves. Timing: 2 to 4 seconds. Timing for the full sequence: 20 seconds. Repeat the sequence four times.

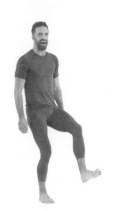

3. Lift your foot off the floor while pointing your toes. Timing: 2 seconds.

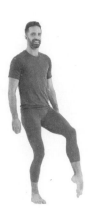

6. Place your feet flat on the floor and straighten both knees. Repeat the complete sequence on the other side.

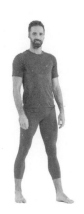

Calf Stretch Sequence

1. Stand with one leg in front of the other, with both knees bent and your back straight. Imagine that you're sitting on your back heel. Timing: 6 seconds.

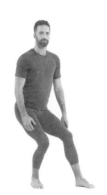

4. Bend your back knee, lift your back heel, and tuck your tailbone under. Timing: 2 seconds.

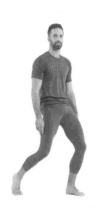

2. Shift your weight forward, straightening your back knee and lifting your heel. Timing: 2 seconds.

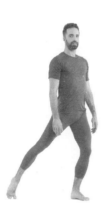

5. Slowly try to put your heel flat on the floor while continuing to tuck your tailbone under. Keep your weight over your front leg. Timing: 8 seconds.

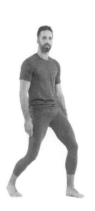

3. Very slowly lower your back heel to the floor, making sure that it's flat on the floor. Timing: 8 seconds.

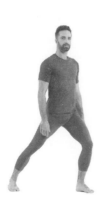

6. Keep your tailbone tucked under and slowly lower your knee toward the floor. The moment you reach your maximum stretch, begin to straighten slowly. Don't stay at the bottom and hold. Timing: 10 seconds. Timing for the full sequence: 36 seconds.

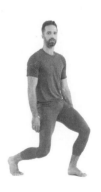

Musketeers Bow—IT Band and Long Adductor Stretch

1. Extend one leg in front, foot flexed, and bend forward from your hips with your hands on your thighs. Timing: 3 seconds.

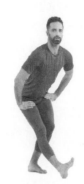

4. Slide your leg to the side and place your foot flat on the floor.

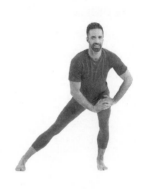

2. Rotate your leg from the hip, turning your leg out while trying to place the outside of your foot on the floor. Timing: 3 seconds.

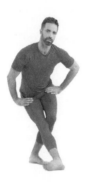

5. Turn your foot out and swing your hips toward the back corner of the room.

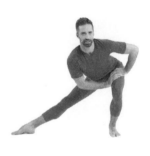

3. Reverse the hip rotation by turning your leg in and trying to put the inside of your foot on the floor. Timing: 3 seconds. Repeat the first three steps twice. Total timing: 18 seconds.

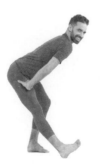

6. Turn your foot back in and stand up straight. Repeat the foot-twisting sequence three times. Timing: 3 seconds per move. Total timing: 18 seconds. Repeat on the other side.

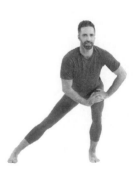

Fluid Spine with Arms

1. Stand with one foot in front of the other in a crunch position. Bend both knees, bend your head, and tuck your elbows in close to your body. Timing: 4 seconds.

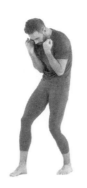

4. Reverse the crunch and rapidly open your arms at shoulder height behind you. Timing: 4 seconds. Repeat three times. Timing for the full sequence: 24 seconds.

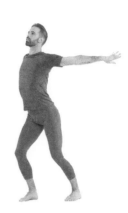

2. Keep your knees bent and arch your upper back while sticking out your buttocks. Shoot your arms down and behind your hips. Timing: 4 seconds. Repeat three times. Timing for the full sequence: 24 seconds. Repeat on the other side.

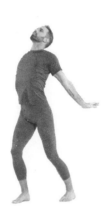

5. Return to the crunch position with your arms tucked in. Timing: 4 seconds.

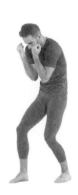

3. Crunch your spine and bend your elbows at shoulder height. Timing: 4 seconds.

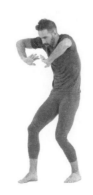

6. Reverse the crunch while rapidly shooting your arms above your head and slightly behind your shoulders. Timing: 4 seconds. Repeat three times. Timing for the full sequence: 24 seconds.

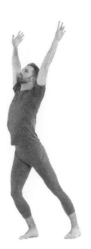

Fluid Spine with Hip Rotation

1. This exercise will loosen the ball-and-socket joint of the hip. Use only your lower back, and don't shift your weight from side to side. Stand with your feet slightly apart, knees bent, tailbone tucked under.

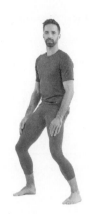

4. Push your buttocks and hips back, arching your lower spine. Timing: 3 seconds.

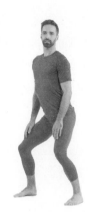

2. Side view.

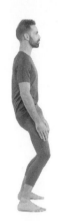

5. Side view of the tuck under. Shift your weight to the other hip and return to the tucked-under position.

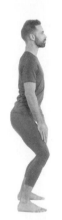

3. Rotate your hips as far as possible to one side. Timing: 3 seconds.

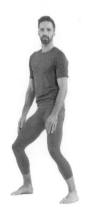

6. Make two complete hip rotations in each direction: buttocks forward, hips to one side, buttocks back, hips to the other side. Timing: 10 to 12 seconds per rotation.

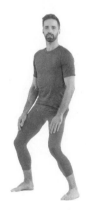

Pliés with Arm Pulls and Presses

1. Stand with your feet comfortably apart, arms above your head and spine straight.

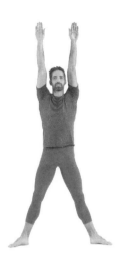

2. Make sure your feet are flat on the floor, not everting or inverting. Bend your knees, keeping them over the arches of your feet. Imagine that you're pulling a stiff elastic down from the ceiling with one hand. Timing: 3 seconds.

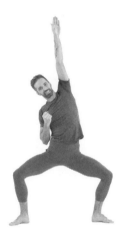

3. Pull your other arm down. Timing: 3 seconds.

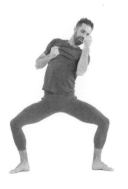

4. Using one arm at a time, push the elastic to the floor, bending your knees. Timing: 3 seconds per arm.

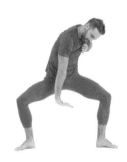

5. Bend forward to touch the floor while lowering your head. Timing: 3 seconds.

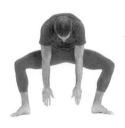

6. Roll up, opening your arms to the side and remaining in a deep plié. Timing: 3 seconds. Timing for the full sequence: 15 seconds. Repeat four times.

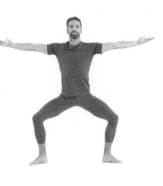

Side Lunges with Arms

1. Stand in a wide, deep plié with your arms across your chest and your hands in fists.

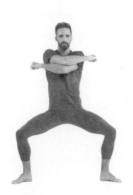

4. Explode into a deep side lunge with your hands in an open flex. Timing: 2 seconds.

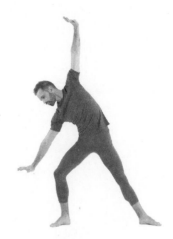

2. Imagine that you're pulling apart a tight strap that's locking your arms in a shortened position. Timing: 2 seconds.

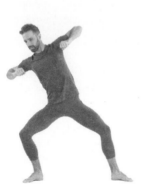

5. Return to your starting position. Timing: 2 seconds. Repeat four times on each side. Timing for the full sequence: 7 to 8 seconds.

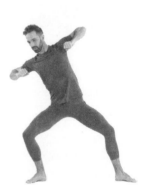

3. Return to your starting position. Timing: 2 seconds.

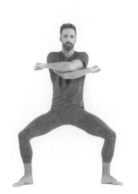

Full-Body Pulling a Cement Ball

1. Stand in a side lunge and imagine that you're holding a cement ball with both hands.

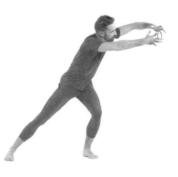

4. Keep pressing the ball toward the floor. Timing: 6 seconds.

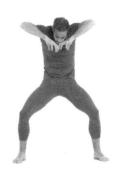

2. Shift your body toward the center and round your upper back as you slowly pull the cement ball toward your middle line. Timing: 6 seconds.

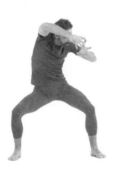

5. Relax at the bottom and prepare to roll up one vertebra at a time. Timing: 3 seconds.

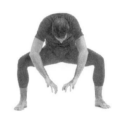

3. Straighten your spine, readjust your arms, and prepare to force the cement ball toward the floor. Imagine you're pushing against a major force as you press the heavy ball downward.

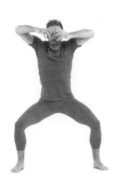

6. Start pushing the cement ball away from your body. Timing: 3 seconds. Total timing for one sequence: 18 to 20 seconds.

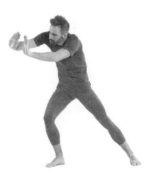

Full-Body Windmill

1. Stand in a wide front lunge with your knees straight. Prepare your arms to do a windmill with one arm stretched to the ceiling and the other to the floor.

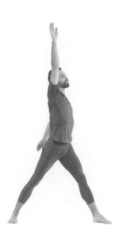

4. Continue in the windmill with one arm sweeping back and the other over your head, keeping your torso and legs straight. Timing: 3 seconds.

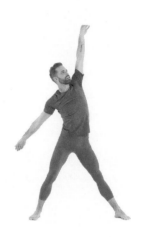

2. Start the windmill movement with your arms. Twist your torso and bend toward the corner of the room. Timing: 4 seconds.

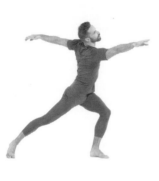

5. You will now have your other arm in front and your legs in a deep lunge, ready to perform a windmill with the other arm. Timing: 3 seconds.

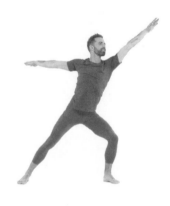

3. Keep your arms moving like the blades of a windmill and sweep them to touch the floor. Balance your weight between your legs. Timing: 3 seconds.

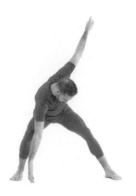

6. Repeat the windmill with the other arm, keeping the same leg in front. Timing: 13 seconds for the full sequence. Repeat, beginning with the other arm.

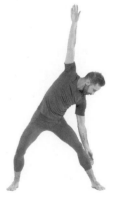

CHAIR/BARRE

Fondu with Kicks

1. Hold the back of a chair. Bend both knees and lift one foot off the floor, toe pointed.

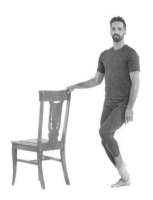

2. Rapidly straighten both legs. Timing: ½ second.

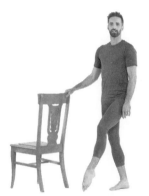

3. Lift the heel of the standing leg. Timing: ½ second.

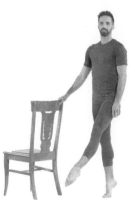

4. Slowly land in a controlled front lunge. Try to touch the floor with your back knee. Keep your back straight while you shift your weight forward in the lunge. Timing: 2 seconds.

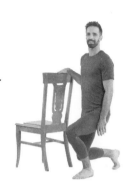

5. Rebound from the lunge, straightening your front leg. Timing: ½ second.

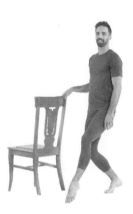

6. Kick your front leg as high as possible, isolating the leg in the hip joint and keeping your back straight. Return to your starting position. Timing: 2 seconds. Timing for the full sequence: 5½ to 7 seconds. Repeat eight times, then repeat the entire sequence on the other leg.

1. Exercise 1: Hold the back of the chair. Start with your feet together, knees bent.

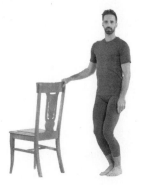

4. Exercise 2: Hold the back of the chair. Start with your feet together. Kick your outside leg to the side, straightening both legs. Timing: 1 second.

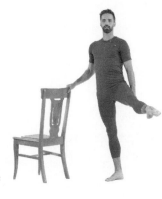

2. Slide your outside leg in front. Keep your foot flat on the floor until your knee straightens and your toes point. Isolate the leg in your hip joint and keep your back straight.

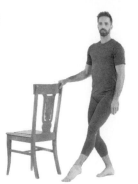

5. Do a controlled fall into a side lunge. Timing: 2 seconds.

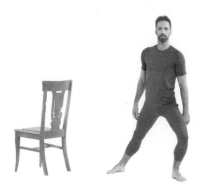

3. Kick your leg without moving your hips or back. Slide your leg to return to the starting position. Repeat eight times. Timing: 2 seconds per kick. Timing for eight kicks: 16 seconds. Repeat on the other side.

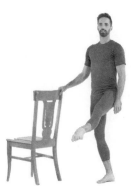

6. Bend both knees and slide your bent leg back into your starting position. Timing: 1 second. Timing for eight kicks into lunges: 32 seconds. Repeat on the other side.

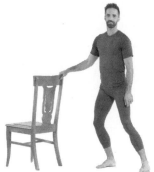

Hip Stretch

1. Stand with your outside leg on the chair and bend your knee.

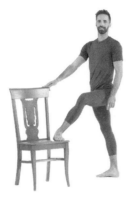

4. Rock your weight forward until it's all on the chair. Timing: 4 seconds.

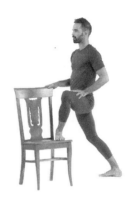

2. Lift your hip. Timing: 4 seconds.

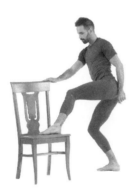

5. Rock your weight back, rounding your spine while bending both knees. Timing: 4 seconds. Repeat two times. Total timing: 16 seconds.

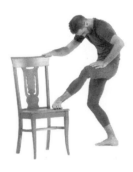

3. Lower your hip. Timing: 4 seconds. Repeat four times. Timing for four hip shifts: 32 seconds.

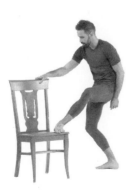

6. Straighten your spine and change legs. Timing: 1 second. Timing for the full sequence: 40 seconds. Repeat the sequence on the other side.

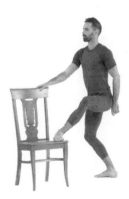

Windmills for Hamstrings

1. Stand with your outside leg on the seat of the chair and bend your standing leg. Keep your back straight and lift your arm straight above your head.

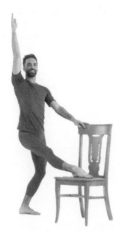

2. Start by reaching as far as you can over your extended leg, as in a windmill rotation. Keep your back as straight as possible. Timing: 5 seconds.

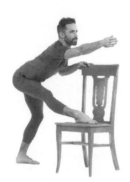

3. Continue the windmill rotation, sweeping your arm toward the floor and trying to lie flat on your front leg. Try to touch the floor with your fingers. Timing: 5 seconds.

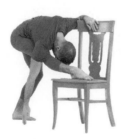

4. Continue the rotation, twisting your spine and sweeping your arm toward the back of the room. Timing: 5 seconds.

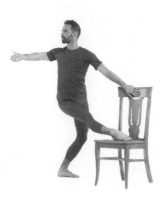

5. Continue the windmill rotation by slowly sweeping your arm above your head. Timing: 5 seconds. Timing for one complete rotation: 20 seconds.

Repeat the sequence on the other side.

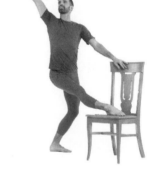

Sweeping over Leg

1. Place the leg closest to the back of the chair on the seat. Reach out and imagine that you're slowly, gently wiping the air with your hand, trying to feel the air going through your fingers.

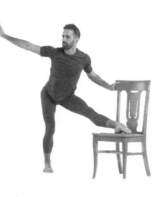

4. Continue wiping the air as you rotate your torso as much as possible. Timing: 7 seconds.

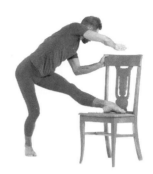

2. Let your torso bend and flow gently forward as you slowly wipe through the air.

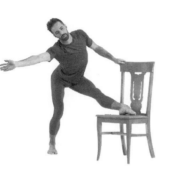

5. Flip your hand so that you can feel the air flowing through your fingers as you reverse the rotation.

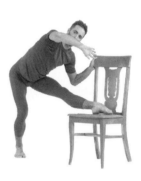

3. Continue wiping the air over your leg.

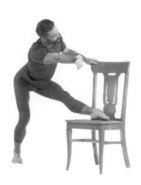

6. Let your body bend and flow throughout this sequence. Timing: 7 seconds. Timing for the full sequence: 14 seconds. Change legs and repeat the sequence.

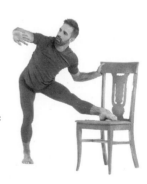

FLOOR WORK

Butterfly Stretch for Hips

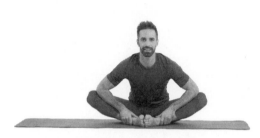

1. Sit with your feet together, bend forward, hold your shins, and place your elbows on your knees. Continue to bend forward gently, using your elbows to push down on your knees. Timing: 8 seconds.

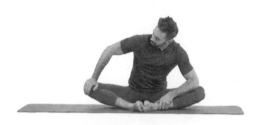

2. Prevent one knee from moving with your elbow. Use the other hand to push your free knee toward the floor in a hip stretch. Timing: 8 seconds.

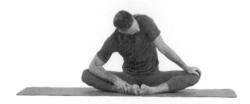

3. Repeat on the other side. Timing: 8 seconds.

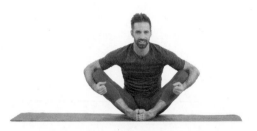

4. Lift both knees high enough to embrace them with your arms. Once you're holding your knees, try to force them open without actually letting them open. This is PNF, a neurological technique used to build tension in the hips. Press for 5 seconds.

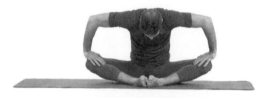

5. Let go of your knees and release them. Breathe slowly and consciously and relax your hips. Push both knees down with your hands to stretch your hips. Timing: 6 seconds. Timing of the full sequence: 35 seconds.

Butterfly for Spine Strength

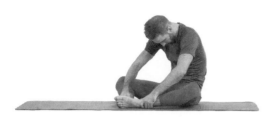

1. Sit with your feet together and, holding both shins, pull away with your arms, dropping your head forward while rounding your spine. Timing: 6 seconds.

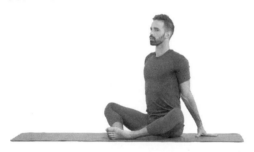

2. Place your hands behind your hips to aid in fully straightening your spine. Timing: 5 seconds.

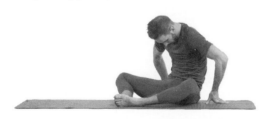

3. Round your spine, still supporting your weight with your hands on the floor. Timing: 5 seconds.

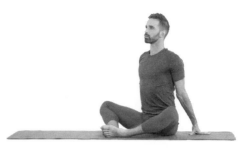

4. Roll up one vertebra at a time and hold your spine straight. Try to let your fingers just touch the floor. Timing: 5 seconds.

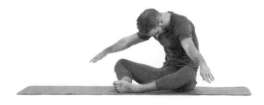

5. Round your spine again and extend your arms to the side. Timing: 5 seconds.

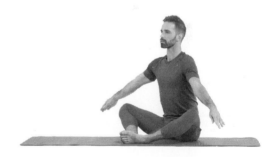

6. Roll up, straightening your spine, and, using only the muscles of the spine, keep your arms extended to the side. Timing: 6 seconds. Timing for the full sequence: 32 seconds.

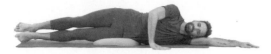

1. Lie on your side. Rest your head on your lower arm and set your other arm as a brace in front of your chest. For better positioning of your legs, use a hemorrhoid cushion under your hips.

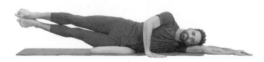

2. Hold your ankles together and raise and lower your legs. Timing: 1 second for each raising and lowering. Repeat eight to sixteen times.

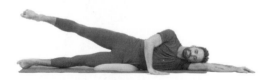

3. Scissor your legs by holding your top leg in place and rapidly lifting your lower leg to join your upper leg. Timing: 1 second for each raising and lowering. Repeat eight to sixteen times.

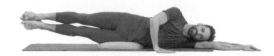

4. Hold your heels together and lift and lower your legs eight times. Timing: 1 second for each raising and lowering.

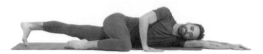

5. Cross your top leg over your lower leg and place your knee on the floor. This will make your body drop forward slightly.

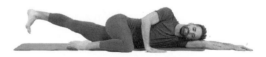

6. Lift your lower leg eight times. Timing: 1 second for each raising and lowering. Turn onto your other side and repeat.

Sit-Ups

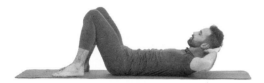

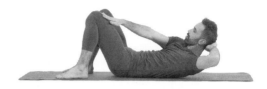

1. These are not rapid sit-ups. Lie flat on the floor with your arms bent behind your head and your hands touching but not supporting your head. Use only your abdominal muscles to lift your shoulders and upper back. Keep your elbows pointing to the side. Take 2 to 3 seconds per sit-up. Repeat eight to sixteen times.

3. Extend your arm and try to touch the opposite knee with each sit-up. Repeat eight times per arm, taking 2 to 3 seconds per sit-up.

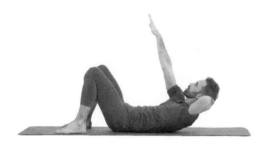

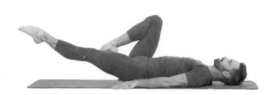

2. Extend one arm and try to touch the ceiling with each sit-up. Repeat eight times per arm, taking 2 to 3 seconds per sit-up.

4. Bicycle your legs slowly, finishing each rotation with your leg fully extended and your toes pointed. Repeat eight to sixteen times, taking 2 to 3 seconds per bicycle.

Baby Stretch for Hips and Lower Back

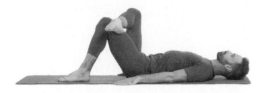

1. Lie on your back and bend one leg, keeping your foot flat on the floor. Cross your other leg over your bent leg, resting your ankle on the thigh of the other leg.

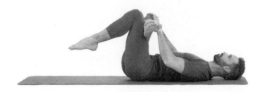

4. Keep shifting your hips, sliding them toward and away from your shoulders. Don't lift your hips off the floor. Repeat four times. Total timing for four shifts: 16 seconds.

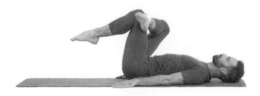

2. Lift your lower leg off the floor. Timing: 8 seconds.

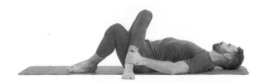

5. Slowly move your foot across your torso and try to place it on the floor. Timing: 10 seconds. Timing for the full sequence: 36 to 40 seconds.

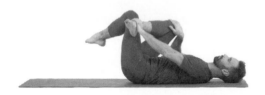

3. Shift your hips, sliding them toward and away from your shoulders. Don't lift your hips off the floor. Timing: 3 seconds per side.

Supine: Hamstrings

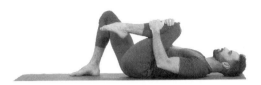

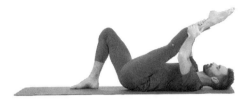

1. Lie flat on the floor and bend one leg, keeping your foot flat on the floor. Bring your other knee as close to your chest as possible. Wiggle your hips six times to relax your glutes. Timing: 6 to 8 seconds.

4. Repeat again, trying to pull your leg even closer to your chest, with your foot pointed. Timing: 6 to 8 seconds.

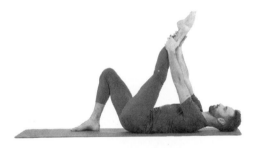

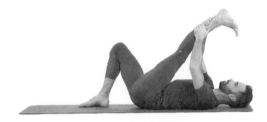

2. Hold your leg with your hands or a resistance band and slowly pull it toward your chest with your foot pointed. Timing: 6 to 8 seconds.

5. Repeat with your foot flexed. Timing: 6 to 8 seconds.

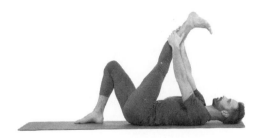

3. Repeat with your foot flexed. Timing: 6 to 8 seconds.

Supine Long Adductor and IT Band Stretch

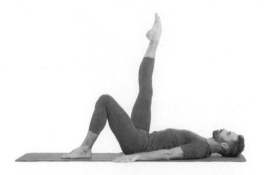

1. Lie flat on your back and bend one leg, keeping your foot flat on the floor. Lift your other leg, keeping it straight and pointing your toes.

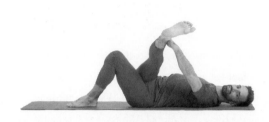

4. Drop your leg across your torso and, using your other arm, try to pull your leg farther across your body. Timing: 6 to 8 seconds.

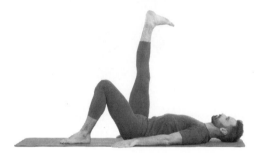

2. Flex and point your foot. Repeat four times. Timing: 4 seconds.

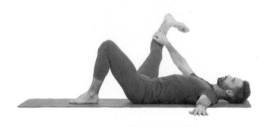

5. Open your leg to the other side, using the arm on the same side to deepen the stretch. Repeat the sequence on the other side.

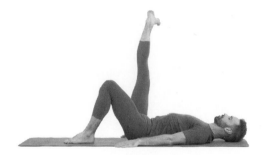

3. Rotate your leg within the hip joint, turning it out and in several times. Timing: 2 seconds per rotation.

Superman for Spine

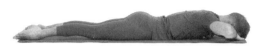

1. Lie on your stomach with your elbows open and your hands under your forehead.

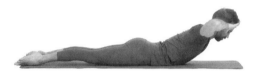

2. Slowly and carefully lift your shoulders as high as you can. Hold for 2 seconds. With control, slowly lower yourself back down to the floor. Timing: 6 seconds. Repeat four times.

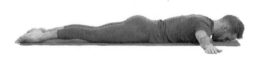

3. Stretch your arms out to the side in line with your shoulders.

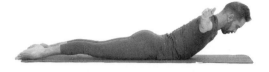

4. Slowly and with complete control lift your upper back. Hold for 2 seconds, then lower yourself to the floor. Repeat two to four times.

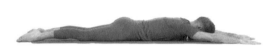

5. Stretch your arms above your head.

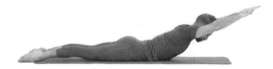

6. Slowly and with complete control lift your upper back. Hold for 2 seconds, then lower yourself to the floor. Repeat two to four times.

Superman for Psoas

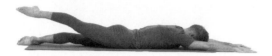

1. Lie on your stomach with your arms stretched out in front. Lift one leg and hold it for 3 seconds, then lower the leg and relax your glutes and back muscles for 3 seconds before lifting your other leg.

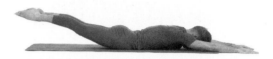

3. Lift both legs together and hold for 3 seconds. Lower your legs and relax your back and glutes for 3 seconds before lifting your legs again. Repeat two times. Total timing for three leg lifts: 25 seconds.

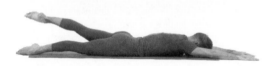

2. Repeat three times, alternating legs and relaxing between each leg lift. Total timing: 30 seconds.

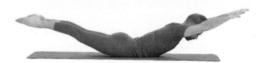

4. Lift both legs and your back simultaneously. Hold for 3 seconds, then lower your legs and back and completely relax your entire body for 6 seconds. Repeat two times. Total timing for three lifts: 30 seconds.

Cat-Cow

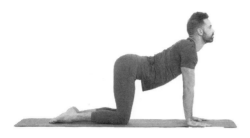

1. Get down on your hands and knees. Your hands should be in line with your shoulders. Try to lengthen your shins and loosen your ankles by flattening the arches of your feet on the floor. Drop your spine into a swayback position. Timing: 5 seconds.

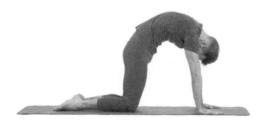

2. Arch your spine as much as possible, like an angry cat. Timing: 5 seconds. Repeat twice.

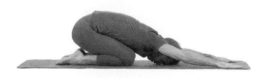

3. Try to sit on your heels while laying your torso flat on your thighs. Elongate your arms in front. Timing: 5 seconds.

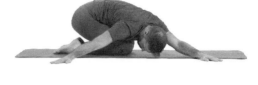

4. Walk your hands around to wrap your arms around one side of your legs.

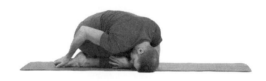

5. Wrap your arms around one side. Timing: 8 seconds. Repeat on the other side.

Seated Hip Stretch with Front Leg Extended

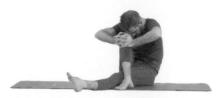

1. Sit on the floor and extend one leg in front of you. Cross your other leg over the extended leg, foot flat on the floor. Hold your knee with both hands. Bend your elbows, lifting them upward, place your forehead on your knee, and pull away from your knee with a rounded back. Timing: 6 seconds.

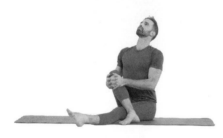

2. Straighten your spine and bring your elbows in close to your body. Pull your chest toward your knee and lift your head, being careful not to drop your head back. Timing: 5 seconds.

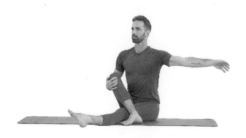

3. Bring your head back. Hold your knee with the arm on the same side and open your other arm to the side. Timing: 1 second.

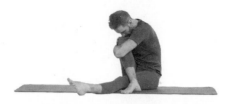

4. Embrace your knee with the opposite arm and pull your knee toward your chest. Bring your head to your knee. Timing: 6 seconds.

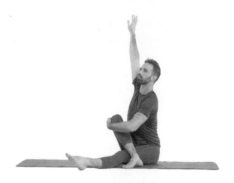

5. Raise your head and the arm on the same side as your bent knee. Keep pulling your knee toward your chest. Timing: 2 seconds.

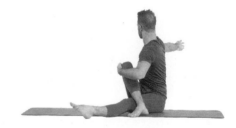

6. Lower your extended arm while twisting your spine toward the back of the room. Use your arm to assist in the rotation. Timing: 6 seconds. Timing of the full sequence: 26 to 30 seconds.

Seated Side Bends for Strength and Hamstring Flexibility

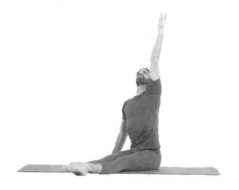

1. Sit on the floor with your legs extended in front, toes pointed. Raise one arm above your head. Reach toward the ceiling, letting your shoulder relax so you can reach higher.

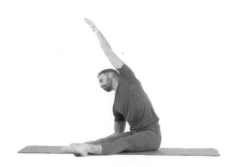

2. Bend slowly to the side and pull your arm as far as it will go, controlling the speed and depth of the side stretch. Timing: 4 seconds.

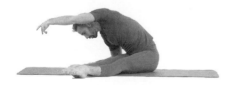

3. Bend as far sideways as possible and slowly sweep both arms toward your legs. Timing: 4 seconds.

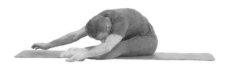

4. When you reach the front, breathe out and relax your back muscles to allow you to reach even farther over your legs.

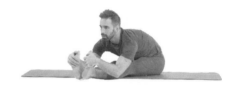

5. Hold the soles of your feet with both hands and try to pull your ankles into a deeper flex. Lie on the front of your legs with your back as straight as possible. Timing: 4 to 6 seconds.

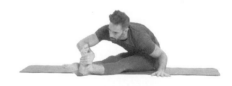

6. Hold the opposite flexed foot for 4 seconds. Repeat, bending to the other side.

AFTERWORD

WE CONTROL OUR FUTURE

In the good old days of hunting and gathering our survival depended on our being physically active and, therefore, physically fit. We definitely don't want to return to those good old days, however. I like having my water come out of the tap and not having to draw it from the nearest well. I like my car, my washing machine, and all my kitchen appliances; I like going to the market and coming home with a basket of fresh food that I didn't have to grow myself. But since today's conveniences mean we no longer need to be as active, in order to keep our bodies as strong, flexible, and healthy as those of our ancestors, we have to replicate the movements that we would have made to fetch heavy buckets of water, dig in the earth, pick apples, or wash and hang laundry.

Being strong and healthy isn't just for the privileged few but for all people. Fitness and energy shouldn't be measured with an index or in miles, muscle mass, or speed; rather, they should be measured by one's ability to move effortlessly, be fully active, and remain pain-free. Being pain-free means being free from chronic pain: our bodies don't hurt as we walk up and down stairs, get into and out of a car, or reach to take something off a high shelf.

When we accept stiffness, pain, and ill health with the attitude that we're victims of natural aging, we embrace the idea that we aren't responsible for our own lives. To admit that we actually *are* responsible for most of our health issues would force us to take action that we don't want to take. We've come to rely on doctors to solve our health problems, but neither medication nor surgery have the power to make our muscles strong and flexible or our bodies fit and toned. There's nothing wrong with the body's design. Muscles were created to be strong, not weak, and mobile, not stiff. Joints were created to move, not be inflexible. Our body was created to be pain-free, not an instrument of torture.

Like petulant teenagers, most adults resent any restrictions on their freedom. I say it's time to grow up and accept responsibility for our magnificent bodies. It's time to exercise regularly and safely, to eat wisely, and to avoid the habits that are killing us, like smoking and excessive alcohol. Before the Industrial Revolution, people were extremely active; they had to be to keep a roof over their heads and food on their tables. Junk food and cheap, sugar-filled drinks didn't exist. As machines replaced manual laborers at home and in business and mechanized transport became more common, people became less and less active.

There is a positive side to these developments: we no longer need to wear out our bodies simply trying to survive. We can enjoy the wonderful technological advancements that have made our lives so much easier, but we still have to pay attention to our bodies. For the first time in history, we have leisure time, access to healthy food, and the knowledge of how to take care of ourselves. We have the ability to live active, healthy, pain-free lives well into our eighties and nineties. The mission of Essentrics is to establish the true meaning of fitness in the world and to help people understand that being healthy, fit, and pain-free is a basic human right.

MEET THE MODELS

AMANDA CYR is an Essentrics Master Trainer, educator, and Essentrics TV workout host. In addition to being a Level 4 Essentrics instructor, she has a bachelor of science degree in biology and is an Ayurve- 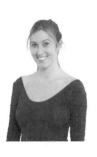 dic wellness practitioner. Amanda has dedicated her life to improving the wellness of others by combining her Essentrics and Ayurvedic practices, but still finds time to enjoy outdoor sports with her rescue dog and husband. She has trained directly under Miranda and has traveled worldwide leading workshops and live events. Amanda has played an important role in the development of other Essentrics trainers and educators, ensuring a strong future for the academic division of Essentrics. She contributed to the creation of this book, with a special focus on building the routines.

ARIANE NEOCEL, OIIAQ, RN, is a registered nurse who specializes in caring for burn victims. She credits her range of motion and strength to a decade of Essentrics classes, 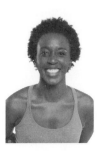 which helps her cope with the physical demands of a career as a trauma nurse. As a member of the flagship Essentrics studio in Montreal, Ariane has a deep understanding of Essentrics techniques and has taken part in creative marketing campaigns showcasing students and instructors. She is dedicated to her nursing career, but still sets time aside to hike and swim.

DR. DAVID LASRY, MD, CCFP (EM), FCFP, Osler Fellow, and trauma team leader, is an emergency physician and professor specializing in trauma care at the McGill University Health Centre and Montreal General 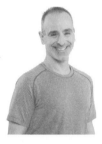 Hospital. Dr. Lasry began practicing Essentrics after a knee injury and chronic back pain began to affect his life. Within days his pain disappeared, and he has been practicing Essentrics daily ever since. Dave is an avid sportsman who enjoys skiing, windsurfing, sailing, hiking, snowboarding, and keeping up with his two young boys.

GAIL GARCEAU is a Level 4 Essentrics instructor, an Essentrics Master Trainer, educator, and Essentrics TV workout host, and holds a bachelor's degree in bio- 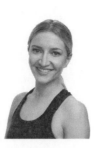 chemistry. She has worked with high-performance athletes including Olympic figure skaters, gymnasts, and the Montreal Canadiens hockey team. She trained directly under Miranda and has traveled worldwide leading workshops and live events. Gail has worked on content and training manuals for Essentrics techniques, participates in scientific research projects, and contributed scientific research and routine-building work to this book. With all that, Gail still finds time to play volleyball, snowboard, and golf with her dad.

JEFF CHEONG has a bachelor's degree in commerce from the University of Toronto and a Master of Business Administration degree from the Schulich School of Business. 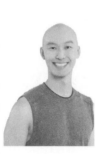 He worked in commercial real estate until he felt a calling to move into the wellness field, and he's never looked back. He has a thriving Essentrics practice and is certified in both Essentrics and Pilates. In his leisure time he plays basketball and volleyball, skis, runs track, and practices martial arts. He is the father of a beautiful daughter named Nori.

PIERRE-LUC GAGNON, PCP, NOCP, is a paramedic technician and outdoor emergency care specialist. Thirteen years ago, he was introduced to Miranda at Joe Beef, one of Montreal's most popular restaurants. It 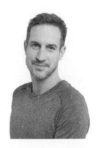 didn't take long for him to become an Essentrics devotee and a good friend of the Essentrics family. Pierre-Luc loves the power of dance and movement and has appeared in several books and campaigns highlighting Essentrics exercises. He uses Essentrics to maintain core strength and flexibility to protect his back while performing his physically demanding job and enjoying adventure travel, mountain biking, and hiking.

RAPHAËL BOUCHARD is a principal dancer with Les Grands Ballets Canadiens, one of Canada's major ballet companies. He was a diver with the Canadian diving team and a gymnast with Cirque 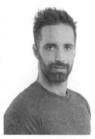 du Soleil before settling on ballet as a career. In 2004 Raphaël joined Les Ballets de Monte Carlo and soon became a principal dancer. In 2015 he returned to North America as a guest performer with the Pacific Northwest Ballet company and joined Les Grands Ballets Canadiens the same year. He is one of the world's most sought-after male dancers.

ROSE-KAYING WOO is an elite Canadian artistic gymnast. She competed at the 2016 Olympic Games in Rio de Janeiro and attended the 2020 Tokyo Olympic Games. She also represented Canada at the 2014

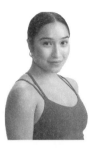

Pacific Rim Championships, where she helped the Canadian team win a silver medal, and most recently claimed the title at the 2022 Canadian Gymnastics Championships. In addition to her athletic success, Rose is completing a bachelor's degree in sociology and is the cofounder of Elegant Woo's gymnastic leotards. Rose uses Essentrics not only as part of her strength and flexibility training but to prevent and heal injuries in a sport that's known to put excessive demand on the joints.

SAHRA ESMONDE-WHITE is one of the cofounders of Essentrics and a head of the Essentrics company. Present since the very first Essentrics class was created by her mother, Miranda, she felt called to help bring Essentrics to the world at large. After completing a bachelor's de-

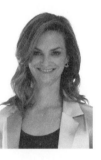

gree in economics and graduate studies in health economics and public health, she gained business experience as a health economist in private firms and at Novartis. Prior to that, she worked in Ireland and Egypt with UNESCO to restore the Great Library of Alexandria. Sahra's personal mission has always been to support women as they age

and to expand the reach of this special technique that allows people to care for their bodies in every decade of their lives. Sahra uses Essentrics to stay fit and healthy for her two miniature wire-haired dachshunds, Rosie and Lincoln.

SHARON CADIZ, EdD, is a retired educator and administrator with expertise in the areas of interpersonal trauma, chemical dependence, child development, and mental health. For over thirty years, Sharon

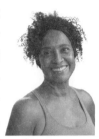

served children, youth, and families in New York City, receiving the highest award from the National Council of Negro Women in 1998 for those services. In 1994 Sharon opened a support production company, 747 Seminars, to serve women in their personal development. Dr. Cadiz overcame debilitating back pain with regular Essentrics workouts. In addition to her daily Essentrics practice, she enjoys yoga, Pilates, aerobics, and long bike rides around New York City.

TROY PERRIN is a strength and conditioning coach and student of the SomaTraining Program. He founded and owns the athletic leisure brand Made Equal and is a rap music producer, singer, and fitness

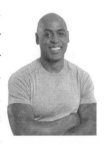

model. He was introduced to Essentrics through classes at his gym. He is the father of two young boys.

ACKNOWLEDGMENTS AND THANKS

A book of this scope and magnitude could never have been written without the participation of a large team. Even though my name is on the cover, let me assure you that there are many people who have also put their hearts, expertise, and energy into making this book a success.

The first people I wish to thank are my two business partners, Melissa Tran and my daughter, Sahra Esmonde-White. Over the past twenty years they've built Essentrics into a thriving international fitness company by nurturing a rapidly growing team of more than fifty employees, both in-house and worldwide, including editors, graphic designers, filmographers, marketers, researchers, lawyers, and much more. They've garnered the endorsements of doctors, physiotherapists, scientists, Olympians, and clients, who have helped to test and retest the validity, safety, and efficacy of Essentrics sequences and routines. So thank you, Sahra and Melissa, from the bottom of my heart for hanging in during those many tough years to help make this book happen.

My next thanks go to Ryan Harbage, my agent. A book cannot make it into the hands of the correct publisher without an agent. This is the fourth book of mine to which Ryan has lent his genius, devotion, and passion. He knows exactly how to best position and represent my work, and I thank my lucky stars for introducing us.

I also thank my lucky stars for the two publishing houses and two editors Ryan found: Leah Miller at Simon & Schuster and Anne Collins at Random House Canada. I'm so honored to have these two women guiding the publication process of this book. I value their input, recommendations, advice, and passionate commitment to delivering this message of health to the world. I can't thank them enough.

Truth be told, I'm not a good writer, which meant I needed a writer-editor to sift through my long-winded manuscript, sort out my thoughts, and put them in order. When Sydny Miner agreed to take on this project, everyone involved breathed a sigh of relief.

This book spent many years in development, and over those years there were three women who made major contributions. Roughly eight years ago, Eléonore (Nelly) Buchet-Deák was a McGill University research assistant investigating posture for this book before returning to her native New York City to work as an actress on Broadway and in film. More recently, Gail Garceau and Amanda Cyr, both Essentrics Master Trainers, helped with research and developing content. Their greatest contribution was helping me design the sixty-plus routines, drawing on their years of experience working with high-performance athletes and people of all ages and levels of fitness. We had a lot of fun building these routines!

I owe enormous gratitude to Lisa Epstein, who joined us as a freelancer to coordinate our massive photo project. Working on an extremely tight timeline under the restrictions created by COVID, Lisa accomplished the impossible and made it look easy. She was given a month to find a photographer and a studio when none were available, then coordinated the schedules of the eleven models who either had full-time jobs or lived out of town, sourced wardrobe items for all the models, and then fed everyone, accommodating their different dietary needs! She pulled it off every day with a big smile and no complaints. She was also responsible for hiring Amy Wetzler, the graphic artist who did an amazing job of transforming complex movements into simple drawings and creating the hundreds of anatomy sketches seen on every sequence page.

No film or photo shoot is possible without a makeup artist, and I have to offer my gratitude to Amélie Bruneau-Longpré, one of Montréal's most sought-after makeup artists. She has worked with us for years, and somehow squeezed our complicated schedule into her packed one.

Due to COVID restrictions, we had to use different photo studios and photographers. I'd like to thank Alex Paskanoi, one of Montreal's leading commercial fashion photographers; Natasha Launi, an independent photographer; and Natasha's assistant, Scott Robert Collins, for the outstanding job they did both in photos delivered and the relaxed but professional atmosphere they created in the studio. Their work in this book speaks for itself.

Next I'd like to give a big shout-out to Allison Fraser, director of marketing and PR at Essentrics. She unofficially acts as my right hand, even though that's not her actual job. She quietly makes sure that, no matter what project we're working on, everyone has what they need. For this book she worked with Lisa Epstein, the photographers, the models, the studio owners, and Amy Wexler, making hotel and travel arrangements and organizing daily COVID testing. She made sure that the models were happy, made-up, warmed up, and standing on set with the cameraman waiting and the music cued— and while all this was going on, a welcome cup of tea magically appeared in my hand. Thanks, Allison, for keeping it all flowing.

I'd like to thank Caitlin Pomeroy for doing exactly what I asked her to do by gluing herself to my side and accurately documenting each of the ten thousand (!) photos taken during the shoot. Her meticulous work made the daunting task of choosing which photos to keep and which to discard much easier.

At a fitness shoot, all the models need to be warmed up and ready to move comfortably when their photo session begins. That responsibility fell to Essentrics trainer Ellyn Ochs, who carefully prepped each model according to their specific needs and then waited for hours for her next model to appear. Good job, Ellyn!

Our in-house production department—director of production Lynda Whyte and videographers and editors Ian Graham and Adam Thompson, all of whom have won international awards in TV production—produced a creative peek behind the scenes and shot inspiring interviews with our models that we'll use in future marketing and promotion campaigns. Thank you all for always being there and doing such an outstanding job.

In addition to everyone listed above, this book required a small army of editors, graphic designers, and anatomy advisors: Allie Barbeau, Julia Bentz, Tanya Escobar, Gail Garceau, Sylvie Lebel, Ellyn Ochs, Tamara Pettman, Marwa Seif, and Kristin Taylor.

And, finally, I cannot thank enough the amazing people who agreed to be models for this book: Gail Garceau, Amanda Cyr, Ariane Neocel, Rose-Kaying Woo, Troy Perrin, Jeff Cheong, Dr. David Lasry, Dr. Sharon Cadiz, Raphaël Bouchard, Pierre-Luc Gagnon, and Sahra Esmonde-White, my beautiful daughter. Please go to the Meet the Models section to learn how accomplished and impressive each one of them is.

NOTES

Introduction: What Is Essentrics?

1 Seper Ekhtiari et al., "Opioid Use in Athletes: A Systematic Review," *Sports Health: A Multidisciplinary Approach* 12, no. 6 (November/December 2020): 534–39; and Christina D. Mack et al., "Epidemiology of Concussion in the National Football League, 2015–2019," *Sports Health: A Multidisciplinary Approach* 13, no. 5 (September/October 2021): 423–30.

2 Jooyoung Kim et al., "Exercise-Induced Rhabdomyolysis Mechanisms and Prevention: A Literature Review," *Journal of Sport and Health Science* 5, no. 3 (September 2016): 324–33.

3 Emilia Patricia T. Zarco et al., "Using Essentrics to Improve the Health of Older Adults," *HSOA Journal of Gerontology & Geriatric Medicine* 8, no. 1 (February 2022).

4 Bruce Elliot and Tim Ackland, "Biomechanical Effects of Fatigue on 10,000 Meter Running Technique," *Research Quarterly for Exercise and Sport* 52, no. 2 (May 1981): 160–66; and H. K. Wang and Thomas Cochrane, "Mobility Impairment, Muscle Imbalance, Muscle Weakness, Scapular Asymmetry, and Shoulder Injury in Elite Volleyball Athletes," *Journal of Sports Medicine and Physical Fitness* 41, no. 3 (September 2001): 403–10.

5 Joseph J. Knapik et al., "Preseason Strength and Flexibility Imbalances Associated with Athletic Injuries in Female Collegiate Athletes," *American Journal of Sports Medicine* 19, no. 1 (January–February 1991): 76–81; and Jean-Louis Croisier et al., "Strength Imbalances and Prevention of Hamstring Injury in Professional Soccer Players: A Prospective Study," *American Journal of Sports Medicine* 36, no. 8 (August 2008): 1469–75.

6 Philip B. Maffetone and Paul B. Laursen, "Athletes: Fit but Unhealthy?" *Sports Medicine—Open* 2, no. 24 (2016), https://doi.org/10.1186/s40798-016-0048-x; and James H. O'Keefe, Barry Franklin, and Carl J. Lavie, "Exercising for Health and Longevity vs. Peak Performance: Different Regimens for Different Goals," *Mayo Clinic Proceedings* 89, no. 9 (September 1, 2014): 1171–75.

7 Tobias Renkawitz, Daniel Boluki, and Joachim Grifka, "The Association of Low Back Pain, Neuromuscular Imbalance, and Trunk Extension Strength in Athletes," *Spine Journal* 6, no. 6 (November–December 2006): 673–83; Roald Bahr et al., "Low Back Pain among Endurance Athletes with and without Specific Back Loading: A Cross-Sectional Survey of Cross-Country Skiers, Rowers, Orienteerers, and Nonathletic Controls," *Spine* 29, no. 4 (February 15, 2004): 449–54; Ardalan Shariat et al., "Effects of Stretching Exercise Training and Ergonomic Modifications on Musculoskeletal Discomforts of Office Workers: A Randomized Controlled Trial," *Brazilian Journal of Physical Therapy* 22, no. 2 (March–April 2018): 144–53; and Carol A. Kennedy et al., "Systematic Review of the Role of Occupational Health and Safety Interventions in the Prevention of Upper Extremity Musculoskeletal Symptoms, Signs, Disorders, Injuries, Claims, and Lost Time," *Journal of Occupational Rehabilitation* 20, no. 2 (June 2010): 127–62.

8 Zarco et al., "Using Essentrics to Improve the Health of Older Adults"; and Emilia Patricia T. Zarco et al., "Perceived Benefits of a Guided Exercise Program among Older Adults," *Gerontology and Geriatric Medicine* 7 (November 2021).

9 University of Birmingham, "A Lifetime of Regular Exercise Slows Down Aging, Study Finds," *ScienceDaily*, March 8, 2018, https://www.sciencedaily.com/releases/2018/03/180308143123.htm.

10 *Aging Backwards: Unlock Your Body's Youth Code*, directed by Lynda Whyte (2015,

Canada), https://essentrics.com/aging-back
wards-1/.

Chapter 1: The Balanced Body

1   James Ashton-Miller, "Soft Tissue Re-
    sponses to Physical Stressors: Muscles,
    Tendons, and Ligaments," in *Work-Related
    Musculoskeletal Disorders: Report, Workshop
    Summary, and Workshop Papers* (Washing-
    ton, DC: National Academies Press, 1999).
2   Jules Mitchell, *Yoga Biomechanics: Stretch-
    ing Redefined* (Pencaitland, UK: Handspring
    Publishing, 2019).
3   N. F. N. Bittencourt et al., "Complex Systems
    Approach for Sports Injuries: Moving from
    Risk Factor Identification to Injury Pattern
    Recognition—Narrative Review and New
    Concept," *British Journal of Sports Medicine*
    50, no. 21 (2016): 1309–14.
4   Steve Dischiavi et al., "Biotensegrity and
    Myofascial Chains: A Global Approach to an
    Integrated Kinetic Chain," *Medical Hypothe-
    ses* 110 (January 2018): 90–96.

Chapter 2: Redefining Stretching

1   Alter, *Science of Flexibility*; Schleip and Wilke,
    Fascia in Sport and Movement; and D. R. Mur-
    phy, "A Critical Look at Static Stretching: Are
    We Doing Our Patients Harm?" *Chiropractic
    Sports Medicine* 5 (1991): 67–70.
2   Ibid.; Kim et al., "Exercise-Induced Rhab-
    domyolysis Mechanisms and Prevention";
    and Russell T. Nelson, "A Comparison of
    the Immediate Effects of Eccentric Training
    vs. Static Stretch on Hamstring Flexibility
    in High School and College Athletes," *North
    American Journal of Sports Physical Therapy*
    1, no. 2 (May 2006): 56–61.
3   Gretchen Reynolds, "Stretching the Truth,"
    New York Times, October 31, 2008, https://
    www.nytimes.com/2008/11/02/sports/play
    magazine/112pewarm.html.
4   Gregory R. Waryasz et al., "Personal Trainer
    Demographics, Current Practice Trends and
    Common Trainee Injuries," *Orthopedic Re-
    views* 8, no. 3 (September 2016): 6600.
5   Peter A. Huijing, "Epimuscular Myofascial
    Force Transmission between Antagonistic
    and Synergistic Muscles Can Explain Move-
    ment Limitation in Spastic Paresis," *Journal
    of Electromyography and Kinesiology* 17,
    no. 6 (December 2007): 708–24.
6   I. Javurek, "Experience with Hypermobility
    in Athletes," *Theorie A Praxe Telesne Vy-
    chovy* 30, no. 3 (1982).
7   Schleip and Wilke, *Fascia in Sport and Mov-
    ment*.
8   Stuart McNish, "Conversations That Matter:
    Dr. Langevin on the Science of Stretch,"
    Osher Center for Integrative Medi-
    cine, November 10, 2017, https://osher
    center.org/2017/11/10/conversations-lang
    evin-science-stretch/.
9   Konstantinos Giannakopoulos et al., "Iso-
    lated vs. Complex Exercise in Strengthening
    the Rotator Cuff Muscle Group," *Journal of
    Strength and Conditioning Research* 18, no. 1
    (February 2004): 144–48.

Chapter 3: The Musculoskeletal Trifecta

1   Todd Ellenbecker, Mark De Carlo, and Carl
    DeRosa, *Effective Functional Progressions in
    Sport Rehabilitation* (Champaign, IL: Human
    Kinetics, 2009).
2   Henry G. Davis, *Conservative Surgery, as Ex-
    hibited in Remedying Some of the Mechani-
    cal Causes That Operate Injuriously Both in
    Health and Disease* (New York: D. Appleton
    & Company, 1867).
3   R. B. Jenkins and R. W. Little, "A Constitutive
    Equation for Parallel-Fibered Elastic Tissue,"
    Journal of Biomechanics 7, no. 5 (September
    1974): 397–402.
4   J. Staubesand, K. U. K. Baumbach, and Y. Li,
    "La structure fine de l'aponévrose jambière
    (patients avec insuffisance veineuse chro-
    nique avancée et ulcère de jambe)," *Phlébol-
    ogie* 50, no. 1 (1997): 105–13.
5   Gregory S. Sawicki, Cara L. Lewis, and Dan-
    iel P. Ferris, "It Pays to Have a Spring in Your
    Step," *Exercise and Sport Sciences Reviews*
    37, no. 3 (July 2009): 130–38.
6   Alexandre Fouré, Antoine Nordez, and Chris-
    tophe Cornu, "Effects of Eccentric Training
    on Mechanical Properties of the Plantar

Flexor Muscle-Tendon Complex," *Journal of Applied Physiology (1985)* 114, no. 5 (March 2013): 523–37.

7 Per Renström and Robert J. Johnson, "Overuse Injuries in Sports: A Review," *Sports Medicine* 2, no. 5 (September–October 1985): 316–33.

8 Jon Hyman and Scott A. Rodeo, "Injury and Repair of Tendons and Ligaments," *Physical Medicine and Rehabilitation Clinics of North America* 11, no. 2 (May 2000): 267–88.

Chapter 4: The Poor Posture Epidemic

1 Jackie Middleton, "The Sitting Disease Is Real," *Canadian Living*, July 31, 2013, https://www.canadianliving.com/health/prevention-and-recovery/article/the-sitting-disease-is-real.

2 James Gallagher, " 'Global Epidemic' of Childhood Inactivity," BBC News, November 22, 2019, https://www.bbc.com/news/health-50466061.

3 Regina Guthold et al., "Worldwide Trends in Insufficient Physical Activity from 2001 to 2016: A Pooled Analysis of 358 Population-Based Surveys with 1.9 Million Participants," *Lancet* 6, no. 10 (October 2018): E1077–86.

4 *Physical Activity Guidelines for Americans*, 2nd ed. (Washington, DC: US Department of Health & Human Services, 2018), https://health.gov/sites/default/files/2019-09/Physical_Activity_Guidelines_2nd_edition.pdf.

5 Nicolaas P. Pronk et al., "Reducing Occupational Sitting Time and Improving Worker Health: The Take-a-Stand Project, 2011," *Preventing Chronic Disease* 9 (2012): E154; and James A. Levine, MD, *Get Up! Why Your Chair Is Killing You and What You Can Do About It* (New York: St. Martin's Griffin, 2014).

6 Sir Muir Gray, "A Quest for Clearer Thinking on Ageing," NHS blog, January 3, 2018, https://www.england.nhs.uk/blog/a-quest-for-clearer-thinking-on-ageing/.

7 Mayo Clinic Staff, "Bone Health: Tips to Keep Your Bones Healthy," Mayo Clinic, March 6, 2021, https://www.mayoclinic.org/healthy-lifestyle/adult-health/in-depth/bone-health/art-20045060.

8 Khaled A. Alswat, "Gender Disparities in Osteoporosis," *Journal of Clinical Medicine Research* 9, no. 5 (May 2017): 382–87.

9 Shayla Mueller and Veronique Murphy, "Tai Chi: Fall Prevention and Bone Health," Osteoporosis, February 27, 2020, https://osteoporosis.ca/tai-chi-fall-prevention-and-bone-health/; L. E. Lanyon and C. T. Rubin, "Static vs. Dynamic Loads as an Influence on Bone Remodelling," *Journal of Biomechanics* 17, no. 12 (1984): 897–905; and N. H. Hart et al., "Mechanical Basis of Bone Strength: Influence of Bone Material, Bone Structure, and Muscle Action," *Journal of Musculoskeletal and Neuronal Interactions* 17, no. 3 (September 2017): 114–39.

10 Huijing, "Epimuscular Myofascial Force Transmission between Antagonistic and Synergistic Muscles Can Explain Movement Limitation in Spastic Paresis."

11 *Stedman's Medical Dictionary*, 25th ed. (Baltimore: Williams and Wilkins, 1990).

12 Ibid.

Chapter 5: Neuromuscular Techniques

1 Chris Beardsley, *Strength Is Specific: The Key to Optimal Strength Training for Sports* (Strength and Conditioning Research Ltd., 2018).

2 Venus Joumaa et al., "The Origin of Passive Force Enhancement in Skeletal Muscle," *American Journal of Physiology—Cell Physiology* 294, no. 1 (January 2008): C74–C78.

3 Beardsley, *Strength Is Specific*; and Stéphanie Hody et al., "Eccentric Muscle Contractions: Risks and Benefits," *Frontiers in Physiology* 10 (2019), https://doi.org/10.3389/fphys.2019.00536.

INDEX

abdominals
  Essentrics sequences using, 85–98, 100,
    102–20, 123–26, 128, 131–40, 142–43, 147–53,
    155, 157–58, 160–62, 164–72, 176–81, 184
  warm-ups using, 59–66, 73–74
Abductor and Glutes Strengthening—Floor
  explained, 164
  in lower-body toning routine, 235
  in routine for hip pain, 376
  in speed routine, 243
achilles tendonitis, Essentrics routine for,
  370–73
Advanced Airplane Hamstrings Stretch, 101
Advanced Ankle Strengthening—Chair
  explained, 148
  in lower-body toning routine, 234
  in routine for being on your feet all day,
    343
  in routine for housekeeping, 356
Advanced Clock Sequence
  for ballet and gymnastics routine, 264
  for dance routine, 279
  explained, 111
  for Upper-Body Toning, 231
  in volleyball routine, 335
advanced flexibility routine, 224–26
Advanced Pulling Sacks of Rice
  in basketball routine, 272
  explained, 100
  in volleyball routine, 336
Advanced Shin Stretch—Floor
  explained, 181
  in routine for being on your feet all day,
    343
Advanced Side Strengthening with Scissor Arms,
  109
Advanced Side Strengthening with Side Presses,
  110
Advanced Sit-Ups with Extended Legs—Floor
  explained, 172
  in upper-body toning routine, 232
Advanced Spine Stretching and Strengthening
  Using Arms Variation #1—Floor, 165

Advanced Spine Stretching and Strengthening
  Using Arms Variation #2—Floor, 166
Advanced Trapeze Strengthening with Quad
  Raisers—Floor
  explained, 167
  in speed routine, 243
  in yoga and Pilates routine, 340
agility, routine for, 244–46
agonist muscle group, 43–44
alignment
  clean load path and, 49–50
  posture and, 25, 37–38
American football, Essentrics routine for,
  259–61
ankle(s)
  eversion or inversion of, 52
  incorrect rolling of, 53
Ankle, Calf, and Shin Stretch
  in basketball routine, 270
  explained, 144
  in explosive power routine, 238
  in knee pain routine, 367
  in racket sports routine, 307
  in routine for balance, 250
  in routine for being on your feet all day,
    341
  in routine for fibromyalgia and IBS,
    381
  in routine for flight attendants, 351
  in routine for foot and calf pain, 372
  in running routine, 313
  in soccer routine, 324
  in routine to stimulate your brain, 209
ankle flexion/extension
  for Essentrics sequences, 136, 140–41,
    143–44, 146–47, 152, 154, 157, 159, 163–65,
    178, 183
  for warm-up, 68
Ankle Mobility with Hip Rotation—Floor
  in beginner flexibility (floor) routine, 219
  explained, 146
  in routine for being on your feet all day,
    343

ankles, Essentrics sequences targeting, 89, 95, 98, 109, 120–22, 136, 140–48, 152, 154, 156–57, 159, 163–65, 177, 179, 183

antagonist muscle group, 43–44

anterior transverse arch of the foot, 31

arch shape, in the human skeleton, 26

arch supports (orthotics), 32

arches of the foot/feet, 31, 32, 38, 51

Arches, Toes, and Ankles (warm-up), 68, 70

Arching the Back Stretches—Floor
    explained, 184
    in spine mobility routine, 257
    in swimming routine, 332

Arm Joints for Shoulder Joint Liberation, in speed routine, 242

Arm Pumps for Pectoral Strength
    in baseball routine, 267
    explained, 133
    in martial arts routine, 302
    in routine for fibromyalgia and IBS, 382
    in routine for hairdressing, 360
    in volleyball routine, 334

Arm Pumps for Posture
    explained, 135
    in upper-body toning routine, 231

Arm Pumps for Shoulder Joint Liberation
    explained, 132
    in manual labor/construction/landscaping routine, 349
    in routine for finger, wrist, and elbow pain, 389
    in yoga and Pilates routine, 337

Arm Pumps for Triceps, 134

arm rotation up and down, 162

Arms Following the Circumference of a Beach Ball—Ceiling to Floor
    in ballet and gymnastics routine, 263
    explained, 85
    in routine to increase your energy, 204

Arms Following the Circumference of a Beach Ball—Ceiling to Waist
    in back pain routine, 365
    explained, 84
    in lower-body toning routine, 233

arms up above the head, Essentrics sequences using, 78, 82

astronauts, weakened bones and, 24

athletes, xi–xii, 7

atlas (C1 vertebra), 28

atrophy
    muscle, 11, 23, 38
    posture and, 391

axis (C2 vertebra), 28

Azar, Alex M. II, 22

Baby Stretch for Hips and Lower Back (posture routine), 420

Baby Stretch with Deep Hip Release—Floor
    in back pain routine, 366
    in cycling routine, 275
    explained, 182
    in figure skating routine, 287
    in hiking routine, 293
    in hockey routine, 295
    in lower-body toning routine, 236
    in routine for cooldown/recovery, 229
    in routine for hip pain, 376
    in routine for stress relief, 200
    in snowboarding routine, 321
    in yoga and Pilates routine, 339

back pain, Essentrics routine for, 363–66

badminton, Essentrics routine for, 305–8

balanced body, 3–7
    stretching and, 9, 14
    through Pilates with Essentrics regime, 10

balance, routine for, 248–51

ballet dancers, 10, 14, 42

ballet, Essentrics routine for, 262–65

banister (chair), 45–46

barre (chair), 45–46

baseball, Essentrics routine for, 266–68

basketball, Essentrics routine for, 269–72

beginner flexibility (chair) routine, 221–23

beginner flexibility (floor) routine, 217–20

bent elbows, Essentrics sequences using, 78–87, 89, 91–100, 103, 105–7, 110, 112–19, 124–25, 132–35, 145, 155, 161, 165–66, 169–71, 175, 177–78

biceps
    eccentric contractions and, 41
    Essentrics sequences using, 78, 79, 83, 85–88, 90–94, 96, 98–100, 103, 105–6, 108–20, 125–26, 128, 131–35, 155, 159, 161, 165–66, 168, 173–78, 180, 184
    warm-ups using, 58–60, 63–67

blocks/risers, 46–47

body, rebalancing the, 3–7

body rotation, 92, 96

body temperature, raising with warm-ups, 57

bone density, 24

bones. *See also* human skeletal system
    in alignment, 25
    of the feet, 30–31
    muscle-fascia interactions and, 16
    physical activity and, 23–24
    rebalancing the body and, 3

Bow and Arrow
    explained, 103
    in routine for agility, 246

brain, Essentrics routine to stimulate your, 208–11

Butterfly for Spine Strength (posture routine), 417

Butterfly Stretch for Hips (posture routine), 416

Butterfly with Deep Hip and Spine Stretch—Floor
in beginner flexibility (floor) routine, 219
explained, 174
in lower-body toning routine, 235
in routine for cooldown/recovery, 228
in routine for hip pain, 376

Butterfly with PNF for Hip Stretch—Floor
in advanced flexibility routine, 225
in ballet and gymnastics routine, 264
in evening routine, 191
explained, 173
in hiking routine, 292
in horseback riding routine, 301
in martial arts routine, 303
in routine for stress relief, 199
in yoga and Pilates routine, 338

C1 vertebra, 28
C2 vertebra, 28
C7 vertebra (vertebra prominens), 28
calf pain, Essentrics routine for, 370–73
Calf Stretch Sequence
in advanced flexibility routine, 225
in American football routine, 260
in ballet and gymnastics routine, 263
in baseball routine, 268
in dance routine, 279
explained, 145
in figure skating routine, 286
in golf routine, 289
in hockey routine, 295
in jumping higher routine, 252
in knee pain routine, 367
in posture routine, 403
in racket sports routine, 306
in routine for balance, 248
in routine for being on your feet all day, 342
in routine for cooldown/recovery, 228
in routine for fibromyalgia and IBS, 384
in routine for flight attendants, 352
in routine for foot and calf pain, 371
in routine for working at a desk all day, 346
in routine to increase your energy, 206
in routine to stimulate your brain, 210
in running routine, 314
in skiing routine, 317
in snowboarding routine, 320
in soccer routine, 325
in speed routine, 242

in surfing routine, 328
in walking the dog routine, 196

Calf Stretch Sequence for Balance
in basketball routine, 271
explained, 149
in routine for balance, 251

canoeing, Essentrics routine for, 309–12

cartilage
function of, 16
in the spine, 27

cartilaginous (partially moveable) joints, 16

Cat and Cow for Spine Flexibility—Floor
for children's routine, 215
for cycling routine, 276
explained, 180
for routine with children, 215
for Spine Mobility routine, 257
for Stress Relief routine, 200

Cat-Cow (posture routine), 425

Ceiling Reach and Open Chest Swan
in beginner flexibility (chair) routine, 221
explained, 114
in manual labor/construction/landscaping routine, 348
in relaxation routine, 201
in routine for cooldown/recovery, 227
in routine for flight attendants, 350
in routine for hairdressing, 358
in routine for working at a desk all day, 344
in travel days routine, 192

Ceiling Reaches, 35

Ceiling Reaches, Embrace Yourself with. *See* Embrace Yourself with Ceiling Reaches

Ceiling Reaches with Overextensions (posture routine), 398

Ceiling Reach with Waist Rotation (warm-up), 60, 70

cell phone use, poor posture and, 33, 35

cervical spine, 27–28

cervical vertebrae, 27–28

chair/barre sequences, 150–62
Deep Hamstring and Spine Stretch with Release—Chair, 154
Deep Side Bend and IT Band Stretch—Chair, 162
Folded Hamstring Stretch—Chair, 160
Four-Directional Hip Stretch—Chair, 151
Hamstring and Spine Stretch—Chair, 159
Hamstring Stretch—Chair, 157
Hip Cleaners—Chair, 150
Hip Flexor and Hamstring Stretch—Chair, 156
Inner and Outer Thigh Rotations: IT Band and Long Adductor Stretch—Chair, 153
Posture Routine, 411–15

chair/barre sequences (*cont.*)
  Preparation: Hip Flexor and Hamstring
    Stretch—Chair, 152
  Pull a Rope IT Band and Hamstring Stretch—
    Chair, 155
  Spine Release—Chair, 161
  Windmill Hamstring and Spine Stretch—Chair,
    158
chair, for exercises, 45, 46
children, Essentrics routine for, 212–15
chin, correct and incorrect positioning of, 49
chronic disease, physical activity and, 22
chronic pain routines
  back pain, 363–66
  fibromyalgia and IBS, 381–84
  finger, wrist, and elbow pain, 388–89
  foot and calf pain, 370–73
  hip pain, 374–77
  knee pain, 367–69
  neck pain, 385–87
  shoulder pain, 378–80
clavicle, 27, 29
clean alignment and, 25
coccyx, 27, 35
collagen, 13
complex movements, 12
computer use, poor posture and, 33, 35
concentric contractions, 41, 42–43
connective tissue, xiii. *See also* cartilage; fascia
  Essentrics and, 13
  healthy, 17
  importance of health, 13–14
  interdependent relationship with muscular
    system, 33
  rebalancing the body and, 3
  skeletal system and, 25
  working in harmony with muscles and joints, 11
construction work, Essentrics routine for,
    347–49
contractions. *See* muscle contraction(s)
Cooldown routine, 227–29
crimps, 17
cross-body rotation, 92
cuboid bone, 31
cuneiform bones, 31
curved spine. *See* spine curved
cycling, Essentrics routine for, 273–76

daily habits, poor posture and, 34
dance, Essentrics routine for, 277–80
dance warm-ups, 73–75
Deep Diagonal Reaches at Three Heights
  explained, 95
  in routine for agility, 244

Deep Hamstring and Spine Stretch with
    Release—Chair
  in American football routine, 261
  in basketball routine, 271
  in beginner flexibility (chair) routine, 223
  explained, 154
  in martial arts routine, 304
Deep Hamstring, Long Adductor, and IT Band
    Stretch—Floor
  in advanced flexibility routine, 226
  in back pain routine, 366
  in ballet and gymnastics routine, 265
  in cycling routine, 275
  explained, 183
  in figure skating routine, 287
  in hiking routine, 293
  in routine for hip pain, 377
  in routine for stress relief, 200
  in snowboarding routine, 322
  in yoga and Pilates routine, 339
Deep Hip Flexor Stretch—Floor
  in advanced flexibility routine, 226
  in ballet and gymnastics routine, 264
  explained, 178
  in figure skating routine, 287
  in routine for recovery/cooldown, 229
  in swimming routine, 332
  in yoga and Pilates routine, 339
Deep Lunges Washing a Large Round Table
  in American football routine, 260
  explained, 98
  in explosive power routine, 239
  in lower-body toning routine, 233
Deep Side Bend and IT Band Stretch—Chair, 162
Deep Side Lunge Washes
  in beginner flexibility (chair) routine, 222
  explained, 106
  in routine for balance, 250
  in routine for foot and calf pain, 371
  in routine to increase your energy, 205
  in skiing routine, 316
  in swimming routine, 330
deltoids
  Essentrics sequences using, 78–83, 85–88,
    90–94, 96–109, 111–20, 126, 131–35, 149,
    154–55, 159, 161, 165–66, 168, 173–80, 184
  warm-ups using, 58–67
desk work, Essentrics routine for, 344–46
Diagonal Presses at Various Heights
  in basketball routine, 270
  in evening routine, 189
  explained, 93
  in golf routine, 289
  in hiking routine, 291

in racket sports routine, 306
in relaxation routine, 202
in routine for flight attendants, 351
in routine for housekeeping, 355
in routine for working at a desk all day, 345
in snowboarding routine, 319
Diagonal Twists (warm-up), 63, 70
discs, of the spine, 27
diving, Essentrics routine for, 281–84
"donut" cushion, 45, 47–48
Double-Arm Figure Eights
in baseball routine, 266
in beginner flexibility (floor) routine, 218
explained, 119
in routine for shoulder pain, 378
in speed routine, 241
in swimming routine, 330
in travel days routine, 192
Double-Arm Half-Body Rotation
explained, 108
in upper-body toning routine, 231
Double-Arm Pulling Ropes to the Floor
in diving routine, 282
explained, 94
in explosive power routine, 240
in martial arts routine, 303
in routine for fibromyalgia and IBS, 383
Double-Arm Shoulder Rotations
explained, 131
in horseback riding routine, 299
in morning routine, 187
in routine for finger, wrist, and elbow pain, 389
in routine for shoulder pain, 380
Double-Arm Swings, Side to Side (warm-up)
explained, 61
in routine for finger, wrist, and elbow pain, 388
in routine for neck pain, 387
in warm-up routine, 70
dropped arches of the foot, 32

eccentric contractions, 41–42
eccentric training, xiv
elbow hinge
Essentrics sequence using, 82
for warm-ups, 58–59, 63–65, 73
elbow pain, Essentrics routine for, 388–89
elbow rotation, for Simple Side-to-Side Steps
warm-up, 58
elbows, Essentrics sequences targeting, 79–83,
91–94, 103–6, 112–16, 119, 124–25, 132–35,
155, 161
elbows bent. See bent elbows
Embrace a Ball Overhead—Swaying Side to Side,
86

Embrace a Ball with Diagonal Movements
in advanced flexibility routine, 224
explained, 87
in routine for spine mobility, 256
Embrace Yourself with Ceiling Reaches
explained, 82
in morning routine, 186
in routine for children, 212
Embrace Yourself with Single-Arm Extensions
in beginner flexibility (floor) routine, 217
explained, 81
in routine for neck pain, 385
Embracing a Beach Ball, 35
energy, routine to increase your, 204–7
equipment, 45–48
erector spinae
Essentrics sequences using, 78, 80–83, 89–90,
95–96, 101, 103–11, 114, 122, 125–26, 128,
151–53, 155–58, 160–62, 165–76, 179–84
warm-ups using, 59, 60, 61, 62, 63, 64, 65, 67, 74
Essentrics
about, xi, xiv
added to yoga practice, 10
appearing as an easy workout, 7–8
benefits of, 12
and connective tissue, 13–14
creation of, xiii
Pilates as complement to, 10
rebuilding crimp through, 17
slowness of sequences, 14
weight-bearing exercises with, 24
Essentrics routines
about, 185
advanced flexibility, 224–26
for agility, 244–47
American football, 259–61
for back pain, 363–66
for balance, 248–51
ballet and gymnastics, 262–65
baseball, 266–68
basketball, 269–72
beginner flexibility (chair), 221–23
beginner flexibility (floor), 217–20
for children, 212–15
cooldown/recovery, 227–29
cycling, 273–76
dance, 277–80
diving, 281–84
evening routine, 189–91
explosive power, 237–40
for fibromyalgia and IBS, 381–84
figure skating, 285–87
for finger, wrist, and elbow pain, 388–89
for foot and calf pain, 370–73

Essentrics routines (*cont.*)
  golf, 288–90
  hiking, 291–93
  for hip pain, 374–77
  hockey, 294–97
  horseback riding, 298–301
  to increase your energy, 204–7
  jumping higher, 252–54
  for knee pain, 367–69
  lower-body training, 233–36
  martial arts, 302–4
  morning routine, 186–88
  for neck pain, 385–87
  for posture, 392–427
  racket sports, 305–8
  relaxation, 201–3
  rowing, kayaking, canoeing, 309–12
  running, 313–15
  for shoulder pain, 378–80
  skiing, 316–18
  snowboarding, 319–22
  soccer, 323–25
  for speed, 241–43
  for spine mobility, 255–57
  to stimulate your brain, 208–11
  stress relief, 198–200
  surfing, 326–29
  swimming, 330–33
  travel days, 192–94
  upper-body toning, 230–32
  volleyball, 334–36
  for the workplace, 341–61
  yoga and Pilates, 337–40
Essentrics sequences, 77. *See also individual*
  names of sequences
  ankle, calf, and shin stretch, 144–49
  chair/barre stretching, 150–62
  floor strengthening, 163–72
  floor stretching, 173–84
  full body—diagonal spine rotation, 88–101
  full-body figure eights, 117–20
  full body—forward flexion—arms in front,
    78–87
  full body—side to side, 102–11
  hands, arms, and shoulders, 129–35
  legs and hips, 136–43
  pliés, 121–28
  upper-body extension, 112–16
evening routine, 189–91
exercise, premature aging of the body and, xi–xii
explosive power, routine for, 237–40
external weights
  avoiding while doing Essentrics, xiv
  eccentric training with, 42

external weights, avoiding, xiv
extreme physical activity, 6–7

Fan Kicks with Lunges
  in baseball routine, 267
  in dance routine, 280
  explained, 139
  in explosive power routine, 239
  in routine for agility, 245
  in routine for balance, 249
  in routine for fibromyalgia and IBS, 382
  in routine for foot and calf pain, 372
  in routine to stimulate your brain, 210
  in surfing routine, 327
  in travel days routine, 193
  in volleyball routine, 336
fascia, xiv. *See also* connective tissue
  about, 16
  and connective tissue workout, 13
  hardening or gluing, 17–18, 33
  importance of hydrated, 18–19
  of inactive or sedentary people, 17
  within our legs, 17
  poor posture and, 28
  sedentary lifestyle and, 17
  standing/walking on the full sole of the foot
    and, 32
fascia sleeve, 17
Fast Pliés with Full Arm Circle (warm-up), 67,
  72
feet, ankle, and calves, sequences for, 144–49
feet/foot
  alignment beginning with the, 38
  anatomy, 30–31
  arches of, 31
  correct positioning for butterfly stretch, 52
  correct positioning of, 51
  importance of well-aligned, 31–32
  positioning in pliés, 53–54
  positioning of, 51
  posture and, 25
  retraining yourself to stand/walk on full sole of
    the, 32
  reversing flat, 32–33
femur, 25, 30, 34
fibromyalgia, Essentrics routine for, 381–84
fibrous (immovable) joints, 15
figure skating, Essentrics routine for, 285–87
finger pain, Essentrics routine for, 388–89
fingers, Essentrics sequences targeting,
  129–30
Fingers Walking Down the Arm
  explained, 107
  in routine for hairdressing, 359

fist open/closed
   Essentrics sequences using, 100, 103, 112
   for warm-ups, 58
fitness myths, 13
flat feet, 32–33
flight attendants, Essentrics routine for, 350–53
floor sequences
   Abductor and Glutes Strengthening—Floor, 164
   Advanced Shin Stretch—Floor, 181
   Advanced Sit-Ups with Extended Legs—Floor, 172
   Advanced Spine Stretching and Strengthening Using Arms Variation #1—Floor, 165
   Advanced Spine Stretching and Strengthening Using Arms Variation #2—Floor, 166
   Advanced Trapeze Strengthening with Quad Raisers—Floor, 167
   Ankle Mobility with Hip Rotation—Floor, 146
   Arching the Back Stretches—Floor, 184
   Arms Following the Circumference of a Beach Ball—Ceiling to Floor, 85
   Baby Stretch with Deep Hip Release—Floor, 182
   Butterfly with Deep Hip and Spine Stretch—Floor, 174
   Butterfly with PNF for Hip Stretch—Floor, 173
   Cat and Cow for Spine Flexibility—Floor, 180
   Deep Hamstring, Long Adductor, and IT Band Stretch—Floor, 183
   Deep Hip Flexor Stretch—Floor, 178
   Double-Arm Pulling Ropes to the Floor, 94
   Long Adductor Stretch with Figure Eight—Floor, 179
   posture routine, 416–27
   Row the Boat with Hamstring and Spine Stretch—Floor, 177
   Seated Hamstring and Glute Stretch—Floor, 175
   Seated Hip Stretch with Spine Rotation—Floor, 176
   Sit-Ups with a Waist Twist—Floor, 170, 171
   Sit-Ups with Single-Leg Kicks—Floor, 171
   Slow Sit-Ups with Arm Variations—Floor, 169
   Strengthening Quad Raiser—Floor, 163
   strengthening sequences, 163–72
   stretching sequences, 173–84
   Superman Spine Strengthening—Floor, 168
Fluid Spine
   in dance routine, 278
   explained, 113
   in routine for hip pain, 374
   in spine mobility routine, 255
Fluid Spine with Arms (posture routine), 405

Fluid Spine with Hip Rotation (posture routine), 406
Folded Hamstring Stretch—Chair
   in diving routine, 284
   explained, 160
   in surfing routine, 329
Fondu with Kicks (posture routine), 411
football, Essentrics routine for American, 259–61
foot pain, Essentrics routine for, 370–73
forward flexion. *See also* Neutral C spine movement
   correct and incorrect, 50–51
   pliés and, 54
Four-Directional Hip Stretch—Chair
   in back pain routine, 365
   in baseball routine, 268
   in beginner flexibility (chair) routine, 223
   explained, 151
   in hockey routine, 296
   for jumping higher routine, 254
   in manual labor/construction/landscaping routine, 349
   in routine for flight attendants, 352
   in rowing routine, 311
   in snowboarding routine, 321
   in travel days routine, 194
Full-Body Diagonal Reaches (posture routine), 395
Full Body—Diagonal Spine Rotation sequences, 88–101
Full-Body Figure Eights, 117–20, 401
Full Body—Forward Flexion—Arms in Front sequences, 78–87
Full-Body Lift: Heavy Weights (posture routine), 400
Full-Body Pulling a Cement Ball (posture routine), 409
full-body range of motion, 9, 11
Full Body—Side to Side sequences, 102–11
Full-Body Windmill (posture routine), 410
full-body workouts, 9, 10, 11

gastrocnemius
   Essentrics sequences using, 85–89, 91–96, 98–100, 103–10, 113, 115, 118, 120–24, 126–27, 136–49, 151–57, 159–60, 163, 165, 175, 177–79, 183
   warm-ups using, 58–68, 73
gluteus muscles, 7
   Essentrics sequences using, 78–81, 89, 95, 97, 99–111, 116–17, 119–28, 136–43, 145–46, 148, 150–59, 162, 164, 167–68, 173–77, 179–83
   warm-ups using, 58–67, 73, 74
Golden Medium, 4, 5–6, 14

golf, Essentrics routine for, 288–90
gracilis, 7
    Essentrics sequences using, 97, 102, 110, 150, 152, 179
Gray, John Armstrong Muir, 23
gymnastics, Essentrics routine for, 262–65

hairdressing, Essentrics routine for, 358–61
Hamstring and Spine Stretch—Chair. *See also* Deep Hamstring and Spine Stretch with Release—Chair; Windmill Hamstring and Spine Stretch—Chair
    in diving routine, 283
    explained, 159
    in jumping higher routine, 254
    in racket sports routine, 308
    in routine for housekeeping, 356
    in rowing routine, 312
    in running routine, 315
    in skiing routine, 318
    in travel days routine, 194
hamstrings, 7, 12
    Essentrics sequences using, 78–79, 82, 83, 85–88, 91–101, 103–4, 106–8, 110, 113, 115–28, 136–44, 147, 149–61, 163–68, 175–81, 183
    warm-ups using, 58, 61–67, 73–74
Hamstring Stretch—Chair. *See also* Folded Hamstring Stretch—Chair; Hip Flexor and Hamstring Stretch—Chair; Pull a Rope IT Band and Hamstring Stretch—Chair
    explained, 157
    in walking the dog routine, 197
Hands, Fingers, and Wrists Mobility Sequence #1
    in basketball routine, 269
    in evening routine, 190
    explained, 129
    in horseback riding routine, 300
    in manual labor/construction/landscaping routine, 347
    in routine for finger, wrist, and elbow pain, 389
    in routine to stimulate your brain, 210
    in walking the dog routine, 196
    in yoga and Pilates routine, 337
Hands, Fingers, and Wrists Mobility Sequence #2
    in beginner flexibility (floor) routine, 219
    in cycling routine, 274
    explained, 130
    in manual labor/construction/landscaping routine, 347
    in routine for fibromyalgia and IBS, 382
    in routine for finger, wrist, and elbow pain, 389
    in routine for hairdressing, 359
    in walking the dog routine, 196

hands: fists open, closed, Essentrics sequences using, 99, 110, 112
hands open and closed, Essentrics sequences using, 92, 94, 96, 155
hands open, Essentrics sequences using, 89, 135
hands, Washing a Small Round Table targeting the, 89
head
    correct and incorrect positioning of, 49
    cushion for the, 48
    nodding the, 28
    shaking or rotating the, 28
health
    compressed organs and, 30
    physical activity and, 22
    poor posture and, 21–22
    posture and, 24
heel lift, for warm-ups, 66, 68
heel lift with toe flexion, Essentrics sequences using, 89, 98, 120, 122, 142, 144–45, 148, 156, 160
hemorrhoid "donut" cushion, 47–48
high-impact activities, xi, 6
hiking, Essentrics routine for, 291–93
hip
    isolating from leg when lifting leg, 54–56
    unbalanced, 7
hip adductors
    Essentrics sequences using, 95–96, 100–101, 121–28, 139, 141, 143, 151, 153, 173–74, 179, 182–83
    warm-ups using, 58, 64, 67
hip ball joint rotation, 98
hip bones, 27
Hip Cleaners—Chair
    in beginner flexibility (chair) routine, 222
    explained, 150
    in routine for agility, 246
    in routine for foot and calf pain, 372
    in routine for relaxation, 203
    in skiing routine, 318
    in soccer routine, 323
    in travel days routine, 193
Hip Flexor and Hamstring Stretch—Chair
    in American football routine, 261
    in basketball routine, 271
    in cycling routine, 275
    in diving routine, 283
    explained, 156
    in hockey routine, 296
    in horseback riding routine, 301
    in jumping higher routine, 254
    in knee pain routine, 368
    in martial arts routine, 304

in racket sports routine, 307
in routine for flight attendants, 353
in rowing routine, 311
in snowboarding routine, 321
in soccer routine, 325
in surfing routine, 328
in walking the dog routine, 197
hip flexors
    Essentrics sequences using, 85–87, 92, 95–96,
        98, 103, 119, 131, 137–40, 142–43, 145, 147,
        149–50, 153, 155–56, 158, 163–64, 167–68,
        170–74, 178–80, 183–84
    warm-ups using, 58–59, 62–67, 74
hip hinge
    for Essentrics sequences, 95, 101, 137–38, 140,
        143–46, 148, 152, 153–54, 155, 157–59, 163,
        165–67, 169–83
    warm-ups, 62, 64, 65
hip hinge back, Essentrics sequences using, 136,
    168
hip hinge for wide stance, Essentrics sequences
    using, 92–94, 96, 100, 103, 106, 108
hip hinge front, Essentrics sequences using, 151,
    164
hip hinge to open legs, 173
hip hinge to the side, Essentrics sequences
    using, 141, 143, 153, 154, 164, 179, 182
hip pain, Essentrics routine for, 374–77
hips, 30
    blocks/risers for elevating, 46–47
    Essentrics sequences targeting, 79–82, 84–89,
        91–101, 103–10, 113, 115–28, 136–43, 145–46,
        149–68, 173–84
    lifting the leg with the, 56
    unbalance in the, 34
Hips and Legs, sequences for, 136–43
Hip Stretch (posture routine), 413
hip sway, for dance warm-ups, 73–74
hockey, Essentrics routine for, 294–97
horseback riding, Essentrics routine for,
    298–301
housekeeping, Essentrics routine for, 354–57
human skeletal system, xii, 25
    agonist/antagonist muscles in, 43–44
    arch shape in, 26
    cervical vertebrae, 27–28
    clavicle of, 29
    diagram, 30
    feet, 30–31
    hips, 30
    scapula of, 29
    skull and spine of, 27
    thoracic spine of, 29
hyperkyphosis, 28

IBS, Essentrics routine for, 381–84
ilium, 27, 30
immobility crisis, 22–24
injuries, xi–xii
    Pilates and, 10–11
    recovery of crimp after, 17
    repetitive strain, 18
    yoga practice and, 10
Inner and Outer Thigh Rotations: IT Band and
    Long Adductor Stretch—Chair
    in American football routine, 261
    in baseball routine, 268
    in beginner flexibility (chair) routine, 223
    in diving routine, 283
    explained, 153
    in golf routine, 290
    in hockey routine, 296
    in horseback riding routine, 301
    in jumping higher routine, 254
    in knee pain routine, 369
    in martial arts routine, 304
    in racket sports routine, 307
    in routine for housekeeping, 356
    in rowing routine, 311
    in running routine, 315
    in skiing routine, 318
    in soccer routine, 325
    in surfing routine, 329
intercostals
    Essentrics sequences using, 78–83, 85–87, 95,
        104–7, 110–11, 149, 162, 179
    warm-ups using, 60–61, 63
ischium, 27, 30
isometric contractions, 41, 43
isotonic contractions, 41, 43
IT band, 7

joints
    benefits of improving range of motion of, 12
    number of, 15
    range of motion of, 7–8, 11
    target training unbalancing the, 13
    three main types of, 15–16
    unbalanced. See unbalanced joints
jumping higher routine, 252–54

Karate Kicks to the Front—Chair
    in children's routine, 214
    explained, 137
    in routine for working at a desk all day, 346
    in rowing routine, 310
Karate Kicks to the Side—Chair
    in children's routine, 214
    explained, 138

Karate Kicks to the Side—Chair (*cont.*)
   in lower-body toning routine, 235
   in martial arts routine, 303
   in routine for agility, 246
   in routine for working at a desk all day, 346
   in routine to increase your energy, 206
kayaking, Essentrics routine for, 309–12
Kicking for Explosive Strength (posture routine), 412
knee alignment, 32
Knee Kicks while Twisting (posture routine), 396
Knee Kicks with Spine Twists (warm-up), 64, 70
knee pain, Essentrics routine for, 367–69
knees
   Essentrics sequences targeting, 78–89, 91–100, 102–10, 113, 115–28, 137–42, 144–45, 147–57, 159–61, 164–65, 170, 173–76, 178–82, 184
   positioning in pliés, 53–54
knees bent
   Essentrics sequences using, 78–83, 87, 89, 91–100, 102–10, 113, 115–18, 121–28, 137–38, 140–42, 144–45, 147–48, 151–52, 156–61, 164, 166, 169–73, 175–76, 178–79, 182–83
   for warm-ups, 58, 59, 61, 62, 63, 64, 65, 66, 67, 68, 69, 73, 74
kyphosis, 28, 49

landscaping work, Essentrics routine for, 347–49
Langevin, Helene M., 13
Large Full-Body Figure Eights with Rotation
   in ballet and gymnastics routine, 263
   in baseball routine, 266
   in diving routine, 282
   explained, 120
   in figure skating routine, 286
   in routine for balance, 249
   in running routine, 315
   in soccer routine, 323
   in yoga and Pilates routine, 338
Large Single-Arm Figure Eights
   in advanced flexibility routine, 224
   explained, 118
   in speed routine, 241
lateral arch of the foot, 31
lateral flexion, 37
latissimus dorsi
   Essentrics sequences using, 79–83, 85–88, 90–120, 123–26, 128, 131, 136–40, 143, 149, 151–53, 155–62, 164–81, 184
   warm-ups using, 58–67, 73
Legs and Hips, sequences for, 136–43
Levine, James, 23

Lift Imaginary Weights Above Your Head
   in American football routine, 259
   explained, 116
   in routine for flight attendants, 351
   in rowing routine, 310
lifting leg(s)
   correct and incorrect positioning for, 54–56
   to the front, 55
   with the hips, 56
   isolating hip joint when, 54–56
   to the side, positioning for, 56
load path of the body, 26
   correct and incorrect positioning of, 49
   the feet and, 30, 31
   kyphosis and, 28
   Neutral C spine movement and, 35, 36, 37, 50–51
   Neutral Elongation and, 35
   posture and, 49
   through the thighs, knees, and shins, 30
long adductors, 7
Long Adductor Stretch with Figure Eight—Floor
   in advanced flexibility routine, 226
   in evening routine, 191
   explained, 179
   in routine for cooldown/recovery, 229
   in swimming routine, 333
lower-body toning routine, 233–36
Low Rapid Kicks
   explained, 136
   in explosive power routine, 238
   in hiking routine, 292
   in lower-body toning routine, 234
   in routine for balance, 249
   in routine for fibromyalgia and IBS, 383
Lullaby and Lower a Blanket
   in evening routine, 190
   explained, 80
   in routine for shoulder pain, 379
   in upper-body toning routine, 231
lumbar spine, 27, 35
Lunge Hip Mobility Sequence
   explained, 141
   in jumping higher routine, 253
   in routine for agility, 244
   in routine for hip pain, 375
lunges. *See* Squash Lunges

manual labor, Essentrics routine for, 347–49
martial arts, Essentrics routine for, 302–4
mat, 48. *See also* floor sequences
McHugh, Malachy, 9–10
medial arch of the foot, 31
midfoot arch, 31

morning routine, 186–88
muscle atrophy, 4, 11, 23, 38
muscle contraction(s), 41–43
    concentric, 42–43
    eccentric, 41–42
    fascia sleeve and, 17
    isometric, 43
    isotonic, 43
muscle flexibility
    improving range of motion in joints and, 11
    isolated targeted stretching and, 12
    range of motion in the joint and, 14
    rebalancing the joints and, 11
muscles, xii–xiii. *See also* specific muscles
    agonist/antagonist pairs, 43–44
    balanced body and, 3, 4
    connective tissue and, xiii, 33
    fascia training versus training of the, 18
    goal of stretching *all*, xiv
    imbalances, 3, 6
    and improving range of motion for joints, 7
    rebalancing the body and, 3
    redefining stretching of, 9–14
    releasing tension from, 43
    skeletal system and, 25
    targeted training of, 13
    unbalanced, 15, 25
    unbalanced hip joint and, 7
    working in harmony with connective tissue
        and joints, 11
muscle training, fascia training versus, 18
muscular relaxation, 43
musculoskeletal system, xii–xiii
    posture and, 22, 25
    rebalancing the, 3
    trifecta of, 11, 15–19
Musketeers Bow—IT Band and Long Adductor
    Stretch
    explained, 143
    in knee pain routine, 368
    in morning routine, 188
    in posture routine, 404
    in routine for balance, 250
    in routine for recovery/cooldown, 228
    in routine to increase your energy, 207
    in routine to stimulate your brain, 211
myths, fitness, 13

National Ballet of Canada, xii
navicular bone, 31
neck, correct and incorrect positioning of, 49
neck pain, Essentrics routine for, 385–87
neck rotation left and right, 175
neuromuscular signaling from the brain, 9–10

neuromuscular techniques
    agonist/antagonist pairs, 43–44
    concentric contractions, 42–43
    eccentric contractions, 41–42
    isometric contractions, 43
    isotonic contractions, 43
Neutral C spine movement
    correct and incorrect, 50
    correct forward flexion and, 36
    function of, 50
    incorrect positioning, 37
    purpose of, 35
    shifting between Neutral Elongation and, 35–36
Neutral Elongation spine movement
    purpose of, 35
    shifting between Neutral C movement and,
        35–36
neutral spine, warm-ups using a, 58–59, 61–67
Nicholas Institute of Sports Medicine and
    Athletic Trauma, 9–10
Nielsen study (2018), 33
no joint, 28

obliques
    Essentrics sequences using, 78–82, 85–98,
        100–111, 113, 115, 118, 123–28, 131, 137–39,
        143, 149, 151, 155, 158, 162, 164, 167, 169–72,
        175–76, 179–80, 184
    warm-ups using, 60–66, 73, 74
180° arm rotation, for warm-ups, 59, 61
Open Chest Swan. *See also* Ceiling Reach and
    Open Chest Swan
    in back pain routine, 364
    in dance routine, 277
    explained, 112
    in routine for foot and calf pain, 370
orthotics, 32
osteoporosis, 24

pain and injuries, xi–xii, xiii
pectorals
    Essentrics sequences using, 79–82, 85–88,
        90–98, 100–120, 123–26, 128, 131–35, 155,
        158–59, 161–62, 165, 167–76, 178–81, 184
    warm-ups using, 58–67
pelvic tuck, for dance warm-ups, 73–74
peri-fascia, 3, 13
physical activity
    bone health and, 24
    health outcomes and, 22–23
    Zone Three (extreme or high-performance
        living) and, 6
Physical Activity Guidelines for Americans (HHS),
    22

physiotherapy exercises, 10–11
pickleball, Essentrics routine for, 305–8
Pilates, 10
    Essentrics routine for, 337–40
Pilates, Joseph, 10
piriformis, 7
plantar fasciitis, Essentrics routine for, 370–73
plantar flexion, for warm-ups, 58, 63, 67
pliés
    foot and knee positioning in, 53–54
    spine positioning in, 54
Pliés with Deep Side Bends
    in American football routine, 260
    explained, 125
    in morning routine, 187
    in routine for balance, 248
Pliés with Hip and Groin Stretch
    explained, 127
    in golf routine, 290
    in hiking routine, 292
    in horseback riding routine, 300
    in knee pain routine, 368
    in routine for hip pain, 375
    in rowing routine, 310
    in snowboarding routine, 320
Pliés with Quadriceps Strengthening
    in ballet and gymnastics routine, 262
    explained, 121
    in figure skating routine, 285
    in jumping higher routine, 252
    in lower-body toning routine, 234
    in racket sports routine, 306
    in soccer routine, 324
    in surfing routine, 327
    in volleyball routine, 335
Pliés with Side-Bend Arm Reaches
    in dance routine, 279
    explained, 128
    in explosive power routine, 238
    in posture routine, 407
    in running routine, 313
Pliés with Single-Arm Figure Eights
    in basketball routine, 270
    in beginner flexibility (floor) routine, 218
    explained, 124
    in routine for agility, 245
Pliés with Single-Arm Full-Body Rotation
    explained, 123
    in routine for spine mobility, 256
    in skiing routine, 317
Pliés with Single-Arm Half-Body Rotation
    explained, 126
    in jumping higher routine, 253
    in martial arts routine, 302

    in routine for fibromyalgia and IBS, 381
    in yoga and Pilates routine, 338
Pliés with Squeeze an Orange under Your Heel
    in children's routine, 213
    in cycling routine, 274
    explained, 122
    in hockey routine, 294
    in routine to increase your energy, 205
    in speed routine, 242
poor posture, 21–25, 28, 29, 30
    reversing, 390–91
position(s)/positioning. *See also* pliés
    ankle, 52–53
    feet/foot, 51
    foot and knee, in pliés, 53–54
    head and neck, 49
    Neutral C (curving the spine), 50–51
    spine, in pliés, 54
    standing straight, 49–50
    when lifting the leg, 54–56
positive (concentric) training, 42–43
posture, 21–38
    alignment and, 25, 37–38
    bad habits and poor, 34
    correct and incorrect positioning of the neck/
        chin and, 49
    daily habits and poor, 34
    epidemic of poor, 21–22
    Essentrics improving, xiv
    fascia and, 33, 35
    health and, 24, 30
    kyphosis and poor, 28
    load path and, 49
    Neutral C spine movement and correct, 36
    physical activity and, 22–23
    prevalence of poor, 21
    qualities of good, 24–25, 35
    reversing poor, 390–91
    role of fascia in, 33, 35
    techniques for good, 37–38
    way of standing on the feet and, 30
Posture Routine
    about, 390, 391
    chair/barre sequences, 411–15
    floor sequences, 416–27
    sequences, 392–427
    standing sequences, 397–410
    warm-ups, 392–96
Preparation: Hip Flexor and Hamstring Stretch—
    Chair
    in back pain routine, 365
    in baseball routine, 268
    in beginner flexibility (chair) routine, 222
    explained, 152

in routine for hip pain, 375
in running routine, 314
in travel days routine, 194
in volleyball routine, 336
psoas, 7
pubis, 27, 30
Pull a Rope IT Band and Hamstring Stretch—
   Chair
in basketball routine, 272
explained, 155
in hockey routine, 297
Pulling Out, 38
Pulling Up, 38
Push a Piano and Pull a Donkey
in cycling routine, 273
explained, 99
in routine for foot and calf pain, 371
in routine to stimulate your brain, 209

quadratus lumborum, 12
Essentrics sequences using, 79–80, 82–83,
   85–88, 95, 99, 101–12, 114, 117, 119–20,
   125–28, 136–40, 149, 151–52, 155–62, 166–68,
   174–76, 179–82
warm-ups using, 59–63, 65, 73–74
quadriceps, 7, 12
Essentrics sequences using, 78–83, 85–89,
   91–110, 113, 115–28, 136–42, 147–53, 155,
   157–61, 163–67, 170–74, 178–81, 183–84
pliés and, 53, 54, 55
warm-ups using, 58–59, 61–67, 73, 74

racket sports, Essentrics routine for, 305–8
racquetball, Essentrics routine for, 305–8
range of motion
balanced body and, 3
benefits of, 12
connective tissue and, 13
Essentrics using full-body, 11
full-body regimens and, 11
and Golden Medium (Zone Two), 5
improving for each joint, 7
muscle flexibility and, 11
stretching and, 9
yoga and, 10
recovery, routine for, 227–29
relaxation, muscular, 43
relaxation, routine for, 201–3
Relaxed Washes (posture routine), 394
Remove a Sweater
in back pain routine, 364
explained, 115
in explosive power routine, 237
in relaxation routine, 202

in routine for spine mobility, 255
in skiing routine, 316
resistance bands, 47
rhomboids
Essentrics sequences using, 78–83, 85–94,
   96–101, 103–10, 113–15, 117–20, 123–26, 128,
   131–35, 154, 158–59, 161, 165–66, 169–76,
   178–81, 184
warm-ups using, 58–67
ribs, 27, 29
Essentrics sequences targeting, 81, 83, 95, 97,
   101, 110–11
risers/blocks, 46–47
Rock the Baby
explained, 79
in routine for hairdressing, 360
rolling
of your ankles, 53
of your feet, 51
rotation in the hip joint, 89, 120, 139, 150, 153
rowing, Essentrics routine for, 309–12
Row the Boat with Hamstring and Spine
   Stretch—Floor
in beginner flexibility (floor) routine, 220
in evening routine, 191
explained, 177
in swimming routine, 333
running, Essentrics routine for, 313–15

sacrum, 27
sartorius, Essentrics sequences using, 97,
   99–100, 121–28, 141, 143, 147, 149, 179, 182
scapula, 27, 29
scar tissue, hardened fascia and, 18, 33
Seated Hamstring and Glute Stretch—Floor, 175
Seated Hip Stretch with Front Leg Extended
   (posture routine), 426
Seated Hip Stretch with Spine Rotation—Floor
in beginner flexibility (floor) routine, 220
explained, 176
Seated Side Bends for Strength and Hamstring
   Flexibility (posture routine), 427
sedentary lifestyle, 4–5, 17
Shin and Ankle Flexibility (posture routine), 402
shins, correct positioning of the, 52
Shin Stretching and Strengthening—Chair
in advanced flexibility routine, 225
in ballet and gymnastics routine, 262
in cycling routine, 274
in diving routine, 282
explained, 147
in figure skating routine, 285
in jumping higher routine, 253
in knee pain routine, 369

Shin Stretching and Strengthening—Chair (*cont.*)
in martial arts routine, 303
in routine for agility, 246
in routine for being on your feet all day, 342
in routine for foot and calf pain, 373
in routine to increase your energy, 206
in skiing routine, 317
in surfing routine, 328
in swimming routine, 331
in volleyball routine, 336
shoulder arm rotation, Essentrics sequences
using, 83, 90, 92, 95, 97, 102–4, 117–18, 120,
124, 126, 131, 158, 172, 179
shoulder arm rotation toward ceiling, 169
shoulder arm rotation up, Essentrics sequences
using, 94–95, 108, 111, 125, 128, 149, 159,
165–68
Shoulder Blasts, 35
in baseball routine, 267
in basketball routine, 269
in dance routine, 277
in diving routine, 281
explained, 83
in golf routine, 288
in hiking routine, 291
in racket sports routine, 305
in routine for hairdressing, 358
in routine for neck pain, 385
in routine for shoulder pain, 378
in routine for working at a desk all day, 344
in rowing routine, 309
in snowboarding routine, 319
in stress relief routine, 199
in surfing routine, 326
in upper-body toning routine, 230
shoulder lift, warm-ups using, 60, 64
shoulder pain, Essentrics routine for, 378–80
shoulder rotation arms up, Essentrics sequences
using, 105–9, 111
Shoulder Rotations. *See* Double-Arm Shoulder
Rotations
Shoulder Rotations (posture routine), 392
shoulders, Essentrics sequences targeting,
78–120, 123–26, 128, 131–35, 149, 154–55,
158–59, 161–62, 165–81, 184
shoulders up, Essentrics sequences using, 78,
83
side hip hinge, for warm-up, 58
Side Leg Lifts
hemorrhoid cushion for, 47–48
for posture routine, 418
Side Lunges with Arms (posture routine),
408
Simple Side-to-Side Steps (warm-up), 58, 69

Simple Windmill—Feet Parallel
in American football routine, 259
explained, 90
in hockey routine, 295
in horseback riding routine, 299
in routine for housekeeping, 355
in routine for manual labor/construction/
landscaping, 348
in routine for shoulder pain, 379
in rowing routine, 309
in snowboarding routine, 320
Single-Arm Pulling a Rope
explained, 92
in routine for children, 213
in upper-body toning routine, 230
Single-Arm Rotations (warm-up), 62, 70
Single-Arm Sweeps into Celebration Arms
in beginner flexibility (chair) routine, 221
explained, 102
in routine for children, 213
in routine for hairdressing, 360
Single-Arm Swings (posture routine), 393
sitting, physical health and, 23
Sit-Ups (posture routine), 419
Sit-Ups with a Waist Twist—Floor
explained, 170
for speed routine, 243
Sit-Ups with Single-Leg Kicks—Floor, 171
skeleton. *See* human skeletal system
skiing, Essentrics routine for, 316–18
skull, 26, 27, 49
inability of joints to move, 15
occipital bone of the, 28
sleeve, fascia, 17
Slow Sit-Ups with Arm Variations—Floor
explained, 169
in upper-body toning routine, 232
Small Single-Arm Figure Eights
in dance routine, 278
explained, 117
in hockey routine, 294
in racket sports routine, 305
in routine for flight attendants, 350
in routine for neck pain, 386
in routine for shoulder pain, 380
in stress relief routine, 198
in volleyball routine, 334
in walking the dog routine, 195
snowboarding, Essentrics routine for,
319–21
soccer, Essentrics routine for, 323–25
soleus
Essentrics sequences using, 85–89, 91–96,
98–100, 103–10, 113, 115, 118, 120–24,

126–27, 136–49, 151–55, 157, 159–60, 163, 165, 175, 177–79, 183

warm-ups using, 58–59, 61–63, 65–68, 73

spasms, 12

speed, routine for, 241–43

spinal rotation, for warm-ups, 62–66

spine

basic movements, 35–37

cervical, 27–28

Essentrics sequences targeting the, 78–115, 117–20, 121–26, 128, 137–40, 143, 149, 151–62, 164–81, 183–84

five parts of, 27

lateral flexion of the, 37

Neutral C movement of, 35–36

Neutral Elongation movement and, 35–36

positioning in pliés, 54

posture and, 25, 391

rotation of the, 37

S curve of, 27

stressing, when lifting legs, 55

thoracic, 29

vertebrae of, 27

spine circle

for Essentrics sequences, 94, 108, 111, 149

for warm-ups, 60

spine curved

Essentrics sequences using, 78–84, 79, 80, 81, 82, 83, 86–87, 92–93, 99, 102–3, 105–6, 112, 117–18, 120, 152, 154, 156–57, 159, 161–62, 176

for warm-ups, 59, 61, 62, 65, 66

spine leaning back, Essentrics sequences using, 161, 168, 176, 179–81, 180–81, 184

spine leaning forward, Essentrics sequences using, 82, 85, 87, 91, 93, 96, 101, 158, 174, 177, 179–81

spine mobility routine, 255–57

Spine Release—Chair

in back pain routine, 363

explained, 161

in golf routine, 290

in hiking routine, 293

in manual labor/construction/landscaping routine, 349

in relaxation routine, 203

in routine for hairdressing, 361

in routine for housekeeping, 357

in routine for shoulder pain, 380

in rowing routine, 312

spine side to side, Essentrics sequences using, 79–82, 162, 167, 169

spine toe touch, Essentrics sequences using, 80, 83, 160

squash, Essentrics routine for, 305–8

Squash Lunges

in American football routine, 260

explained, 140

in routine for agility, 245

in routine for being on your feet all day, 342

in routine to increase your energy, 205

in running routine, 314

in soccer routine, 324

in speed routine, 242

in walking the dog routine, 196

Standing Quad Stretch

explained, 142

in morning routine, 188

in routine for flight attendants, 352

in swimming routine, 331

standing sequences, posture routine, 397–410

standing straight, correct and incorrect position for, 49–50

static stretching, 9–10

straight spine, Essentrics sequences using, 78, 80–83, 88, 90, 95, 97, 101–2, 109, 112, 114, 125–26, 131–35, 137–40, 144–48, 150, 152, 154–60, 162, 165–66, 169–71, 174, 184

Strengthening Quad Raiser—Floor

explained, 163

in lower-body toning routine, 236

stress relief routine, 198–200

stretching

balanced body and, 14

combined with strengthening, 13

full-body range of motion and, 9

not sticking with programs for, 11–12

redefining, 12, 15

traditional static, 9–10

Superman for Psoas (posture routine), 424

Superman for Spine (posture routine), 423

Superman Spine Strengthening—Floor

in ballet and gymnastics routine, 265

explained, 168

in figure skating routine, 286

in routine for children, 214

in spine mobility routine, 257

in upper-body toning routine, 232

Supine: Hamstrings (posture routine), 421

Supine Long Adductor and IT Band Stretch (posture routine), 422

surfing, Essentrics routine for, 326–29

Sweeping behind Head into Cutting the Air

in beginner flexibility (chair) routine, 222

explained, 104

in horseback riding routine, 299

in relaxation routine, 202

Sweeping behind Head into Cutting the Air
      (*cont.*)
   in spine mobility routine, 256
   in walking the dog routine, 195
Sweeping over Leg (posture routine), 415
swimming, Essentrics routine for, 330–33
Swinging Both Arms Forward and Back
      (warm-up)
   in Essentrics warm-up routine, 69
   explained, 59
   in routine for finger, wrist, and elbow pain, 388
   in routine for neck pain, 386
synovial (freely moveable) joints, 16

Tai Chi, 24
Tai Chi Spine Rotations (warm-up)
   in Essentrics warm-up routine, 70
   explained, 66
   in routine for neck pain, 387
tendons, 16
tennis, Essentrics routine for, 305–8
tennis players, 23–24
TheraBands, 47
thigh bone, 30
thoracic spine, 27, 29
360° arm rotation, for warm-ups, 62, 66
Throw a Frisbee (warm-up), 65, 70
tibia, 30
tibialis anterior
   Essentrics sequences using, 122, 136, 140–48,
      152–54, 156–57, 159, 163–65, 177–81, 183, 184
   warm-up using, 68
tibialis posterior
   Essentrics sequences using, 121–22, 136,
      140–42, 144–46, 149, 152, 156–57, 159, 163,
      165, 177–79, 183
   warm-up using, 68
toe flexion and extension. *See also* heel lift with
      toe flexion, Essentrics sequences using
   Essentrics sequence using, 144
   warm-up using, 68
toes, Essentrics sequences targeting, 120,
      144–45, 147–48, 156, 160
torso, isolating when lifting legs, 54–55
torso rotation, 90, 91, 95, 101
towel, for seated or leg-on-the-barre stretches, 47
traditional static stretching, 9–10
trapezius (upper back) muscles
   Essentrics sequences using, 78–83, 85–120,
      123–26, 128, 131–35, 155, 158–61, 165–81,
      184
   and neck/head positioning, 49
   warm-ups using, 58–67
Travel Days routine, 192–94

Tremblay, Mark, 21
triceps
   Essentrics sequences using, 78, 79, 83, 85–94,
      96–100, 102–20, 125–26, 128, 131–35, 149,
      154–55, 159, 161, 165–66, 168, 173–80, 184
   warm-ups using, 58, 59, 60, 63, 64, 65, 66, 67
Triceps Stretch into Windmills
   explained, 97
   in explosive power routine, 239
   in morning routine, 187
   in routine for balance, 250
   in routine for working at a desk all day, 345

unbalanced hips, 34
unbalanced joints
   and door hinge analogy, 15
   pain from, 7
   static stretching and, 9, 10
   targeted training and, 13
   yoga and, 10
unbalanced muscles, 15, 25
University of Australia, 9
University of Nevada, 9
Upper-Body Extension, 112–16
upper body rotation, Essentrics sequences
      using, 175–76
Upper-Body Toning routine, 230–32
upper body twist, Essentrics sequences using,
      158, 162
upper torso rotation, Essentrics sequences
      using, 170
US Department of Health and Human Services,
      22

vertebrae
   about, 27
   C7, 28
   cervical, 27–28
   Neutral C and, 36, 50
   rotation of the spine and, 37
   thoracic, 29
volleyball, Essentrics routine for, 334–36

Waist Rotations. *See also* Ceiling Reach with
      Waist Rotation (warm-up)
   in beginner flexibility (floor) routine, 218
   in dance routine, 278
   explained, 88
   in horseback riding routine, 298
   in posture routine, 399
   in routine for housekeeping, 354
   in routine for shoulder pain, 379
   in routine to stimulate your brain, 208
walking the dog routine, 195–97

warm-ups, 57–68
  Arches, Toes, and Ankles, 68
  Ceiling Reach with Waist Rotation, 60
  dance sequences, 73–75
  Diagonal Twists, 63
  Double-Arm Swings, Side to Side, 61
  Fast Pliés with Full Arm Swing, 67
  Knee Kicks with Spine Twists, 64
  posture routine, 392–96
  routine for, 69–72
  Simple Side-to-Side Steps, 58
  Single-Arm Rotations, 62
  Swinging Both Arms Forward and Back, 59
  Tai Chi Spine Rotations, 66
  Throw a Frisbee, 65
Washing a Small Round Table
  in evening routine, 190
  explained, 89
  in explosive power routine, 237
  in golf routine, 289
  in manual labor/construction/landscaping
    routine, 348
  in routine for fibromyalgia and IBS, 383
  in routine for housekeeping, 355
  in routine to stimulate your brain, 209
  in spine mobility routine, 255
  in stress relief routine, 199
Washing Windows above the Shoulders
  in advanced flexibility routine, 224
  in cycling routine, 273
  explained, 105
weight-bearing exercise, bone loss and, 24
Windmill Hamstring and Spine Stretch—Chair
  explained, 158
  in routine for flight attendants, 353
Windmills for Hamstrings (posture routine),
  414
Windmills, Triceps Stretch. *See* Triceps Stretch
  into Windmills
Windmill with Spine Flexion
  in cooldown/recovery routine, 228
  explained, 96
  in surfing routine, 327

  in swimming routine, 331
  in travel days routine, 193
  in volleyball routine, 335
workplace routines, 341–61
Wraparound Arms
  in back pain routine, 364
  explained, 91
  in golf routine, 289
  in horseback riding routine, 300
  in routine for hip pain, 374
  in routine for neck pain, 386
  in routine for working at a desk all day, 345
wrist extension, 132
wrist pain, Essentrics routine for, 388–89
wrists, Essentrics sequences targeting, 110, 116,
  129–30, 132–35

yes joint, 28
yoga
  Essentrics routine for, 337–40
  static poses used by, 10

Zombie
  in children's routine, 212
  in cooldown/recovery routine, 227
  in diving routine, 281
  in evening routine, 189
  explained, 78
  in golf routine, 288
  in horseback riding routine, 298
  in morning routine, 186
  in relaxation routine, 201
  in routine for foot and calf pain, 370
  in routine for housekeeping, 354
  in routine to increase your energy, 204
  in routine to stimulate your brain, 208
  in stress relief routine, 198
  in surfing routine, 326
Zombie and Open Chest Swan (posture routine),
  397
Zone One, 4–5
Zone Three, 6–7
Zone Two, 5–6

ABOUT THE AUTHOR

MIRANDA ESMONDE-WHITE is one of North America's greatest educators on healthy aging, injury prevention in sports, and pain-free living. She is best known for her PBS fitness series *Classical Stretch*, which debuted in 1999 and is the #1 fitness show on the network. A classically trained ballerina formerly with the National Ballet of Canada, Esmonde-White created the Essentrics technique, which uses low-intensity strengthening and stretching exercises to relieve pain, prevent injury, and tone the body. Based in Montreal, she works with professional and Olympic athletes and celebrities and teaches classes to thousands of students worldwide. She is the author of *Aging Backwards*, a *New York Times* and *Globe and Mail* bestseller that sparked an award-winning PBS documentary of the same name. Her subsequent bestseller, *Forever Painless*, also became a PBS pledge-documentary hit.